Hepatobiliary Imaging

Editors

BENJAMIN M. YEH
FRANK H. MILLER

RADIOLOGIC CLINICS
OF NORTH AMERICA

www.radiologic.theclinics.com

Consulting Editor
FRANK H. MILLER

September 2022 • Volume 60 • Number 5

ELSEVIER

1600 John F. Kennedy Boulevard • Suite 1800 • Philadelphia, Pennsylvania, 19103-2899

http://www.theclinics.com

RADIOLOGIC CLINICS OF NORTH AMERICA Volume 60, Number 5
September 2022 ISSN 0033-8389, ISBN 13: 978-0-323-84924-1

Editor: John Vassallo (j.vassallo@elsevier.com)
Developmental Editor: Karen Solomon

Radiologic Clinics of North America (ISSN 0033-8389) is published bimonthly by Elsevier Inc., 360 Park Avenue South, New York, NY 10010-1710. Months of issue are January, March, May, July, September, and November. Periodicals postage paid at New York, NY and additional mailing offices. Subscription prices are USD 529 per year for US individuals, USD 1335 per year for US institutions, USD 100 per year for US students and residents, USD 624 per year for Canadian individuals, USD 1362 per year for Canadian institutions, USD 717 per year for international individuals, USD 1362 per year for international institutions, USD 100 per year for Canadian students/residents, and USD 315 per year for international students/residents. To receive student and resident rate, orders must be accompanied by name of affiliated institution, date of term and the signature of program/residency coordinatior on institution letterhead. Orders will be billed at individual rate until proof of status is received. Foreign air speed delivery is included in all *Clinics* subscription prices. All prices are subject to change without notice. **POSTMASTER:** Send address changes to *Radiologic Clinics of North America*, Elsevier Health Sciences Division, Subscription Customer Service, 3251 Riverport Lane, Maryland Heights, MO63043. **Customer Service: Telephone: 1-800-654-2452** (U.S. and Canada); **1-314-447-8871** (outside U.S. and Canada). **Fax: 1-314-447-8029. E-mail: journalscustomerservice-usa@elsevier.com (for print support); journalsonlinesupport-usa@elsevier.com (for online support).**

Reprints. For copies of 100 or more of articles in this publication, please contact the Commercial Reprints Department, Elsevier Inc., 360 Park Avenue South, New York, New York 10010-1710. Tel.: +1-212-633-3874; Fax: +1-212-633-3820; E-mail: reprints@elsevier.com.

Radiologic Clinics of North America also published in Greek Paschalidis Medical Publications, Athens, Greece.

Radiologic Clinics of North America is covered in *MEDLINE/PubMed (Index Medicus), EMBASE/Excerpta Medica, Current Contents/Life Sciences, Current Contents/Clinical Medicine, RSNA Index to Imaging Literature, BIOSIS, Science Citation Index,* and *ISI/BIOMED.*

Contributors

CONSULTING EDITOR

FRANK H. MILLER, MD, FACR, FSAR, FSABI
Lee F. Rogers, MD, Professor of Medical Education, Chief, Body Imaging Section and Fellowship, Medical Director, MRI, Professor, Department of Radiology, Northwestern Memorial Hospital, Northwestern University Feinberg School of Medicine, Chicago, Illinois, USA

EDITORS

BENJAMIN M. YEH, MD, FSAR, FSABI
Professor of Radiology, Director of Contrast and CT Research Laboratory, Department of Radiology and Biomedical Imaging, University of California, San Francisco, San Francisco, California, USA

FRANK H. MILLER, MD, FACR, FSAR, FSABI
Lee F. Rogers, MD, Professor of Medical Education, Chief, Body Imaging Section and Fellowship, Medical Director, MRI, Professor, Department of Radiology, Northwestern Memorial Hospital, Northwestern University Feinberg School of Medicine, Chicago, Illinois, USA

AUTHORS

EMRE ALTINMAKAS, MD
Department of Diagnostic, Molecular and Interventional Radiology, BioMedical Engineering and Imaging Institute, Icahn School of Medicine at Mount Sinai, New York, New York, USA; Department of Radiology, Koc University School of Medicine, Istanbul, Turkey

AMIR A. BORHANI, MD
Associate Professor of Radiology – Abdominal Imaging, Department of Radiology, Northwestern University Feinberg School of Medicine, Medical Director, NMH Computed Tomography, Northwestern Medicine, Chicago, Illinois, USA

CHRISTOPHER BUROS, MD
Assistant Professor, Department of Radiology, University of Pittsburgh Medical Center, Pittsburgh, Pennsylvania, USA

ROBERTA CATANIA, MD
Department of Radiology, Northwestern University Feinberg School of Medicine, Chicago, Illinois, USA

JONATHAN R. DILLMAN, MD, MSc
Professor, Department of Radiology, Cincinnati Children's Hospital Medical Center, University of Cincinnati College of Medicine, Cincinnati, Ohio, USA

KHALED M. ELSAYES, MD
Department of Abdominal Imaging, The University of Texas MD Anderson Cancer Center, Houston, Texas, USA

DAVID T. FETZER, MD
Associate Professor, Department of Radiology, UT Southwestern Medical Center, Dallas, Texas, USA

ALICE FUNG, MD
Department of Diagnostic Radiology, Oregon
Health & Science University, Portland, Oregon,
USA

ALESSANDRO FURLAN, MD
Associate Professor, Department of Radiology,
University of Pittsburgh Medical Center,
Pittsburgh, Pennsylvania, USA

ROSSANO GIROMETTI, MD
Associate Professor, Institute of Radiology,
Department of Medicine, University Hospital
Santa Maria Della Misericordia, Udine, Italy

SERGIO GROSU, MD
Department of Radiology and Biomedical
Imaging, University of California, San Francisco,
San Francisco, California USA; Department of
Radiology, University Hospital, LMU Munich,
Marchioninistr, Munich, Germany

DAE WOOK HWANG, MD, PhD
Division of Hepatobiliary and Pancreatic
Surgery, Department of Surgery, University
of Ulsan College of Medicine, Asan
Medical Center, Seoul, Republic of
Korea

KARTIK JHAVERI, MD, FRCPC, DABR
Professor, CME Director, JDMI University
Health Network, Department of Medical
Imaging, University of Toronto, Clinician-
Scientist, UHN Director, Abdominal MRI,
Toronto, Ontario, Canada

ASHLEY KALOR, MD
Assistant Professor, Department of Radiology,
University of Pittsburgh Medical Center,
Pittsburgh, Pennsylvania, USA

NANDAN KESHAV, MD, MS
Department of Radiology and Biomedical
Imaging, University of California San Francisco,
San Francisco, California, USA

ANDREA SIOBHAN KIERANS, MD
Assistant Professor, Weill Cornell Medicine,
Weill Greenberg Center, New York, New York,
USA

DONG WOOK KIM, MD, PhD
Department of Radiology and Research
Institute of Radiology, University of Ulsan
College of Medicine, Asan Medical Center,
Seoul, Republic of Korea

SO YEON KIM, MD, PhD
Department of Radiology and Research
Institute of Radiology, University of Ulsan
College of Medicine, Asan Medical Center,
Seoul, Republic of Korea

MICHAEL J. KING MD
Department of Diagnostic, Molecular and
Interventional Radiology, Icahn School of
Medicine at Mount Sinai, New York, New York,
USA

SERGIO P. KLIMKOWSKI, MD
Department of Abdominal Imaging, The
University of Texas MD Anderson Cancer
Center, Houston, Texas, USA

INDIRA LAOTHAMATAS MD
Department of Diagnostic, Molecular and
Interventional Radiology, Icahn School of
Medicine at Mount Sinai, New York, New York,
USA

SARA LEWIS, MD
Department of Diagnostic, Molecular and
Interventional Radiology, BioMedical
Engineering and Imaging Institute, Icahn
School of Medicine at Mount Sinai, New York,
New York, USA

ALAIN LUCIANI, MD, PhD
Medical Imaging, Henri Mondor University
Hospital, Faculté de Médecine, Universite
Paris Est Creteil, France

EKTA MAHESHWARI, MD
Assistant Professor, Department of Radiology,
University of Pittsburgh Medical Center,
Pittsburgh, Pennsylvania, USA

MIKAIL MALIK
McMaster University, Hamilton, Ontario,
Canada

MICHAEL A. OHLIGER, MD, PhD
Department of Radiology and Biomedical
Imaging, University of California San Francisco,
Department of Radiology, Zuckerberg
San Francisco General Hospital,
San Francisco, California, USA

CHRISTINE O. MENIAS, MD
Department of Radiology, Mayo Clinic,
Scottsdale, Arizona, USA

CIARA O'BRIEN, MB, BCh, BAO, FFRRCSI
Staff Radiologist, Abdominal Division, JDMI
University Health Network, Mt. Sinai Hospital,
Women's College Hospital Assistant Professor,
Department of Medical Imaging, University of
Toronto, Toronto, Ontario, Canada

FRANK H. MILLER, MD, FACR, FSAR, FSABI
Lee F. Rogers, MD, Professor of Medical
Education, Chief, Body Imaging Section and
Fellowship, Medical Director, MRI, Professor,
Department of Radiology, Northwestern
Memorial Hospital, Northwestern University
Feinberg School of Medicine, Chicago, Illinois,
USA

SÉBASTIEN MULÉ, MD, PhD
Associate Professor, Medical Imaging, Henri
Mondor University Hospital, Faculté de
Médecine, Universite Paris Est Creteil,
France

PAUL E. NOLAN, MD
Department of Radiology, Northwestern
University Feinberg School of Medicine,
Chicago, Illinois, USA

MICHAEL C. OLSON, MD
Assistant Professor, Department of Radiology,
Mayo Clinic, Rochester, Minnesota, USA

ROSA ALBA PUGLIESI, MD
Resident, Department of Radiology,
Ludwigsburg's Hospital, Ludwigsburg,
Germany

ARTHI REDDY, MD
Department of Diagnostic, Molecular and
Interventional Radiology, Icahn School of
Medicine at Mount Sinai, New York, New York,
USA

SCOTT B. REEDER, MD, PhD
Professor, Department of Radiology, University
of Wisconsin-Madison, Madison, Wisconsin,
USA

EDOUARD REIZINE, MD
Medical Imaging, Henri Mondor University
Hospital, Faculté de Médecine, Universite
Paris Est Creteil, France

JUDY H. SQUIRES, MD
Associate Professor, Department of Radiology,
UPMC Children's Hospital of Pittsburgh,

University of Pittsburgh School of Medicine
PUH, Pittsburgh, Pennsylvania, USA

JOHNATHON STEPHENS, MD
Radiology, Brigham and Women's Hospital,
Boston, Massachusetts, USA

BACHIR TAOULI, MD, MHA
Department of Diagnostic, Molecular and
Interventional Radiology, BioMedical
Engineering and Imaging Institute, Icahn
School of Medicine at Mount Sinai, New York,
New York, USA

JENNIFER W. UYEDA, MD
Assistant Professor of Radiology, Brigham and
Women's Hospital, Boston, Massachusetts,
USA

CAMILA LOPES VENDRAMI, MD
Department of Radiology, Northwestern
University Feinberg School of Medicine,
Chicago, Illinois, USA

SUDHAKAR K. VENKATESH, MD
Professor, Department of Radiology, Mayo
Clinic, Rochester, Minnesota, USA

REBECCA WAX, MD
Department of Diagnostic, Molecular and
Interventional Radiology, Icahn School of
Medicine at Mount Sinai, New York, New York,
USA

CHRISTOPHER L. WELLE, MD
Assistant Professor, Department of Radiology,
Mayo Clinic, Rochester, Minnesota, USA

BENJAMIN M. YEH, MD, FSAR, FSABI
Professor of Radiology, Director of Contrast
and CT Research Laboratory, Department of
Radiology and Biomedical Imaging, University
of California, San Francisco, San Francisco,
California, USA

CHANGHOON YOO, MD, PhD
Department of Oncology, University of Ulsan
College of Medicine, Asan Medical Center,
Seoul, Republic of Korea

HEI SHUN YU, MD
Instructor of Radiology, Brigham and Women's
Hospital, Boston, Massachusetts, USA

Contents

Contrast-enhanced liver MR imaging is an important diagnostic tool for many different liver diseases with the sensitivity and specificity in diagnosing liver diseases typically far exceeding other imaging modalities. The safety profile of GBCA is excellent with minimal adverse events. Both extracellular and hepatobiliary contrast agents offer unique advantages and potential limitations. ECA is excellent for obtaining high-quality arterial phase imaging and can be particularly useful for the evaluation of hepatocellular carcinoma (HCC) in cirrhotic patients. In contrast, hepatobiliary agent (HBA) can help distinguish FNH from adenomas, detect liver metastases, and provide biliary imaging due to their uptake within normal hepatocytes and biliary excretion.

Abbreviated magnetic resonance imaging (AMRI) approach became a hot topic in liver imaging recently. Different AMRI protocols including noncontrast AMRI (NC-AMRI), hepatobiliary-AMRI (HBP-AMRI) using gadoxetic acid, and dynamic-AMRI (Dyn-AMRI) using extracellular contrast agent, have been described in the literature. In this review, the use of these AMRI approaches in various indications including hepatocellular carcinoma (HCC) screening and surveillance in chronic liver disease; fat, iron, and fibrosis screening and assessment in nonalcoholic fatty liver disease (NAFLD); and finally liver metastasis screening and surveillance in patients with colorectal cancer are summarized.

Chronic liver disease (CLD) is a large and ever-growing problem in both the US and world health care systems. While histologic analysis through liver biopsy is the gold standard for hepatic parenchymal evaluation, this is not feasible in such a large population of patients or as a way of monitoring change over time. This review discusses MRI-based techniques for assessing hepatic fibrosis, hepatic steatosis, and hepatic iron content, with discussions of both current techniques and future advancements

Contrast-enhanced ultrasound (CEUS) is increasingly performed for focal liver lesion evaluation because of its high safety profile and ability to yield a definitive diagnosis in many patients, obviating multiphase CT or MRI. CEUS uses specific ultrasound contrast agents (UCAs) that are exceedingly safe, without the risk of renal or liver toxicity. UCAs are cleared rapidly from the body, allowing for multiple injections during a single examination, with no potential for deposition in the patient. This review highlights the performance of CEUS for liver lesion evaluation and illustrates the imaging appearance of common liver lesions in children and adults.

> Dual-energy computed tomography (DECT) increases confidence in hepatobiliary computed tomography (CT) evaluation by boosting visible iodine enhancement and differentiating between materials based on relative attenuation of 2 different X-ray energy spectra. Image reconstructions from DECT scans improve the detection and characterization of focal liver lesions, allows for quantification of diffuse liver disease, and reveals gallstones that may be missed on standard CT imaging. Our article aims to illustrate the basic concepts of DECT and types of image reconstruction relevant for the assessment of hepatobiliary diseases. We then review literature on the use of DECT for evaluating focal and diffuse hepatobiliary diseases.

> The liver is one of the most commonly injured organ in the abdomen and pelvis. Hepatobiliary trauma is best assessed by contrast-enhanced CT in hemodynamically stable patients. Prompt and accurate diagnosis of hepatobiliary traumatic injuries and associated vascular injuries guides management and allows for successful nonsurgical management of the traumatic injuries. CT can accurately detect and characterize hepatobiliary traumatic injuries and the associated vascular injuries in addition to evaluating delayed complications. We will review hepatobiliary trauma and associated vascular injuries as well as their associated complications.

> Focal hepatic lesions are frequently discovered incidentally on cross-sectional imaging or abdominal ultrasound, and in the general population, a vast majority of those incidental findings are benign entities. However, the formal diagnosis of benign liver lesions is not always straightforward and may require advanced imaging modalities, such as MRI with hepatobiliary contrast agent or contrast-enhanced ultrasound (CEUS). This review presents the typical features of the main benign liver lesions, including focal nodular hyperplasia (FNH), hepatocellular adenoma (HCA), hepatic cysts, hemangioma, angiomyolipoma, and pseudotumors, such as inflammatory pseudotumors or hepatic granulomas. However, beyond the specific and classical MRI features, some lesions may present atypical patterns. Moreover, arterial phase hyperenhancement, often present in benign liver lesions, can be seen in malignant lesions such as hepatocellular carcinoma. Hence, accurate analysis of clinical and biological contexts is mandatory to optimize our diagnostic performance. The objective of this investigation was, therefore, to review the specific presentations of benign liver tumors and to illustrate their diagnostic pitfalls.

> Atypical liver malignancies can either be uncommon presentations of commonly encountered liver malignancies or rare tumors infrequently seen in clinical practice and often pose a challenge in diagnostic imaging interpretation. These lesions tend to be highly variable in their imaging appearance and are less well discussed in the literature. Commonly, an inter-disciplinary approach incorporating clinical information, imaging data, and histopathology is needed to reach an accurate diagnosis. The diagnostic radiologist's knowledge of such liver malignancies can aid the clinical team in reaching the correct diagnosis and enabling appropriate

management. In this article, we review certain technical considerations and focus on the unusual appearances of common primary and secondary malignant liver lesions, uncommon malignant liver lesions, with emphasis on computed tomography (CT) and magnetic resonance imaging (MRI).

Focal nodular hyperplasia-like (FNH-like) nodules are hepatocellular lesions with similar radiologic and pathologic features as typical FNH but occur within an abnormal liver. They arise due to alteration of hepatic vasculature at both the microscopic and macroscopic levels. Although these nodules are not thought to have malignant potential, their imaging features overlap with premalignant and malignant lesions including hepatocellular carcinoma (HCC) and arise in patients who may be at risk for HCC, posing a diagnostic and management dilemma. It is important to consider these benign entities when reviewing liver imaging of patients at risk for HCC to reduce unnecessary interventions.

The gallbladder is a source of common disease processes with a wide variety of presentations. Common pathologies include acute or chronic cholecystitis, adenomyomatosis, cancer, polyps, and postoperative complications. Accurate imaging assessment of the gallbladder can be very challenging and fraught with potential pitfalls. Ultrasound is the imaging modality of choice for the initial evaluation of patients who present with right upper quadrant pain. CT is often used as part of a broader evaluation of patient's abdominal pain if nongallbladder pathologies are also suspected. MRI/MRCP is typically reserved for problem-solving and evaluating patients who present with cholestatic presentation. We discuss common pitfalls, diagnostic challenges, and problem-solving approaches to the imaging evaluation of common gallbladder patho logies.

Biliary cancer, also known as cholangiocarcinoma, is a primary malignant epithelial neoplasm arising in the bile duct. Cholangiocarcinoma can be classified into intrahepatic, perihilar, and distal cholangiocarcinoma according to anatomic location. Multiphase thin-section computed tomography is the primary imaging modality for diagnosis and treatment planning. MR imaging with magnetic resonance cholangiopancreatography provides additional information for differential diagnosis, complex biliary anatomy, and tumor extent. For preoperative assessment of extrahepatic cholangiocarcinoma, longitudinal tumor extent, vascular involvement, lymph node and distant metastasis, and remnant liver volume are the key features. The adoption of recent advances in imaging techniques enables enhanced image quality and helps to offer optimal treatment options.

Sclerosing cholangitis is characterized by irregular and ill-defined inflammation, fibrosis, and stricturing of the bile ducts and may be primary or secondary in cause. It causes progressive destruction of the biliary tree, progressive parenchymal cirrhosis, hepatic failure, and malignancy such as cholangiocarcinoma. The sub-types of sclerosing cholangitis can be broken down into primary sclerosing cholangitis (PSC), immune-mediated sclerosing cholangitis, infectious cholangitis, and ischemic cholangitis with other causes including metastatic disease and chemotherapy change. MR imaging is the gold standard test to investigate and differentiate PSC and other types of cholangitis.

Nandan Keshav and Michael A. Ohliger

The liver's unique blood supply facilitates multiple important physiologic roles. Liver vascular disorders have distinct appearances on imaging examinations and may mimic other pathologies. This article reviews the imaging appearances of vascular disorders from a multimodality perspective. Liver vascular pathologies are categorized by how they affect liver inflow, liver outflow, and those with abnormal arterial-venous connections. By understanding the physiologic and pathologic underpinnings of the hepatic vasculature, the radiologist is well positioned to positively affect patient care.

FDA-approved labelling. This information is intended solely for CME and is not intended to promote off-label use of these medications. If you have any questions, contact the medical affairs department of the manufacturer for the most recent prescribing information.

TO ENROLL

To enroll in the *Radiologic Clinics of North America* Continuing Medical Education program, call customer service at 1-800-654-2452 or sign up online at http://www.theclinics.com/home/cme. The CME program is available to subscribers for an additional annual fee of USD 356.00.

METHOD OF PARTICIPATION

In order to claim credit, participants must complete the following:
1. Complete enrolment as indicated above.
2. Read the activity.
3. Complete the CME Test and Evaluation. Participants must achieve a score of 70% on the test. All CME Tests and Evaluations must be completed online.

CME INQUIRIES/SPECIAL NEEDS

For all CME inquiries or special needs, please contact elsevierCME@elsevier.com.

RADIOLOGIC CLINICS OF NORTH AMERICA

THE CLINICS ARE AVAILABLE ONLINE!
Access your subscription at:
www.theclinics.com

RADIOLOGIC CLINICS OF NORTH AMERICA

FORTHCOMING ISSUES

November 2022
Imaging of Diffuse Lung Disease
Stephen B. Hobbs, Editor

Hot Topics in Emergency Radiology
Jennifer W. Uyeda and Scott D. Steenburg, Editors

March 2023
Imaging of the Lower Limb
Alberto Bazzocchi and Giuseppe Guglielmi, Editors

RECENT ISSUES

July 2022
Imaging of the Older Population
Frank Chang and Christine B. Chung, Editor

Imaging of Thoracic Infections
Loren Ketai, Editor

March 2022
Imaging of Bone and Soft Tissue Tumors and Simulators
Hillary W. Garner, Editor

THE CLINICS ARE AVAILABLE ONLINE!
Access your subscription at:
www.theclinics.com

Preface
Compendium of Hepatobiliary Imaging Reviews

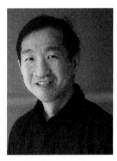
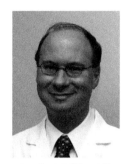

Benjamin M. Yeh, MD   Frank H. Miller, MD
Editors

Although accounting for less than 10% of the overall mass of the abdomen and pelvis, the liver and biliary tract command outsized attention at medical imaging. Many systemic and organ-specific diseases influence the imaging appearance of the hepatobiliary system, and key radiological findings in these organs often prove critical for patient triage, disease monitoring, and preprocedural planning. The complexity of hepatobiliary imaging is influenced by the dual blood supply of the liver, its central role in metabolism and processing of blood from the gastrointestinal tract, and its propensity for developing both metastatic and primary tumors. Effective hepatobiliary imaging involves the integration of advances in imaging technology with new understandings of both diffuse and focal disease.

To serve you, our readers, we assembled a panel of expert radiologists to provide practical snapshots of current state-of-the-art liver and biliary tract imaging. These focused articles are curated to provide a solid overview of the breadth of concerns that are faced by radiologists who image the liver. We review key advances in MR imaging, computed tomography (CT), and ultrasound technology and aimed toward practical daily implementation and troubleshooting of technical issues to benefit everyday radiology. Key points are highlighted along with image examples and references.

The technical topics include tips on rapid MR imaging in different clinical scenarios, pros and cons of different contrast agents for imaging the liver and bile ducts, advances in dual-energy CT as it applies to focal and diffuse liver disease, and an update on contrast-enhanced ultrasound usage and interpretation. These descriptions include methods to minimize imaging artifacts in different clinical scenarios.

A major issue with hepatobiliary imaging is the high frequency of benign and incidental disease that is seen in daily practice. As such, our articles include reviews of liver-specific and biliary-specific topics that explore daily interpretive considerations for common benign disease, whether they be incidental or life-threatening. The appearances of common and uncommon focal benign liver lesions are reviewed. Critical considerations for patient triage in the setting of hepatobiliary blunt and penetrating trauma are included with attention to imaging options for the efficient workup of liver injury.

In-depth discussions are provided to explore entities that are often confusing in appearance and may mimic more concerning lesions. These include focal regenerative nodules, also known as focal nodular hyperplasia-like lesions, and vascular disorders of the liver, both of which may be diagnosed in the correct clinical context with attention to typical imaging features and avoiding undue workup.

Radiol Clin N Am 60 (2022) xv–xvi
https://doi.org/10.1016/j.rcl.2022.06.001
0033-8389/22/© 2022 Published by Elsevier Inc.

Benign and malignant pathologies of the biliary tract and gallbladder are reviewed for each cross-sectional modality with emphasis on image acquisition and interpretation pitfalls. Given the increased recognition of the importance of diffuse liver disease on patient outcomes, we provide a dedicated review on diffuse liver disease quantification, including steatosis, fibrosis, and iron deposition.

Regrettably, given practical limitations in space, it is not possible to provide in-depth review of all essential topics of hepatobiliary imaging. We therefore did not include reviews of hepatocellular carcinoma screening systems, local treatment, and disease monitoring, which in and of themselves would consume more than an entire issue, and which continue to evolve rapidly. For similar reasons, we also do not include a review of molecular hepatobiliary imaging.

Our review is intended to serve radiologists in practice, trainees, as well as imaging technologists. It may be useful for casual reading, and as a reference in the reading room to be utilized as challenging cases are encountered.

Sincerely,

Benjamin M. Yeh, MD
Department of Radiology and
Biomedical Imaging
University of California–San Francisco
505 Parnassus Avenue, M391, Box 0628
San Francisco, CA 94143-0628, USA

Frank H. Miller, MD
Department of Radiology
Northwestern Memorial Hospital
Northwestern University Feinberg School of
Medicine
676 North Saint Clair Suite 800
Chicago, IL 60611, USA

E-mail addresses:
Benjamin.Yeh@ucsf.edu (B.M. Yeh)
Frank.Miller@nm.org (F.H. Miller)

Update on MR Contrast Agents for Liver Imaging
What to Use and When

Ashley Kalor, MD[a], Rossano Girometti, MD[b], Ekta Maheshwari, MD[a],
Andrea Siobhan Kierans, MD[c], Rosa Alba Pugliesi, MD[d],
Christopher Buros, MD[a], Alessandro Furlan, MD[a],*

KEYWORDS

- Gadolinium-based contrast agent • Extracellular contrast agent • Hepatobiliary agent
- Hepatobiliary phase • Magnetic resonance imaging • Contrast media • Hepatobiliary excretion
- Metastasis

KEY POINTS

- Gadolinium is highly paramagnetic leading to shortening of the T1 relaxation time; this property is used as a signal enhancement on contrast-enhanced MR studies.
- Extracellular contrast agents are eliminated almost entirely through glomerular filtration. Hepatobiliary agents (HBA) are eliminated via glomerular filtration and biliary excretion; this property is advantageous for biliary imaging.
- Focal nodular hyperplasia is typically iso- to hyperintense on hepatobiliary phase (HBP) imaging although adenomas are typically hypointense.
- HBP imaging offers increased sensitivity for the detection of most hepatic metastases.
- The determination of use of ECA versus HBA in the setting of chronic liver disease (CLD) should take into consideration the patient's liver reserve and regional and institutional factors.

INTRODUCTION

Contrast-enhanced MR imaging plays a key role in the evaluation of patients with liver disease. Since the first contrast-enhanced liver MRI using gadopentate dimeglumine more than 30 years ago, the list and the applications of MR contrast agents significantly expanded.[1] Contrast-enhanced images represent the central component of a liver MR imaging study and provide valuable information including characterization of focal liver lesions, vessel patency, vascular and biliary anatomy, and organ function.

Gadolinium-based contrast agents (GBCA) are the mainstay contrast agents for MR liver imaging. Due to its seven unpaired electrons, the gadolinium

ion Gd^{3+} is highly paramagnetic, thus shortening the T1, T2, and T2* relaxation times of water protons in nearby tissues (ie, relaxivity). This property is advantageous in T1-weighted imaging (T1WI) and is seen as a signal enhancement, which is the basis of contrast-enhanced MR studies.[2] As contrast enhancement is due to the effect on the nearby tissue and not the single gadolinium molecule, GBCA create an amplification effect. In comparison, iodinated contrast molecules used for CT are imaged directly. For this reason, MRI is more sensitive than CT and the dose of contrast given with MRI can be much lower.[3] Six GBCAs are currently available for use in the United States, which can be classified as extracellular or hepatobiliary based on their distribution (**Table 1**).

[a] Department of Radiology, University of Pittsburgh Medical Center, Radiology Suite 200 E Wing, 200 Lothrop Street, Pittsburgh, PA 15213, USA; [b] Department of Medicine, Institute of Radiology, University Hospital Santa Maria Della Misericordia, p.le S. Maria della Misericordia, 15, Udine 33100, Italy; [c] Weill Cornell Medicine, Weill Greenberg Center, 1305 York Avenue, 3rd Floor, New York, NY 10021, USA; [d] Department of Radiology, Ludwigsburg's Hospital, Posilipostrasse 4, Ludwigsburg 71640, Germany
* Corresponding author.
E-mail address: furlana@upmc.edu

Radiol Clin N Am 60 (2022) 679–694
https://doi.org/10.1016/j.rcl.2022.04.005
0033-8389/22/© 2022 Elsevier Inc. All rights reserved.

radiologic.theclinics.com

Abbreviations	
MR	magnetic resonance
GBCA	Gadolinium-based contrast agent
ECA	Extracellular contrast agent
FNH	Focal nodular hyperplasia

In this article, we will review the characteristics of the available GBCA, the recommendations for their use in liver MR imaging, as well as suggestions on the contrast agent to be used according to the clinical indication.

EXTRACELLULAR AND HEPATOBILIARY GADOLINIUM-BASED CONTRAST AGENTS
Pharmacokinetics

The majority of GBCA agents are classified as extracellular because of their distribution within the extracellular space, which includes the vascular space and the interstitial space (Fig. 1). The GBCA enters the liver via the hepatic artery and portal vein, and it then quickly distributes from the blood pool (sinusoids) into the interstitial (peri-sinusoidal) space.[4] These agents are then eliminated almost entirely via glomerular filtration via the kidneys. In patients with normal renal function, 98% of the contrast is eliminated in 24 h. There are currently four approved extracellular contrast agents: gadodiamide (Gd-DTPA-BMA; Omniscan, GE Healthcare), gadoteridol (Gd-HP-DO3A; ProHance, Bracco Diagnostics), gadobutrol (Gd-DO3A-butriol;

Gadavist, Bayer Healthcare), and gadoterate meglumine (Gd-DOTA meglumine; Dotarem, Guerbet Group; Clariscan, GE Healthcare) (see Table 1). Gadoversetamide and gadopentate dimeglumine were recently removed from the market. The recommended dose of gadolinium-based extracellular agents is 0.1 mmol/kg of body weight (0.2 mL/kg) at a flow rate of 2 to 3 mL/s with a max dose of 20 mL.

Hepatobiliary agents (HBA) combine the pharmacokinetics of extracellular agents with hepatocellular uptake and biliary excretion.[5] The hepatobiliary phase (HBP) is characterized by increased T1-weighted signal intensity of healthy liver parenchyma or focal liver lesions with functional hepatocytes following a delay in contrast administration.[6,7] Focal or diffuse abnormalities containing no hepatocytes or nonfunctional hepatocytes will appear hypointense in relation to the hepatic parenchyma.[6,8] At optimal peak enhancement, hepatic parenchyma is hyperintense to the hepatic vessels. Currently available HBA are linear ionic gadolinium-based molecules with high relaxivity, namely gadoxetic acid, also known as gadoxetate disodium (Gd-EOB-DTPA; Eovist, Primovist, Bayer Healthcare), and gadobenate dimeglumine (Gd-BOPTA; Multihance, Bracco Diagnostics). Gadoxetic acid is administered at a 0.025 mmol/kg dose (0.1 mL/kg), with approximately 50% renal excretion and 50% biliary excretion, causing earlier and more intense parenchymal enhancement. A typical 10 to 20 min delay is necessary to achieve appropriate HBP.8. *The commonly used dosage of gadobenate*

Table 1
Gd-based contrast agents and their properties

Generic Name (Trade Name)	Kinetics	Manufacturer	Structure/ Ionicity	ACR Group
Gadodiamide (Omniscan)	Extracellular	GE Healthcare	Linear/nonionic	Group I
Gadoteridol (ProHance)	Extracellular	Bracco Diagnostics	Macrocyclic/ nonionic	Group II
Gadobutrol (Gadavist)	Extracellular	Bayer Healthcare	Macrocyclic/ nonionic	Group II
Gadoterate meglumine (Dotarem; Clariscan)	Extracellular	Guerbet Group; GE Healthcare	Macrocyclic/ ionic	Group II
Gadobenate dimeglumine (MultiHance)	Hepatobiliary	Bracco Pharmaceuticals	Linear/ionic	Group II
Gadoxetic acid (Primovist or Eovist)	Hepatobiliary	Bayer Pharmaceuticals	Linear/ionic	Group III

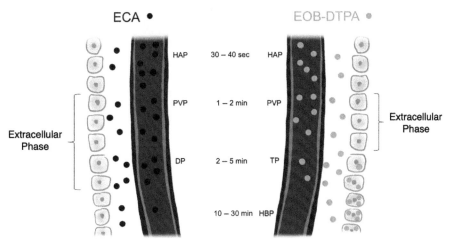

Fig. 1. Extracellular agents (ECA) are confined to the vascular and interstitial spaces, although hepatobiliary agents (such as EOB-DTPA) combine the pharmacokinetics of ECA with hepatocellular uptake. DP, delayed phase; EOB-DTPA, gadoxetic acid; HAP, hepatic arterial phase; HBP, hepatobiliary phase; PVP, portal venous phase; TP, transitional phase.

dimeglumine is 0.1 mmol/kg (0.2 mL/Kg), with about 3% to 5% hepatobiliary uptake and excretion leading to a HBP peak enhancement between 90 and 120 min after contrast injection. The pharmacodynamics of HBA is mediated by membrane transporters unique to hepatocytes organic anion-transporting polypeptides B1/B3 (OATPB1/B3) at the interface between sinusoid and hepatocyte, and multidrug resistance-associated proteins 2 and 3 (MRP2, MRP3) at the interface between hepatocyte and biliary canaliculi[9–11] (**Fig. 2**). The magnitude of contrast uptake-related enhancement depends on the presence of hepatocytes, their density and relative volume of the interstitial compartment, and degree of expression and function of the transporters as well as patency of the biliary system and/or presence of fibrotic stroma causing nonhepatocellular contrast retention.[4,7]

Protocol considerations

Three-dimensional gradient-echo, fat-suppressed T1WI is the recommended sequence for dynamic, multiphasic contrast-enhanced liver MRI imaging.

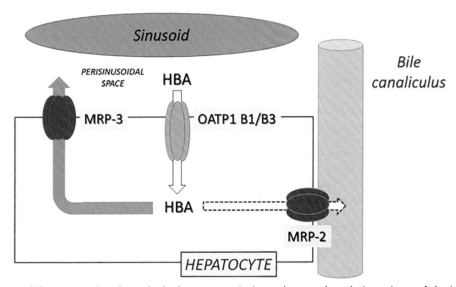

Fig. 2. Hepatobiliary agent (HBA) uptake by hepatocytes is dependent on the relative volume of the interstitial compartment, degree of expression/function of the transporter proteins, patency of the biliary system, and presence of fibrotic stroma. MRP, multidrug resistance-associated proteins; OATP, organic anion-transporting polypeptides.

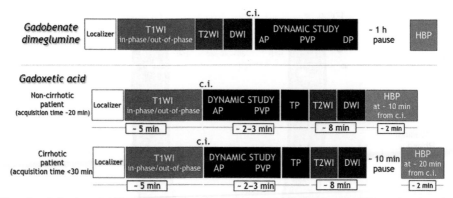

Fig. 3. MR protocols for hepatobiliary agents. Note how timing of the HBP (hepatobiliary phase) varies depending on the agent used. AP, arterial phase; c.i., contrast injection; DP, delayed phase; DWI, diffusion-weighted imaging; PVP, portal venous phase; T1WI, T1-weighted imaging; T2WI, T2-weighted imaging; TP, transitional phase.

Typically, this includes the late arterial phase, portal venous phase, and delayed phase (or extracellular phase). In a properly acquired late hepatic arterial phase, enhancement should be visualized within the hepatic artery and branches as well as within the portal veins with no or faint hepatic vein enhancement. This is in contrast to an early hepatic arterial phase where contrast is in the hepatic artery and not in the portal veins. A late arterial phase can be acquired using a bolus-tracking technique or a fixed delay followed by multiarterial acquisition. The portal venous phase begins immediately after the late arterial phase and ends around 2 min postinjection. A delayed phase is generally acquired 3–5 min postcontrast injection.[4]

Most of a HBA-based liver MRI protocol is unchanged compared with one using extracellular agents in terms of field strength, coils, sequence types, acquisition parameters, and timing of postcontrast dynamic phases.[4,12,13] Dual contrast elimination enables the acquisition of a liver MRI combining a multiphasic dynamic study with the acquisition of a delayed HBP.[6] Due to the slow clearance from the extracellular space, gadobenate dimeglumine has similar kinetic properties of an extracellular contrast agent in the first few minutes after contrast injection. However, when using gadoxetic acid, accumulation of contrast in the hepatic parenchyma begins 1 to 2 min postinjection. The extracellular phase with gadoxetic acid is therefore shorter than with gadobenate dimeglumine and limited to the portal venous phase. When injecting gadoxetic acid, the interval time between the portal venous phase and the HBP is referred to as the transitional phase. In this period, typically 2 to 5 min postinjection, contrast is present within the extracellular space (vascular and interstitial) and within the hepatocytes (see Fig. 1).

The timing of the HBP depends on which HBA is used (Fig. 3). In the case of gadobenate dimeglumine, the HBP is acquired 90 to 120 min after the dynamic multiphasic study, with the patient usually waiting outside the magnet before acquiring the HBP images. For gadoxetic acid, most institutions adopt an optimized protocol where T2-weighted imaging (T2WI) and diffusion-weighted imaging (DWI) are performed after the dynamic postcontrast sequences. However, T2-weighted magnetic-resonance cholangiopancreatography (MRCP) should be obtained before gadoxetic acid injection. The reason for this is that in normal functioning livers, the contrast can be taken up by the hepatocytes and excreted in the bile ducts within the first 2 to 5 min after injection, thus shortening the T2 signal of the bile and obscuring the visualization of the ducts. Additionally, the timing for the HBP may vary depending on the presence (or not) of liver cirrhosis to account for potentially delayed parenchymal enhancement (see Fig. 3). A 10-min delay is assumed to be adequate for diagnosis in most subjects without chronic liver disease. This strategy minimizes costs and patient discomfort within one single MRI scan while having no detrimental effect on the diagnostic capability of T2WI and DWI.[13]

Advantages and disadvantages

The choice of an extracellular or hepatobiliary contrast agent depends on multiple factors including clinical indication, liver function, history of allergic reactions, preference of the institution, and level of expertise of the reader. Table 2 summarizes the main advantages and disadvantages of HBA versus ECA.

Safety considerations

The safety profile of GBCA is excellent. Most adverse events are mild with allergic reactions requiring hospitalization occurring in less than

Table 2
Advantages and disadvantages inherent to hepatobiliary agents (HBA)

Advantage	Consequences	Examples of Clinical Use
Increased contrast-to-noise ratio between nonhepatocellular hypointense liver lesions and hyperintense background parenchyma	• Better lesion conspicuity • Diagnosis of additional lesions	• Small colorectal cancer metastases • Cholangiocarcinoma
Signal intensity of focal hepatic lesions on HBP images	• Improved characterization of liver abnormalities • Contribution to the differential diagnosis of focal liver lesions	• Benign vs malignant focal liver lesions • Primary hepatocellular lesions vs nonhepatocellular lesions • Differentiation of hepatocellular lesions (eg, focal nodular hyperplasia or hepatocellular adenoma) • Hypervascular focal liver lesions vs arterial-enhancing pseudolesions • Imaging features unique to HBP (eg, targetoid appearance) • Ancillary features for diagnosing hepatocellular carcinoma or other malignancy using LI-RADS • Additional information in evaluating diffuse and vascular liver disease
Signal intensity of HCC on HBP images	• Decreased levels of OATP1 B1/B3 expression make HCC hypointense in the HBP compared with parenchymal hyperenhancement, thus increasing lesion conspicuity • Hepatocellular uptake declines in less differentiated HCC, although it is preserved in well-differentiated HCC	• Improved diagnosis of early HCC • Differential diagnosis of HCC vs cholangiocarcinoma or combined HCC-cholangiocarcinoma • Prediction of tumor differentiation • Prediction of microvascular invasion (under investigation) • Prognostic information (under investigation)
Hyperintensity of the bile ducts on HBP images	Possibility of acquiring contrast-enhanced magnetic resonance cholangiography during the HBP (Gd-EOB-DTPA recommended)	• Biliary anatomy • Iatrogenic and noniatrogenic injuries of the bile ducts • Biliary leakage
Potential for functional studies (Gd-EOB-DTPA)	Still under investigation, not for routine use	• Quantification of liver function • Quantification of biliary drainage • Assessment of hepatocarcinogenesis

Disadvantage	Consequences	Potential solution(s)
Higher costs and longer acquisition time than extracellular agents, especially Gd-EOB-DTPA	Need for cost-effectiveness considerations on a per-institutional basis	Abbreviated liver MRI protocols (under investigation)
HBP sensitive to increased concentration of bilirubin, which is a physiologic ligand competing for OATP1 B1/B3	Suboptimal and delayed HBP	Avoiding HBA in patients with hyperbilirubinemia
HBA uptake reduced in advanced chronic liver disease/cirrhosis	Suboptimal and delayed HBP	Delaying the timing of the HBP acquisition in cirrhotic patients (see "technical/protocol considerations")
Occurrence of transient severe motion artifact (especially using Gd-EOB-DTPA), supposed to relate to "acute transient dyspnea"[a]	Impaired image quality of the arterial phase because of phase-encoded stripe artifacts overlapping abdominal organs and extending beyond the abdominal wall into the background	• Use of bolus tracking/fluoroscopic triggering techniques to tailor the timing of the arterial phase • Multi-arterial phase technique • Shortening the scanning time
Occurrence of truncation artifacts from temporal mismatch between short data acquisition time and narrow arterial peak caused by low volume contrast volume (especially with Gd-EOB-DTPA)	Impaired image quality of the arterial phase because of intra-abdominal stripes artifacts, more intense on the phase-encode direction, not extending beyond the abdominal wall, which remains well delineated	• Contrast dilution (eg, to 50% at 2 mL/s) • Low injection rates (1 mL/s) on nondiluted contrast
Low-contrast dose can reduce peak arterial enhancement of lesions, and decrease vessels-to-background liver contrast (Gd-EOB-DTPA)	• Less pronounced arterial hyperenhancement • Lower sensitivity for neoplastic and nonneoplastic portal vein thrombosis	Use of Gd-BOPTA or an extracellular agent
Delayed phase replaced by transitional phase (TP) when using Gd-EOB-DTPA	In patients with preserved liver function, TP starts at 2–5 min after contrast injection, being characterized by mixed enhancement deriving from both extracellular contrast and intracellular uptake (vessels isointense to liver parenchyma)	• Caution in qualifying lesion-to-parenchyma hypointensity in the TP as extracellular "washout" following arterial hyperenhancement, as this appearance might derive from decreased intracellular uptake • Use of proper criteria for image interpretation accounting for the TP (LI-RADS)
Difficult assessment of enhancing "capsule" when evaluating HCC with Gd-EOB-DTPA	Liver enhancement in the PVP or TP obscuring capsule enhancement.	• Use of proper criteria for image interpretation (LI-RADS) • Use of a different contrast agent

Abbreviations: AP, arterial phase; Gd-BOPTA, gadobenate dimeglumine; Gd-EOB-DTPA, gadoxetic acid; HBA, hepatobiliary agents; HBP, hepatobiliary phase; HCC, hepatocellular carcinoma; LI-RADS, liver reporting and data system; MRI, magnetic resonance imaging; OATP, organic anion transporter protein 1; PVP, portal venous phase; TP, transitional phase.
   Table references: advantages[4,5,7,12,14,17,23]; consequences:[4–6,14,17].
 [a] Risk factors: male sex, higher body mass index, higher contrast dose, previous similar episodes, chronic obstructive pulmonary disease.

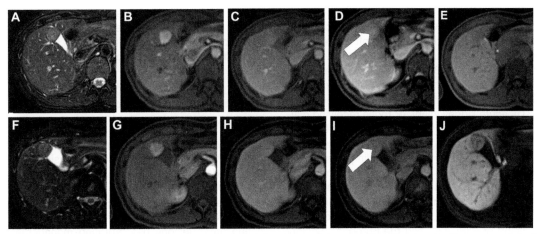

Fig. 4. Comparison of focal nodular hyperplasia (FNH) using gadobenate dimeglumine (*A–E*) versus gadoxetic acid (*F–J*) contrast. Note how in the transitional phase the central scar is hyperintense with gadobenate dimeglumine (*D, arrow*) and hypointense with gadoxetic acid (*I, arrow*).

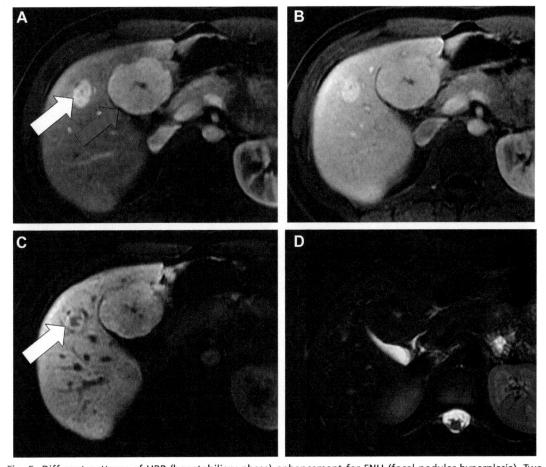

Fig. 5. Different patterns of HBP (hepatobiliary phase) enhancement for FNH (focal nodular hyperplasia). Two separate FNH lesions (*red* and *white arrows*) demonstrate arterial phase hyperenhancement (*A*), isointense/hyperintense signal on portal venous phase (*B*), retention of contrast on HBP (*C*), and central T2 hyperintense scar (*D*). Note how the smaller lesion (*white arrow*) demonstrates more peripheral hyperintensity and central hypointensity on HBP (*C*).

0.01% of injections.[14] Nephrogenic systemic fibrosis (NSF) is a very rare, late complication due to the accumulation of Gd in soft tissues leading to progressive skin thickening. The risk is highest with a group I GBCA in patients with a severe renal impairment, which includes GFR less than 30 mL/min/1.73 m², chronic kidney disease (CKD), acute kidney injury, or those receiving dialysis. The risk of NSF following administration of a standard dose of a group II GBCA is extremely low; however, it may rarely occur in patients with stage 5 or 5D CKD.[15] The American College of Radiology has stated that group II agents can be used in patients with renal impairment and GFR screening is optional. Although the Canadian Association of Radiology and the European Society of Urogenital Radiology agree to expanding the use of group II agents in patients with renal impairment, they also advise "caution" when using these agents in patients with a GFR less than 30 mL/min per 1.73 m². As for group III agents, there is currently insufficient data to determine the risk of NSF; therefore, screening should be performed for patients receiving group III agents.[14] More recent concern over the accumulation of Gd in

the brain, bone, and other soft tissue organs seems to be higher in linear agents compared with more stable macrocyclic agents.[16] The long-term effects of Gd deposition are unknown.

GBCA-ENHANCED MRI FOR CHARACTERIZATION OF A LIVER LESION IN A NONCIRRHOTIC, NONONCOLOGY PATIENT

GBCA-enhanced MR imaging plays a critical role in the characterization of focal liver lesions incidentally detected on CT and ultrasound.

Focal nodular hyperplasia and hepatocellular adenoma. Although FNH and HCA generally occur in a similar population (ie, young women), differentiating these lesions has profound management implications. FNH, the second most common benign liver tumor, is made of multiple monoacinar nodules of normal-functioning hepatocytes occurring in a normal liver. FNH may increase in size but does not evolve into malignancy, and, in the absence of symptoms, FNH is typically managed conservatively.[17] HCA is rarer than FNH. HCA is a benign hepatocellular lesion with different molecular subgroups associated with various risks

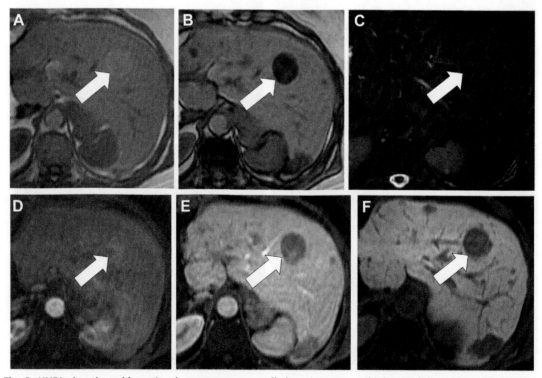

Fig. 6. HNF1α-inactivated hepatic adenomas are generally hypointense on the hepatobiliary phase (*F*). Another characteristic imaging feature (due to intracellular fat) is signal drop-out on out-of-phase sequence (*B*) relative to in-phase (*A*). Lesions are isointense to mildly hyperintense on T2-weighted sequence (*C*), mildly hyperenhancing on arterial phase (*D*), and less likely to have persistent enhancement on portal venous phase (*E*). Note the multiple adenomas with similar imaging characteristics.

and complications.[17] The most recent molecular classification defines eight different HCA subgroups[18] including HNF1α-inactivated (HNF1A) HCA, inflammatory HCA, β-catenin-activated HCA, mixed β-catenin-activated and inflammatory HCA, sonic hedgehog-activated HCA, and unclassified HCA. The highest risk of malignant transformation is in the β-catenin-activated subtype and in the mixed β-catenin-activated and inflammatory subtype. Due to the risk of hemorrhage and malignant transformation, surgery is typically the management option for lesions greater than 5 cm, lesions increasing in size, or lesions occurring in men.[17]

Contrast-enhanced liver MRI with an ECA can differentiate most cases of FNH from HCA. FNH has characteristic imaging features[17] including homogeneous appearance, iso-intensity to the liver parenchyma on precontrast T1-weighted and T2-weighted images, marked arterial phase hyperenhancement that becomes isointense on portal venous phase, central scar, and no capsule. However, the central scar is seen in less than half of the cases of FNH. When present, it typically appears hyperintense on T2-weighted and delayed phase images obtained after the injection of an extracellular or a predominantly extracellular (ie, gadobenate dimeglumine) GBCA given the accumulation of contrast in the extracellular space of the fibrotic scar. When using gadoxetic acid, the scar may appear hypointense in the transitional phase given the contrast uptake in the hepatocytes of the lesion and in the hepatic parenchyma (Fig. 4). On the other hand, the MR imaging appearance of HCA depends on the molecular subtype and includes key features such as washout on the extracellular phase (HNF1A), intralesional fat (HNF1A), or increased T2-signal intensity (inflammatory).[19] GBCA-enhanced MRI with HBA has a high accuracy in differentiating FNH from HCA and is particularly useful in cases where the diagnosis remains indeterminate on a contrast-enhanced MRI obtained with an ECA.[20,21] The appearance of FNH and HCA on the HBP images depends on the OATP1 B1/B3 hepatocyte transporter expression. In FNH, OATP1 B1/B3 expression is equal to or greater than the surrounding liver parenchyma, whereas the transporter is not present in about 70% of HCA.[22] For this reason, most FNHs are homogeneously iso- or hyperintense to the surrounding parenchyma or present with a peripheral hyperintensity and a central scar with iso- or hypointensity on HBP imaging[23] (see Fig. 4; Fig. 5). In contrast, most HCA will appear as hypointense on the HBP images (Fig. 6). The expression of hepatocyte transporters depends on the HCA

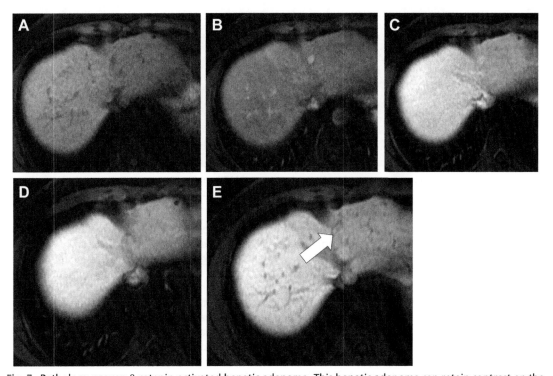

Fig. 7. Pathology-proven β-catenin-activated hepatic adenoma. This hepatic adenoma can retain contrast on the hepatobiliary phase (E, arrow). Lesion demonstrates T1 hypointensity (A), arterial phase hyperenhancement (B), and retention of contrast on portal venous/delayed phases (C, D).

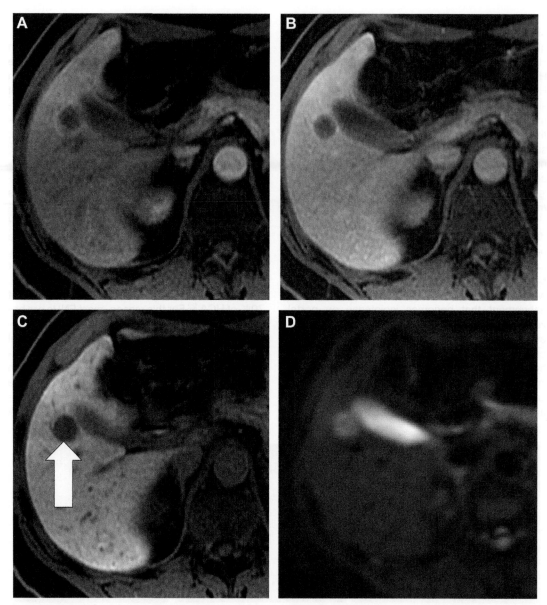

Fig. 8. Metastasis from lung cancer on gadoxetic acid-enhanced MR imaging shows rim enhancement on arterial (*A*) and portal venous (*B*) phases. Lesion does not demonstrate contrast uptake on the hepatobiliary phase (*C, arrow*) and shows restricted diffusion (*D*).

molecular subtype.[22] Although 100% of the HNF1A subtype are hypointense on HBP images, iso- or hyperintensity of HCA on HBP images has been reported in 83% of β-catenin-activated HCA (**Fig. 7**) and 19% of inflammatory HCA.[24] Differentiating these HCA subtypes from FNH can therefore be problematic even when using HBA. In these cases, it is important to rely on other imaging features typical for FNH (eg, a central scar) or features more commonly seen in HCA such as the atoll sign in inflammatory HCA or heterogeneous T1- and T2-signal intensity in the β-catenin-activated HCA.[25]

Hemangioma. Hepatic hemangioma, the most common benign liver lesion, typically presents with high signal intensity on T2-weighted images and with a characteristic enhancement pattern including peripheral, nodular, discontinuous enhancement, and progressive fill-in on later post-contrast images.[26] When using gadoxetic acid, hemangiomas may appear relatively hypointense to the surrounding liver parenchyma on the transitional phase images,[27] a sign referred to as "pseudo-washout."[28] The appearance may lead to misdiagnosing small flash-filling hemangiomas as hepatic adenomas or metastases. Analysis of

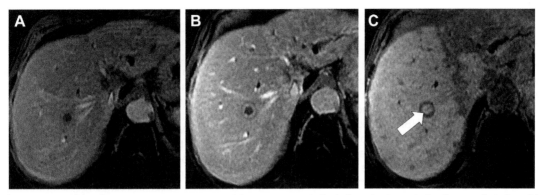

Fig. 9. Targetoid enhancement pattern seen with some metastatic lesions is characterized on gadoxetic acid-enhanced MR images as rim enhancement on arterial and portal venous phases (*A, B*) with central contrast retention on the hepatobiliary phase (*C, arrow*).

the enhancement characteristics on earlier phases and of the signal on T2w images helps in the proper diagnosis.

GBCA-ENHANCED MRI FOR DETECTION OF HEPATIC METASTASES

In many institutions, GBCA-enhanced MRI is the preferred imaging modality for the detection of liver metastasis. Among the available GBCA, hepatobiliary contrast agents, particularly gadoxetic acid, provide the highest sensitivity for the detection of hepatic metastases, especially small lesions.[13,29,30] Most metastases are mildly to moderately hyperintense on T2-weighted imaging and demonstrate restricted diffusion with low signal on ADC maps. Additionally, most are hypointense on precontrast T1WI and hypovascular and hypointense to the liver parenchyma on extracellular postcontrast imaging.[31] However, metastases can have a wide variety of appearances on MRI depending on the primary malignancy. Cystic or necrotic metastases show marked T2 hyperintensity similar to water (eg, metastases from neuroendocrine tumors, cystic

ovarian neoplasms, and sarcoma). Other metastases such as melanoma may demonstrate intrinsic T1 hyperintensity due to intracellular melanin production. Additionally, neuroendocrine, renal, thyroid, and breast cancer metastases are often hyperenhancing on arterial phase imaging.

On the HBP imaging, most metastases are hypointense to the surrounding liver due to the lack of OATP1 B1/B3 transporter expression (**Fig. 8**). However, lesion hyperintensity on HBP imaging post gadoxetic acid administration has been reported with metastases from primary malignancies such as pancreatic ductal adenocarcinoma, colorectal cancer (CRC), and neuroendocrine tumors. A "targetoid" appearance has been described with central enhancement secondary to the accumulation of contrast within the intercellular matrix of the tumor due to necrosis/fibrosis or due to the preserved cellular expression of OATP1 B1/B3[32,33] (**Fig. 9**). In CRC, HBP enhancement correlates with OATP1 B1/B3 expression, and it has been suggested as a prognostic marker that predicts overall survival and treatment response.[34]

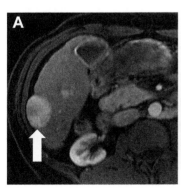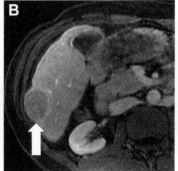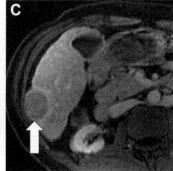

Fig. 10. Hepatocellular carcinoma (*arrow*) in a cirrhotic liver demonstrates arterial phase hyperenhancement (*A*) with washout and enhancing capsule on portal venous (*B*) and delayed phases (*C*).

GBCA-ENHANCED MRI FOR SCREENING AND DIAGNOSIS OF HEPATOCELLULAR CARCINOMA IN CIRRHOSIS

Dynamic contrast-enhanced MRI is critical in the diagnosis, surveillance, and evaluation of treatment response in patients with chronic liver disease (CLD) and hepatocellular carcinoma (HCC)[35] (Fig. 10). Both ECA and HBA are routinely used in patients with CLD for the diagnosis of HCC. Limitations unique to HBA in this patient population include a shorter extracellular phase for evaluation of washout, obscuration of HCC capsule due to the increased contrast uptake in the surrounding liver, transient severe motion artifacts on arterial phase imaging, and a relatively low contrast dose reducing the peak arterial lesion enhancement and the vessels-to-background liver contrast (see Table 2). In cirrhotic patients with liver dysfunction, lack of contrast uptake on HBP images negates the added advantages of this sequence. However, despite these limitations, prior investigations have demonstrated increased sensitivity (86.9%–91.7%) for HCC diagnosis, especially for lesions less than 2 cm in size, with the use of HBA compared with ECA (sensitivity: 74%–82%).[36–39] This finding is likely due to the increased signal-to-noise ratio on the HBP images[40] (Fig. 11). The specificity of HCC diagnosis using HBA is variable with studies demonstrating similar or decreased specificity compared with ECA.[38] This is likely in part due to the variability among HCC diagnosis guidelines in assigning washout appearance. Western guidelines restrict washout to the portal venous phase only[35] although Eastern criteria extend this definition to include washout on transitional phase and HBP[41] in turn leading to decreased specificity.[42] Therefore, the varying diagnostic accuracies of ECA and HBA must be carefully weighed to determine the optimal contrast agent for the patient population at hand.

Although ultrasound has historically been used for HCC screening, given its suboptimal sensitivity, abbreviated MRI has recently been explored. Most investigations involving abbreviated MRI have been performed with HBA.[43] Sensitivities and specificities for HCC detection in a screening/surveillance cohort range from 80% to 91% and 93% to 99%, respectively.[43–45] Only one investigation evaluated abbreviated screening MRI using an ECA and demonstrated sensitivities of 89% to 100% and specificities of 89% to 95%.[46] Further head-to-head comparisons of ECA versus HBA for HCC screening on

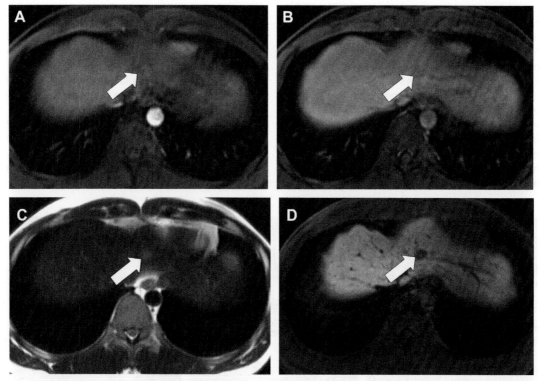

Fig. 11. Hepatobiliary phase (HBP) has been shown to increase sensitivity for small lesions. Note how this left lateral segment hepatocellular carcinoma is much less conspicuous on the arterial (A) and portal venous (B) phase images compared with HBP (D). The lesion is mildly hyperintense on the T2-weighted sequence (C).

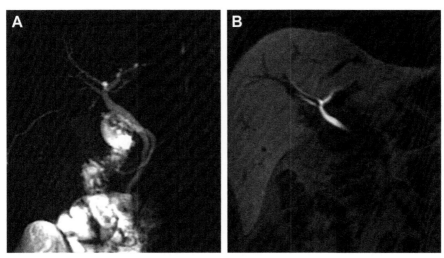

Fig. 12. Living liver donor evaluation is obtained with a combination of T2-weighted MR cholangiography (MRC) (*A*) and contrast-enhanced T1-weighted MRC (*B*) to more clearly demonstrate biliary anatomy. Note the variant biliary anatomy with the right posterior duct draining into the common hepatic duct.

abbreviated MRI are needed to determine the superiority of one over another.

EVALUATION OF LIVING LIVER DONOR CANDIDATE

GBCA-enhanced MRI of liver donor candidates provides relevant information to the transplant surgeon including arterial and venous anatomy, biliary anatomy, and fat and fibrosis content in the liver.[47] In most transplant centers, the evaluation of the biliary anatomy is obtained with a combination of T2-weighted MR cholangiography (MRC) and contrast-enhanced T1-weighted MRC using hepatobiliary contrast agents to increase the diagnostic confidence[48] (**Fig. 12**). The preferred hepatobiliary contrast agent for this task is gadoxetic acid given the higher percentage of contrast excreted through the biliary system and the short interval time to obtain the HBP images. The contrast is injected after obtaining the T2-weighted MRC to avoid signal loss within the bile ducts due to the T2* relaxation of the excreted Gd. At our institution, images are obtained at 10 min postcontrast injection and are repeated at 15 min postinjection if the first set of images demonstrates suboptimal visualization of the intrahepatic biliary branches. Using a larger (25°–40°) flip angle can help the visualization of the intrahepatic biliary branches.[49] When using gadoxetic acid, a number of adjustments have been proposed to improve the quality of the postcontrast images obtained for the evaluation of the vascular anatomy including the use of high-temporal resolution imaging sequences (eg, CAIPIRINHA).[50]

SUMMARY

Contrast-enhanced liver MR imaging is an important diagnostic tool for many different liver diseases by aiding in the detection and characterization of liver lesions, determining vascular and biliary anatomy and patency, and evaluating organ function. Additionally, the safety profile of GBCA is excellent with most adverse events being mild and transient. Both ECA and HBA offer unique advantages and potential limitations. ECA agents are excellent for obtaining high-quality arterial phase imaging and can be particularly useful for the evaluation of HCC in cirrhotic patients. In contrast, the use of HBA is of particular value in distinguishing FNH from HCA, detecting liver metastases, and biliary imaging.

CLINICS CARE POINTS

- Gadolinium-based contrast agents for liver MRI can be categorized as extracellular agent (ECA) and hepatobiliary agent (HBA). The choice of one group over the other depends on a number of factors including the clinical indication, the patient's conditions, and the institution preferences.

- When performing dynamic postcontrast imaging, the late hepatic arterial phase is preferred for the detection of hypervascular lesions compared with early arterial phase; contrast should be present in the hepatic arteries and portal vein but not present (or faintly present) in the hepatic veins.

- HBA are taken up by normal liver parenchyma or lesions with functional hepatocytes via OATP1 B1/B3 hepatocyte transporters. The HBP occurs 10 to 30 min after injection of gadoxetic acid and 90 to 120 min after injection of gadobenate dimeglumine.

- The appearance of hepatocellular adenomas (HCA) on HBP images depends on the molecular subtype and on the expression of OATP1 B1/B3 transporters. Although most HCA are hypointense on HBP images, some inflammatory types and β-catenin-activated HCA may appear iso- to-hyperintense on HBP images.

DISCLOSURE

Alessandro Furlan: Consultant for Bracco Diagnostics

REFERENCES

1. Lohrke J, Frenzel T, Endrikat J, et al. 25 years of contrast-enhanced MRI: developments, current challenges and future perspectives. Adv Ther 2016;33(1):1–28.

2. Bellin M-F, Van Der Molen AJ. Extracellular gadolinium-based contrast media: An overview. Eur J Radiol 2008;66(2):160–7.

3. Gandhi SN, Brown MA, Wong JG, et al. MR contrast agents for liver imaging: What, when, how. RadioGraphics 2006;26(6):1621–36.

4. CT/MRI LI-RADS v2018 | American College of Radiology. Available at: https://www.acr.org/Clinical-Resources/Reporting-and-Data-Systems/LI-RADS/CT-MRI-LI-RADS-v2018. Accessed August 29, 2021.

5. Seale MK, Catalano OA, Saini S, et al. Hepatobiliary-specific MR contrast agents: Role in imaging the liver and biliary tree. RadioGraphics 2009;29(6):1725–48.

6. Welle CL, Venkatesh SK, Reeder SB, et al. Dual contrast liver MRI: A pictorial illustration. Abdom Radiol 2021;46(10):4588–600.

7. Yoneda N, Matsui O, Kitao A, et al. Benign hepatocellular nodules: Hepatobiliary phase of gadoxetic acid–enhanced MR Imaging based on molecular background. RadioGraphics 2016;36(7):2010–27.

8. Ringe KI, Husarik DB, Sirlin CB, et al. Gadoxetate disodium–enhanced MRI of the liver: Part 1, protocol optimization and lesion appearance in the noncirrhotic liver. Am J Roentgenol 2010;195(1):13–28.

9. Leonhardt M, Keiser M, Oswald S, et al. Hepatic uptake of the magnetic resonance imaging contrast agent Gd-EOB-DTPA: Role of human organic anion transporters. Drug Metab Dispos 2010;38(7):1024–8.

10. Nassif A, Jia J, Keiser M, et al. Visualization of hepatic UPTAKE transporter function in healthy subjects by Using gadoxetic acid–enhanced MR Imaging. Radiology 2012;264(3):741–50.

11. Pastor CM, Langer O, Van Beers BE. Liver imaging and hepatobiliary contrast media. Contrast Media Mol Imaging 2018;2018:1–2.

12. Neri E, Bali MA, Ba-Ssalamah A, et al. ESGAR consensus statement on liver MR imaging and clinical use of liver-specific contrast agents. Eur Radiol 2016;26:921–31.

13. Koh DM, Ba-Ssalamah A, Brancatelli G, et al. Consensus report from the 9th international forum for liver magnetic resonance imaging: Applications of gadoxetic acid-enhanced imaging. Eur Radiol 2021;31(8):5615–28.

14. ACR manual on contrast media. Available at: https://www.acr.org/-/media/ACR/Files/Clinical-Resources/Contrast_Media.pdf. Accessed August 29, 2021.

15. Weinreb JC, Rodby RA, Yee J, et al. Use of intravenous gadolinium-based contrast media in patients with kidney disease: Consensus statements from the American College of Radiology and the National Kidney Foundation. Kidney Med 2020;3(1):142–50.

16. Radbruch A, Weberling LD, Kieslich PJ, et al. Gadolinium retention in the Dentate nucleus and globus pallidus is dependent on the class of contrast agent. Radiology 2015;275(3):783–91.

17. European Association for the Study of the Liver (EASL). EASL Clinical Practice Guidelines on the management of benign liver tumours. J Hepatol 2016;65(2):386–98.

18. Nault J-C, Couchy G, Balabaud C, et al. Molecular classification of hepatocellular Adenoma associates with risk factors, bleeding, and malignant transformation. Gastroenterology 2017;152(4):880–94.e6.

19. Van Aalten SM, Thomeer MG, Terkivatan T, et al. Hepatocellular adenomas: Correlation of MR imaging findings with pathologic subtype classification. Radiology 2011;261(1):172–81.

20. Guo Y, Li W, Cai W, et al. Diagnostic value of gadoxetic acid-enhanced MR imaging to distinguish HCA and its subtype from FNH: A systematic review. Int J Med Sci 2017;14(7):668–74.

21. Vanhooymissen IJSML, Thomeer MG, Braun LMM, et al. Intrapatient comparison of the hepatobiliary phase of Gd-BOPTA and Gd-EOB-DTPA in the differentiation of hepatocellular adenoma from focal nodular hyperplasia. J Magn Reson Imaging 2018;49(3):700–10.

22. Sciarra A, Schmidt S, Pellegrinelli A, et al. OATPB1/B3 and MRP3 expression in hepatocellular adenoma predicts Gd-EOB-DTPA uptake and correlates with risk of malignancy. Liver Int 2018;39(1):158–67.

23. Vernuccio F, Gagliano DS, Cannella R, et al. Spectrum of liver lesions hyperintense on hepatobiliary phase: An approach by clinical setting. Insights into Imaging 2021;12(1).

24. Ba-Ssalamah A, Antunes C, Feier D, et al. Morphologic and molecular features of hepatocellular adenoma with gadoxetic acid-enhanced MR Imaging. Radiology 2015;277(1):104–13.

25. Auer TA, Walter-Rittel T, Geisel D, et al. HBP-enhancing hepatocellular adenomas and how to discriminate them from FNH in Gd-EOB MRI. BMC Med Imaging 2021;21(1):28.

26. Mamone G, Di Piazza A, Carollo V, et al. Imaging of hepatic hemangioma: from A to Z. Abdom Radiol 2020;45(3):672–91.

27. Gupta RT, Marin D, Boll DT, et al. Hepatic hemangiomas: difference in enhancement pattern on 3T MR imaging with gadobenate dimeglumine versus gadoxetate disodium. Eur J Radiol 2012;81(10): 2457–62.

28. Doo KW, Lee CH, Choi JW, et al. Pseudo washout" sign in high-flow hepatic hemangioma on gadoxetic acid contrast-enhanced MRI mimicking hypervascular tumor. AJR Am J Roentgenol 2009;193(6): 90–6.

29. Lee KH, Lee JM, Park JH, et al. MR Imaging in patients with suspected live metastases: value of liver-specific contrast agent gadoxetic acid. Korean J Radiol 2013;14(6):894–904.

30. Jhaveri KS, Fischer SE, Hosseini-Nik H, et al. Prospective comparison of gadoxetic acid-enhanced liver MRI and contrast-enhanced CT with histopathological correlation for preoperative detection of colorectal liver metastases following chemotherapy and potential impact on Surgical plan. HPB 2017; 19(11):992–1000.

31. Roth CG, Mitchell DG. Hepatocellular carcinoma and other hepatic malignancies: MR imaging. Radiol Clin North Am 2014;52:683–707.

32. Ha S, Lee CH, Kim BH, et al. Paradoxical uptake of Gd-EOB-DTPA on the hepatobiliary phase in the evaluation of hepatic metastasis from breast cancer: Is the "target sign" a common finding? Magn Reson Imaging 2012;30(8):1083–90.

33. Granata V, Catalano O, Fusco R, et al. The target sign in colorectal liver metastases: An atypical Gd-EOB-DTPA "uptake" on the hepatobiliary phase of MR imaging. Abdom Imaging 2015; 40(7):2364–71.

34. Cheung HM, Karanicolas PJ, Coburn N, et al. Delayed tumour enhancement on gadoxetate-enhanced MRI is associated with overall survival in patients with colorectal liver metastases. Eur Radiol 2018;29(2):1032–8.

35. Marrero JA, Kulik LM, Sirlin CB, et al. Diagnosis, staging, and management of hepatocellular carcinoma: 2018 practice guidance by the American Association for the Study of Liver Diseases. Hepatology 2018;68(2):723–50.

36. Roberts LR, Sirlin CB, Zaiem F, et al. Imaging for the diagnosis of hepatocellular carcinoma: A systematic review and meta-analysis. Hepatology 2018;67(1): 401–21.

37. Ahn SS, Kim MJ, Lim JS, et al. Added value of gadoxetic acid-enhanced hepatobiliary phase MR imaging in the diagnosis of hepatocellular carcinoma. Radiology 2010;255(2):459–66.

38. Kierans AS, Kang SK, Rosenkrantz AB. The Diagnostic performance of dynamic contrast-enhanced MR imaging for detection of small hepatocellular carcinoma measuring up to 2 cm: A meta-analysis. Radiology 2016;278(1):82–94.

39. Min JH, Kim JM, Kim YK, et al. Prospective intraindividual comparison of magnetic resonance imaging with gadoxetic acid and extracellular contrast for diagnosis of hepatocellular carcinomas using the liver imaging reporting and data system. Hepatology 2018;68(6):2254–66.

40. Goodwin MD, Dobson JE, Sirlin CB, et al. Diagnostic challenges and pitfalls in MR imaging with hepatocyte-specific contrast agents. Radiographics 2011;31(6):1547–68.

41. 2018 Korean Liver Cancer Association-National Cancer Center Korea practice guidelines for the management of hepatocellular carcinoma. Korean J Radiol 2019;20(7):1042–113.

42. Kim SY. Diagnosis of hepatocellular carcinoma: Which MRI contrast agent? Which diagnostic criteria? Clin Mol Hepatol 2020;26(3):309–11.

43. Brunsing RL, Chen DH, Schlein A, et al. Gadoxetate-enhanced abbreviated MRI for hepatocellular carcinoma surveillance: Preliminary experience. Radiol Imaging Cancer 2019;1(2):e190010.

44. Tillman BG, Gorman JD, Hru JM, et al. Diagnostic per-lesion performance of a simulated gadoxetate disodium-enhanced abbreviated MRI protocol for hepatocellular carcinoma screening. Clin Radiol 2018;73(5):485–93.

45. Besa C, Lewis S, Pandharipande PV, et al. Hepatocellular carcinoma detection: diagnostic performance of a simulated abbreviated MRI protocol combining diffusion-weighted and T1-weighted imaging at the delayed phase post gadoxetic acid. Abdom Radiol 2017;42(1):179–90.

46. Khatri G, Pedrosa I, Ananthakrishnan L, et al. Abbreviated-protocol screening MRI vs. complete-protocol diagnostic MRI for detection of hepatocellular carcinoma in patients with cirrhosis: An equivalence study using LI-RADS v2018. J Magn Reson Imaging 2020;51(2):415–25.

47. Hecht EM, Wang ZJ, Kambadakone A, et al. Living donor liver transplantation: Preoperative planning and postoperative complications. Am J Roentgenol 2019;213(1):65–76.

48. Cai L, Yeh BM, Westphalen AC, et al. 3D T2-weighted and Gd-EOB-DTPA-enhanced 3D T1-weighted MR cholangiography for evaluation of biliary anatomy in living liver donors. Abdom Radiol 2017;42(3):842–50.

49. Kim S, Mussi TC, Lee LJ, et al. Effect of flip angle for optimization of image quality of gadoxetate disodium–enhanced biliary imaging at 1.5 T. Am J Roentgenol 2013;200(1):90–6.

50. Jhaveri K, Guo L, Guimarães L, et al. Mapping of hepatic vasculature in potential living liver donors: comparison of gadoxetic acid-enhanced MR imaging using CAIPIRINHA technique with CT angiography. Abdom Radiol 2018;43(7):1682–92.

Abbreviated Liver Magnetic Resonance Imaging Protocols and Applications

Emre Altinmakas, MD[a,b,c],*, Bachir Taouli, MD, MHA[a,b]

KEYWORDS

- Abbreviated MRI • Chronic liver disease • Screening • Surveillance • Hepatocellular carcinoma
- NASH • NAFLD • Liver fibrosis

KEY POINTS

- An abbreviated magnetic resonance imaging (AMRI) approach is a faster and cheaper alternative than a complete MRI protocol for HCC surveillance and liver fat/iron/fibrosis quantification.
- Three different types of AMRI protocols have been used for HCC surveillance: noncontrast-AMRI, hepatobiliary phase (HBP)-AMRI, and dynamic-AMRI.
- Further evidence from prospective (multicenter) data is required.

INTRODUCTION

Hepatocellular carcinoma (HCC) is the 3rd cause of cancer death worldwide and the most rapidly rising cause of cancer death in the United States.[1] The European Association for the Study of Liver Disease[2] and the American Association for the Study of the Liver Disease (AASLD) clinical practice guidelines recommend HCC surveillance with ultrasound (US) every 6 months for patients at risk.[2,3] However, US has been shown to have limited sensitivity, especially in patients with obesity, advanced cirrhosis, and fatty liver disease.[4,5] In a metanalysis by Tzartzeva and colleagues, the sensitivity of US for the detection of HCC was found to be 78% and it was as low as 45% for the detection of early HCC.[6] On the other hand, with the recent technological advances, it is now possible to accurately quantify liver fat and iron, and liver fibrosis, making MRI a powerful modality for assessing liver disease. The advantages of MRI include the lack of ionizing radiation and higher diagnostic performance compared with US, which have pushed for its increased use in the evaluation of chronic liver disease. However, due to its relatively long study duration and higher cost, current guidelines do not advocate the use of MRI for HCC screening and surveillance.

To address these limitations, abbreviated magnetic resonance imaging (AMRI) protocols which consist of a few selected MRI sequences, have been proposed for HCC screening/surveillance with promising results. In AMRI protocols, there is a reduction in the number of sequences which shortens the table time and increases patient throughput, while keeping an acceptable diagnostic performance. This also makes MRI more acceptable for claustrophobic patients. Furthermore, having less images/sequences reduces radiologist reporting time which in turn shortens the reporting turn-around time.

[a] Department of Diagnostic, Molecular and Interventional Radiology, Icahn School of Medicine at Mount Sinai, 1470 Madison Avenue, New York, NY 10029, USA; [b] BioMedical Engineering and Imaging Institute, Icahn School of Medicine at Mount Sinai, 1470 Madison Avenue, New York, NY 10029, USA; [c] Department of Radiology, School of Medicine, Koç University, 34450, Istanbul, Turkey
* Corresponding author. Department of Diagnostic, Molecular and Interventional Radiology, Icahn School of Medicine at Mount Sinai, 1470 Madison Avenue, New York, NY 10029.
E-mail address: emre.altinmakas@mountsinai.org

Radiol Clin N Am 60 (2022) 695–703
https://doi.org/10.1016/j.rcl.2022.04.002
0033-8389/22/© 2022 Elsevier Inc. All rights reserved.

Abbreviations	
AASLD	American Association for the Study of the Liver Disease
AMRI	Abbreviated magnetic resonance imaging
AP	Arterial phase
DWI	Diffusion-weighted imaging
Dyn-AMRI	Dynamic-abbreviated magnetic resonance imaging
HBP	Hepatobiliary phase
HBP-AMRI	Hepatobiliary-abbreviated magnetic resonance imaging
HCC	Hepatocellular carcinoma
IP	In phase
MRE	Magnetic resonance elastography
NAFLD	Nonalcoholic fatty liver disease
NASH	Nonalcoholic steatohepatitis
NC-AMRI	Noncontrast-abbreviated magnetic resonance imaging
NPV	Negative predictive value
OP	Out of phase
PDFF	Proton-density fat fraction
PPV	Positive predictive value
PVP	Portal venous phase
TP	Transitional phase
US	Ultrasound

With the abovementioned advantages, in addition to HCC screening and surveillance, AMRI protocols have been proposed for the quantification of liver fat, iron, and degree of fibrosis, as well as metastasis screening in colorectal cancer. In this review, different liver AMRI protocols and their clinical applications are discussed.

Abbreviated Magnetic Resonance Imaging Protocols for Hepatocellular Carcinoma Screening and Surveillance

Three types of AMRI protocols have been proposed in HCC screening/surveillance: noncontrast-abbreviated magnetic resonance imaging (NC-AMRI), hepatobiliary-AMRI (HBP-AMRI) using gadoxetic acid, and dynamic-AMRI (Dyn-AMRI). Due to the lack of dynamic series, the full LI-RADS algorithm cannot be applied to observation on NC-AMRI and HBP-AMRI protocols which may potentially lead to a recall of full contrast-enhanced CT or MRI study in the presence of positive findings on AMRI. However, an adapted version of LI-RADS has been proposed for HBP-AMRI by Brunsing and colleagues.[7]

Dyn-AMRI has the advantage of being both a screening and a diagnostic test by allowing full LI-RADS categorization, without the need for a recall study. In most previous studies, the performance of AMRI was retrospectively assessed based on a reconstructed protocol created by extracting select sequences from a full contrast-enhanced MRI protocol (Table 1). Furthermore, a number of previous studies include potential bias as they include nonscreening population with a higher pretest probability for HCC compared with a screening population. There is a very limited prospective data on the performance of AMRI protocols in HCC screening/surveillance among screening populations.[7,8] Reconstructed NC-AMRI. HBP-AMRI, and dyn-AMRI protocols are detailed in Figure 1.

Noncontrast abbreviated magnetic resonance imaging protocols

As the name implies, NC-AMRI does not warrant contrast material which eliminates the possibility of contrast-related side effects including allergy, gadolinium tissue deposition, and nephrogenic systemic fibrosis (NSF), and makes the protocol

Abbreviated Liver MRI Protocols and Applications

Table 1
Published studies investigating the performance of AMRI in HCC surveillance

Author (Year)	Population	Design	n	% HCC	AMRI Protocol	Sensitivity	Specificity	PPV	NPV
NC-AMRI									
Jalli et al,[9] 2015	NS	R	96	31.2	DWI	76.6%	100%	100%	90.4%
Sutherland et al,[10] 2017	S	P	192	3	DWI	83%	98%	63%	99%
McNamara et al,[11] 2018	NS	R	37	54.1	DWI	78%	88%	85%	83%
Ahmed et al,[12] 2020	S	R	41	26.8	T2WI	86.6%	100%	100%	93.9%
Violi et al,[13] 2020	S	R	237	5.5	T2WI + DWI	61.5%	95.5%	44.4%	97.7%
Ahmed et al,[12] 2020	S	R	41	26.8	T2WI + DWI	100%	100%	100%	100%
Park et al,[8] 2020	S	P	382	11.3	T2WI + DWI	79.1%	97.9%	61.8%	99.1%
Kim et al,[14] 2020	S	R	226	76.5	T2WI + DWI	87.3%	86.8%	95.6%	67.7%
Kim et al,[15] 2014	NS	R	157	85.9	T2WI + DWI + T1WI	91.7%	77.5%	94.7%	68.1%
Jalli et al,[9] 2015	NS	R	96	31.2	T2WI + DWI + T1WI	83.3%	100%	100%	92.9%
Han et al,[16] 2018	NS	R	247	70.8	T2WI + DWI + T1WI	84.6%	81.9%	NA	NA
Chan et al,[17] 2019	NS	R	188	14.3	T2WI + DWI + T1WI	84.5%	92.7%	67%	97.2%
Besa et al,[18] 2017	NS	R	174	35.6	T2WI + DWI + T1 IP/OP	85.5%	94.9%	90.3%	92.%
Kim et al,[14] 2020	S	R	226	76.5	T2WI + DWI + T1 IP/OP	89.6%	79.2%	93.4%	70%
Whang et al,[19] 2020	NS	R	263	53.2	T2WI + DWI + T1 IP/OP	86.1%	92.7%	NA	NA
Jalli et al,[9] 2015	NS	R	96	31.2	T2WI + T1WI	83.3%	84.8%	71.4%	91.8%
HBP-AMRI									
Marks et al,[20] 2015	NS	R	298	16.4	HBP + T2WI	82.6%	93.2%	71%	96.5%
Tillman et al,[21] 2018	NS	R	79	16.5	HBP + T2WI	85.2%	NA	78%	95%
[a]Brunsing et al,[7] 2019	S	R	141	8.5	HBP + T2WI + DWI	92%	91%	48%	99%
Whang et al,[19] 2020	NS	R	263	53.2	HBP + T2WI + DWI	89.7%	92.7%	NA	NA
Violi et al,[13] 2020	S	R	237	5.5	HBP + T2WI + DWI	80.8%	94.9%	47.7%	98.8%
Marks et al,[20] 2015	NS	R	298	16.4	HBP + T2WI + DWI	83.7%	93.2%	71.4%	96.7%
Besa et al,[18] 2017	NS	R	174	35.6	HBP + T2WI + DWI + T1 IP/OP	80.6%	96.1%	92%	90%
Besa et al,[18] 2017	NS	R	174	35.6	HBP + T2WI + T1 IP/OP	89.8%	91.1%	84.8%	94.2%

(continued on next page)

Table 1
(continued)

Author (Year)	Population	Design	n	% HCC	AMRI Protocol	Sensitivity	Specificity	PPV	NPV
Dynamic-AMRI									
Khatri et al,[22] 2020	NS	R	86	32.6	CE-T1WI + T2WI	92.1%	88.6%	NA	NA
Violi et al,[13] 2020	S	R	237	5.5	CE-T1WI + T2WI + DWI	84.6%	99.8%	95.7%	99.1%
[b]Lee et al,[23] 2018	NS	R	156	Unclear	CE-T1WI + T2WI + T1 IP/OP	-	-	-	-
Besa et al,[18] 2017	NS	R	174	35.6	CE-T1WI + T2WI + T1 IP/OP	90.3%	100%	100%	94.9%

CE-T1WI protocol consisted of precontrast, arterial phase, portal venous phase, and transitional phase imaging.

Abbreviations: AMRI, abbreviated magnetic resonance imaging; CE-T1WI, contrast enhanced-T1 weighted imaging; DWI, diffusion-weighted imaging; HBP, hepatobiliary phase; HBP-MRI, hepatobiliary phase-magnetic resonance imaging; IP/OP, in phase/opposed phase; NA, nonavailable; NPV, negative predictive value; NS, nonscreening; P, prospective; PPV, positive; predictive value; R, retrospective; S, screening; T1WI, T1 weighted imaging; T2WI, T2 weighted imaging.

[a] AMRI studies were evaluated prospectively.

[b] High concordance with full MRI.

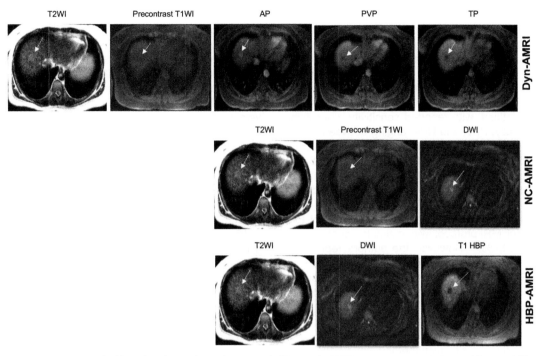

Fig. 1. Reconstructed abbreviated MRI (AMRI) protocols (Dynamic-AMRI, noncontrast-AMRI, and hepatobiliary phase-AMRI) from a complete gadoxetate-enhanced abdominal MRI study obtained in a 45-year-old female with HBV cirrhosis and 1.4 cm pathologically proven HCC in the hepatic dome. The lesion (*arrow*) shows hyperintense signal on T2WI and restricted diffusion on DWI. On dynamic series, there is nonrim arterial phase hyperenhancement with portal venous phase washout and hypointensity on TP and HBP. AP, arterial phase; DWI, diffusion-weighted imaging; HBP, hepatobiliary phase; IP, in phase; OP, out of phase; PVP, portal venous phase; TP, transitional phase.

simpler. Various NC-AMRI protocols including DWI (diffusion-weighted imaging) alone, T2WI (T2-weighted imaging) alone, T2WI + DWI, T2WI + DWI + FS T1WI (fat-suppressed T1WI), T2WI + DWI + T1W-IP/OP (in phase/opposed phase), and T2WI + T1WI have been described for HCC surveillance with sensitivity and specificity ranging between 61.5% and 100% and 77.5% to 100%, respectively.[8–19] In the largest prospective study with 382 screening subjects from Korea, an AMRI protocol consisting of DWI + T2WI was compared with US and sensitivity, specificity, negative predictive value (NPV), and positive predictive value (PPV) were found to be 79.1% versus 27.9%, 97.9% versus 94.5%, 99.1% versus 96.9%, and 61.8% versus 17.7%, respectively, for HCC detection.[8] The mean size of the 48 detected HCCs was 1.6 cm (range 1.0–4.8 cm). Jalli and colleagues compared the performance of different reconstructed NC-AMRI protocols in nonscreening population (n = 96) retrospectively. A 10-min long NC-AMRI protocol which consisted of T2WI + DWI + T1WI showed better diagnostic performance compared with T2WI + T1WI and

DWI alone, with an accuracy of 94.7%.[9] Lastly, in a retrospective study with 237 screening patients, NC-AMRI with T2WI + DWI was found to have low sensitivity (61.5%) and PPV (44.4%), with high specificity (95.5%) and NPV (97.7%).[13]

Hepatobiliary phase-abbreviated magnetic resonance imaging protocols

These protocols are based on T1WI obtained during the hepatobiliary phase postgadoxetic acid injection (typically at 20-min postinjection). In HBP-AMRI, to shorten the acquisition time, contrast material is given outside the MRI room and approximately 20 minutes later, the AMRI protocol is started with T1-HBP followed by other sequences. However, instead of this nonreconstructed protocol, most published studies evaluated the performance of reconstructed HBP-AMRI protocols. Different HBP-AMRI protocols including HBP alone or its combination with T1WI, T2WI, or DWI have been investigated for the detection of HCC.[7,13,18–21] At this point, there is only one published study that used a nonreconstructed HBP-AMRI protocol which has consisted of T2WI + DWI + T1-HBP.[7] In this single-center study, 141 screening patients were included and sensitivity, specificity, and accuracy for HCC detection (n = 12) were all more than 90%. There was no comparison with US. The remainder of the published studies used a reconstructed HBP-AMRI protocol among screening or nonscreening populations, with reported sensitivity, specificity, accuracy, PPV, and NPV ranging between 80.6% and 89.8%, 91.1% and 96.1%, 90.5% and 91.6%, 47.7% and 92%, and 90% and 98.8%, respectively. In the largest study with 298 subjects, an accuracy of 91.6% was achieved with the combination of HBP + T2WI + DWI. The acquisition time of this protocol was half of that of a full MRI protocol, with estimated cost savings was 30.7%.[20] However, the authors reported a relatively high call-back rate (19.3%) as the full LI-RADS algorithm cannot be applied to observations in HBP-AMRI due to lack of dynamic series.[20] To address this limitation, Brunsing and colleagues proposed an adapted LI-RADS classification that can be used in HBP-AMRI.[7] According to this classification method, each HBP-AMRI study can be scored, for example, using a recently published four-point scale: negative, subthreshold, positive, and inadequate results.[7] However, its performance in the detection of HCC has not been well studied yet.

Dynamic-abbreviated magnetic resonance imaging protocols

This protocol relies on dynamic contrast-enhanced T1WI sequences (CE-T1WI) including pre-contrast, arterial, portal venous, and delayed venous phases after the administration of contrast material, typically using an extracellular agent. Unlike the other AMRI protocols, this protocol does not warrant a confirmatory study when an observation is detected as Dyn-AMRI includes all postcontrast sequences that are required for the full LI-RADS algorithm. Different reconstructed combinations have been used in previous studies: CE-T1WI + T2WI, CE-T1WI + T2WI + DWI, and CE-T1WI + T2WI + T1WI IP/OP.[13,18,22,23] For example, Besa and colleagues used CE-T1WI + T2WI + T1WI IP/OP and reported sensitivity, specificity, accuracy, PPV, and NPV of 90.3%, 100%, 96.6%, 100%, and 94.9% for the detection of HCC, respectively.[18]

COMPARISON OF DIFFERENT ABBREVIATED MAGNETIC RESONANCE IMAGING PROTOCOLS FOR HEPATOCELLULAR CARCINOMA SURVEILLANCE

AMRI protocols have their own advantages and disadvantages as discussed above. In a metanalysis combining 15 studies (including screening and diagnostic populations), the overall sensitivity and specificity of AMRI for detecting HCC were found to be 86% and 96%.[24] In subgroup analysis, CE-AMRI (HBP-AMRI and Dyn-AMRI) showed slightly better performance than NC-AMRI with sensitivity and specificity of 94% versus 86% and 94% versus 87%, respectively.[24] In another metanalysis including 10 studies (including only screening population), HBP-AMRI showed a significantly higher sensitivity for detecting HCC compared with NC-AMRI (87% vs 82%), but significantly lower specificity (93% vs 98%).[25] In a retrospective study (n = 237) by Vietti Violi and colleagues, reconstructed HBP-AMRI and Dyn-AMRI (using gadoxetate) showed excellent sensitivity and specificity for HCC detection, whereas NC-AMRI had limited sensitivity (61.5%). In the same study, all AMRI methods were effective compared with semiannual US with the incremental costs were less than $12,000, with population-level life-year gain of 3 to 12 months.[13] Finally, Besa and colleagues compared HBP-AMRI and Dyn-AMRI and concluded that HBP-AMRI has a clinically acceptable sensitivity and NPV for HCC detection.[18] However, in most of these studies, instead of using AMRI protocol prospectively in HCC screening population, reconstructed AMRI protocols were applied retrospectively in screening or non-screening populations. Also, there has only one study in the literature comparing prospective AMRI protocols with US which is the most preferred modality in HCC screening worldwide.[8]

Abbreviated Magnetic Resonance Imaging Protocols for Liver Fat, Iron, and Fibrosis Detection

Nonalcoholic fatty liver disease (NAFLD), which represents a spectrum of diseases ranging from steatosis to nonalcoholic steatohepatitis (NASH), is becoming one of the most common causes of chronic liver disease worldwide. NAFLD may sometimes progress to liver fibrosis and cirrhosis if left untreated. Other than fat, iron accumulation also plays a role in liver fibrosis; therefore, the detection of iron in liver tissue is important. The reference standard for the detection of liver fat and iron accumulation and fibrosis is liver biopsy. However, it is an invasive method, and it only samples a small amount of liver tissue and suffers from interobserver variability. On the other hand, with the recent advances in MRI technology, fat, iron, and fibrosis can be quantified noninvasively. Proton-density fat fraction (PDFF) for fat and R2* for iron quantification and MR elastography

(MRE) for the detection of fibrosis have been adopted in clinical practice. To the best of our knowledge, there is only one study in the literature investigating AMRI in patients with NAFLD.[26] In this study (n = 25), an NC-AMRI protocol consisting of liver fat and iron quantification, MRE, and visceral adipose tissue measurement was found to be a feasible, less expensive, and accessible option for monitoring and screening patients with NAFLD, metabolic syndrome and obesity.[26] When taking the high prevalence of these entities into account, AMRI approach may become a screening tool among this population. Further studies are required to validate these preliminary results and to determine the optimal AMRI protocol in terms of diagnostic performance and cost-effectiveness. **Figure 2** shows a reconstructed AMRI protocol consisted of R2*, PDFF, and MRE images in a patient with NASH.

Abbreviated Magnetic Resonance Imaging Protocols in Colorectal Cancer Liver Metastasis Screening and Surveillance

AMRI protocols have been proposed for the screening and follow-up of liver metastasis in patients with colorectal cancer.[27–29] In a study by Canellas and colleagues, a reconstructed HBP-AMRI protocol (T2WI + DWI + T1W HBP) showed sensitivity and AUC of 93.5% and 0.93, respectively, in the detection of liver metastatic disease (n = 57). No statistically significant differences in sensitivity and AUC for lesion characterization were found between AMRI and the full MRI protocols.[27] In another study, Torkzad and colleagues showed that a reconstructed AMRI (DWI + T1W HBP) had high agreement with complete MRI for the posttreatment follow-up of colorectal cancer liver metastases.[29] Despite these promising results, AMRI is not the standard of care in colorectal cancer surveillance because of its cost and slightly longer acquisition time compared with CT which is the widely accepted modality for follow-up of these patients. To address this limitation, Granata and colleagues investigated the performance of an 8-min-long reconstructed NC-AMRI protocol (T2WI + DWI) in 108 patients with 732 pathologically proven colorectal cancer liver metastases. In that study, HBP-AMRI and full gadoxetic acid MRI were found to be equally accurate in the detection of liver metastasis, with a detection rate of more than 96%.[28] HBP-AMRI protocol in a patinet with colorectal liver metastasis is shown in **Figure 3**.

FUTURE PERSPECTIVES AND LIMITATIONS

An AMRI approach has the potential to become a solid alternative for HCC screening and surveillance in patients with chronic liver disease and could potentially be expanded to other clinical settings such as diffuse liver disease or liver metastasis screening. Shorter table time is the main advantage compared with a complete MRI. Despite the abovementioned promising results, it should be kept in mind that these data predominantly rely on the retrospective application of reconstructed AMRI protocols in nonscreening populations (for HCC). Prospective studies on screening population and cost-effectiveness analysis are lacking. Also, there is a need for adapted interpretation algorithms that can be used in NC-AMRI and HBP-AMRI as these protocols do not contain dynamic series.

On the other hand, AMRI approaches neither have been incorporated in any practice guidelines nor under insurance coverage. Further multicentric and prospective studies in the screening population need to be conducted to investigate the optimal AMRI protocol for different clinical scenarios for clinical adoption.

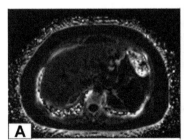 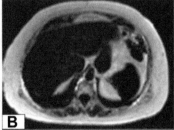 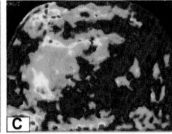

Fig. 2. 69-year-old female patient with NASH and stage 0 liver fibrosis. An AMRI protocol was reconstructed from a complete MRI and consisted of (*A*) R2* map (TR: 14.4 msec/TE: 2.3 msec, 4.7 msec, 7.1 msec, 9.5 msec, 11.9 msec, 14.3 msec, 16.7 msec, and 19.0 msec), (*B*) proton density fat fraction (PDFF) map (TR: 14.4 msec/TE: 2.3 msec, 4.7 msec, 7.1 msec, 9.5 msec, 11.9 msec, and 14.3 msec), and (*C*) MR Elastography. Only mild fat deposition was noted with PDFF of 7% and no iron was detected (3 msec). There was no or mild fibrosis (liver stiffness 3.29 kPa).

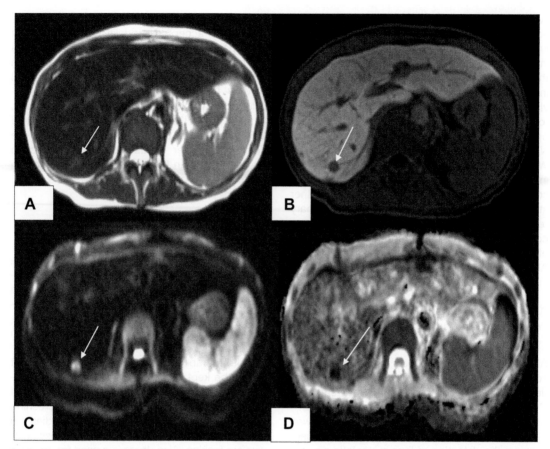

Fig. 3. 59-year-old female with sigmoid colon adenocarcinoma and a newly developed 0.9 cm liver metastasis. A reconstructed HBP-AMRI protocol obtained from a complete gadoxetic acid-enhanced MRI protocol. The lesion (*white arrow*) shows hyperintense signal on T2WI (*A*) and becomes hypointense compared with background liver on HBP imaging (*B*), with restricted diffusion on DWI (*C*), and ADC map (*D*). ADC, apparent diffusion coefficient; DWI, diffusion-weighted imaging; HBP, hepatobiliary phase; T2WI, T2 weighted imaging.

CLINICS CARE POINTS

- An abbreviated magnetic resonance imaging (AMRI) approach is a faster and cheaper alternative than a complete MRI protocol for HCC surveillance and liver fat/iron/fibrosis quantification.

- Three different types of AMRI protocols have been used for HCC surveillance: noncontrast-AMRI, hepatobiliary phase (HBP)-AMRI, and dynamic-AMRI.

- Further evidence from prospective (multicenter) data is required.

DISCLOSURE

B. Taouli: research support from Bayer Health-Care, Regeneron, Takeda, Echosens, Helio Health.

REFERENCES

1. Marrero JA, Kulik LM, Sirlin CB, et al. Diagnosis, staging, and management of h epatocellular carcinoma: 2018 practice guidance by the American Association for the Study of Liver Diseases. Hepatology 2018;68(2):723–50.
2. European Association for the Study of the Liver. Electronic address, e.e.e. and L. European Association for the Study of the, EASL Clinical Practice Guidelines: Management of Hepatocellular Carcinoma. J Hepatol 2018;69(1):182–236.
3. Heimbach JK, Kulik LM, Finn RS, et al. AASLD guidelines for the treatment of hepatocellular carcinoma. Hepatology 2018;67(1):358–80.
4. Samoylova ML, Mehta N, Roberts JP, et al. Predictors of ultrasound failure to detect hepatocellular carcinoma. Liver Transpl 2018;24(9):1171–7.
5. Simmons O, Fetzer DT, Yokoo T, et al. Predictors of adequate ultrasound quality for hepatocellular

carcinoma surveillance in patients with cirrhosis. Aliment Pharmacol Ther 2017;45(1):169–77.

6. Tzartzeva K, Obi J, Rich NE, et al. Surveillance imaging and alpha fetoprotein for early detection of hepatocellular carcinoma in patients with cirrhosis: a meta-analysis. Gastroenterology 2018;154(6): 1706–18.e1.

7. Brunsing RL, Chen DH, Schlein A, et al. Gadoxetate-enhanced abbreviated mri for hepatocellular carcinoma surveillance: preliminary experience. Radiol Imaging Cancer 2019;1(2):e190010.

8. Park HJ, Jang HY, Kim SY, et al. Non-enhanced magnetic resonance imaging as a surveillance tool for hepatocellular carcinoma: comparison with ultrasound. J Hepatol 2020;72(4):718–24.

9. Jalli R, Jafari SH, Sefidbakht S, et al. Comparison of the accuracy of DWI and ultrasonography in screening hepatocellular carcinoma in patients with chronic liver disease. Iranian J Radiol 2015;12(1):e12708.

10. Sutherland T, Watts J, Ryan M, et al. Diffusion-weighted MRI for hepatocellular carcinoma screening in chronic liver disease: direct comparison with ultrasound screening. J Med Imaging Radiat Oncol 2017;61(1):34–9.

11. McNamara MM, Thomas JV, Alexander LF, et al. Diffusion-weighted MRI as a screening tool for hepatocellular carcinoma in cirrhotic livers: correlation with explant data-A pilot study. Abdom Radiol (Ny) 2018;43(10):2686–92.

12. Ahmed NNA, El Gaafary SM, Elia RZ, et al. Role of abbreviated MRI protocol for screening of HCC in HCV related cirrhotic patients prior to direct-acting antiviral treatment. Egypt J Radiol Nucl Med 2020; 51(1):1–7.

13. Violi NV, Lewis S, Liao J, et al. Gadoxetate-enhanced abbreviated MRI is highly accurate for hepatocellular carcinoma screening. Eur Radiol 2020;30(11): 6003–13.

14. Kim JS, Lee JK, Baek SY, et al. Diagnostic performance of a minimized protocol of non-contrast mri for hepatocellular carcinoma surveillance. Abdom Radiol 2020;45(1):211–9.

15. Kim YK, Kim YK, Park HJ, et al. Noncontrast MRI with diffusion-weighted imaging as the sole imaging modality for detecting liver malignancy in patients with high risk for hepatocellular Carcinoma. Magn Reson Imaging 2014;32(6):610–8.

16. Han S, Choi JI, Park MY, et al. The diagnostic performance of liver mri without intravenous contrast for detecting hepatocellular carcinoma: a case-controlled feasibility study. Korean J Radiol 2018; 19(4):568–77.

17. Chan MV, McDonald SJ, Ong YY, et al. HCC screening: assessment of an abbreviated non-contrast MRI Protocol. Eur Radiol Exp 2019;3(1):49.

18. Besa C, Lewis S, Pandharipande PV, et al. Hepatocellular carcinoma detection: diagnostic performance of a simulated abbreviated MRI protocol combining diffusion-weighted and t1-weighted imaging at the delayed phase post gadoxetic acid. Abdom Radiol (Ny) 2017;42(1):179–90.

19. Whang S, Choi MH, Choi JI, et al. Comparison of diagnostic performance of non-contrast MRI and abbreviated MRI using gadoxetic acid in initially diagnosed hepatocellular carcinoma patients: a simulation study of surveillance for hepatocellular carcinomas. Eur Radiol 2020;30(8):4150–63.

20. Marks RM, Ryan A, Heba ER, et al. Diagnostic per-patient accuracy of an abbreviated hepatobiliary phase gadoxetic acid-enhanced MRI for hepatocellular carcinoma surveillance. AJR Am J Roentgenol 2015;204(3):527–35.

21. Tillman BG, Gorman JD, Hru JM, et al. Diagnostic per-lesion performance of a simulated gadoxetate disodium-enhanced abbreviated MRI protocol for hepatocellular carcinoma screening. Clin Radiol 2018;73(5):485–93.

22. Khatri G, Pedrosa I, Ananthakrishnan L, et al. Abbreviated-protocol Screening MRI vs. Complete-protocol diagnostic MRI for detection of hepatocellular carcinoma in patients with cirrhosis: an equivalence study using LI-RADS v2018. J Magn Reson Imaging 2020; 51(2):415–25.

23. Lee JY, Huo EJ, Weinstein S, et al. Evaluation of an abbreviated screening MRI protocol for patients at risk for hepatocellular carcinoma. Abdom Radiol (NY) 2018;43(7):1627–33.

24. Gupta P, Soundararajan R, Patel A, et al. Abbreviated MRI for hepatocellular carcinoma screening: a systematic review and meta-analysis. J Hepatol 2021;75(1):108–19.

25. Kim DH, Choi SH, Shim JH, et al. Meta-analysis of the accuracy of abbreviated magnetic resonance imaging for hepatocellular carcinoma surveillance: non-contrast versus hepatobiliary phase-abbreviated magnetic resonance imaging. Cancers (Basel) 2021; 13(12):2975.

26. Cunha GM, Villela-Nogueira CA, Bergman A, et al. Abbreviated mpMRI protocol for diffuse liver disease: a practical approach for evaluation and follow-up of NAFLD. Abdom Radiol (NY) 2018; 43(9):2340–50.

27. Canellas R, Patel MJ, Agarwal S, et al. Lesion detection performance of an abbreviated gadoxetic acid-enhanced MRI protocol for colorectal liver metastasis surveillance. Eur Radiol 2019;29(11):5852–60.

28. Granata V, Fusco R, Avallone A, et al. Abbreviated MRI protocol for colorectal liver metastases: how the radiologist could work in presurgical setting. PLoS One 2020;15(11):e0241431.

29. Torkzad MR, Riddell AM, Chau I, et al. Clinical performance of abbreviated liver mri for the follow-up of patients with colorectal liver metastases. AJR Am J Roentgenol 2021;216(3):669–76.

Magnetic Resonance Imaging of Liver Fibrosis, Fat, and Iron

Christopher L. Welle, MD[a], Michael C. Olson, MD[a],
Scott B. Reeder, MD, PhD[b], Sudhakar K. Venkatesh, MD[a],*

KEYWORDS

- Hepatic fibrosis • Hepatic steatosis • Hepatic iron • MR elastography • Proton density fat fraction
- R2*

KEY POINTS

- Chronic liver disease (CLD) is a large and increasing problem in the world, and noninvasive imaging modalities are needed for assessment and long-term monitoring.
- MR elastography is the predominant noninvasive MR method for detecting and staging hepatic fibrosis and shows high accuracy and reproducibility.
- Multiple additional MR techniques are being researched for the assessment of hepatic fibrosis.
- Recent advances in hepatic fat and iron measurement using quantitative chemical shift-encoded MRI have made measuring hepatic iron and fat straightforward and accessible.

Abbreviations	
MRE	Magnetic resonance elastography
PDFF	Proton density fat fraction

INTRODUCTION

Chronic liver disease (CLD) is an increasing concern for both the US and world health care systems, with approximately 2 million people dying each year worldwide from CLD.[1] Importantly, this problem is not going away or lessening. While the prevention and treatment of viral hepatitis have significantly improved over the past few decades, the growing global problem of obesity and type 2 diabetes has led to a continued increase in CLD, particularly due to nonalcoholic fatty liver disease (NAFLD).[1,2]

With more and more patients with CLD, it is imperative to develop methods to screen and monitor for disease progression efficiently and effectively. Although histologic analysis through liver biopsy remains the gold standard,[3] practical limitations such as availability, cost, and risk of complications limit its utility as a widespread or long-term solution. Therefore, noninvasive imaging, both underlying etiology (eg, hepatic steatosis and iron deposition) and the end result (hepatic fibrosis), has and will continue to be an important part of CLD management. In the past, imaging assessment of CLD was typically limited to somewhat rudimentary qualitative assessment, such as evaluating liver morphology as a sign of fibrosis or decreased hepatic attenuation on computed tomography (CT) as a sign of hepatic steatosis. However, advances in magnetic resonance (MR) imaging have allowed for accurate noninvasive assessment of CLD. In this review, we will discuss

[a] Department of Radiology, Mayo Clinic, Rochester, MN 55902, USA; [b] Department of Radiology, University of Wisconsin, Madison, WI 53792, USA
* Corresponding author.
E-mail address: venkatesh.sudhakar@mayo.edu

Radiol Clin N Am 60 (2022) 705–716
https://doi.org/10.1016/j.rcl.2022.04.003

current MR techniques for the evaluation of hepatic fibrosis, steatosis, and iron content as well as future avenues for advancement currently being studied.

MAGNETIC RESONANCE IMAGING OF LIVER FIBROSIS
Routine or Morphologic-based Assessment

Advanced fibrosis or cirrhosis has long been identified on cross-sectional imaging by macro-alterations to the liver morphology and architecture. For instance, surface nodularity, caudate and left lateral lobe hypertrophy with right and left medial lobe atrophy, widening of the fissures, and increased parenchymal reticulation on pre and postcontrast MR images are all signs of advanced fibrosis.[4,5] However, these features are typically only present on advanced fibrosis cases when it may be too late for effective treatment and to prevent progression of CLD.[5] Secondary effects of hepatic fibrosis such as sequela of portal hypertension (eg, ascites, splenomegaly, and upper abdominal varices) are mostly seen in advanced cases and are also more nonspecific, as they can be seen in nonfibrotic processes such as nodular regenerative hyperplasia (NRH).[6] Therefore, while these morphologic signs can be used to indicate advanced fibrosis, they are not suitable for the diagnosis or monitoring of liver fibrosis.

Magnetic Resonance Elastography

MR elastography (MRE) is the primary MR technique currently used to evaluate hepatic fibrosis. The increased extracellular matrix and collagen deposition that occurs with hepatic fibrosis lead to increased liver stiffness (LS).[7] This increased stiffness can be measured using MRE, allowing for indirect but accurate fibrosis assessment. Examples of MRE examinations in different stages of fibrosis are shown in **Figs. 1–3**.

Currently, two-dimensional (2D) MRE is the predominant technique for clinical evaluation. MRE can be performed as a standalone examination or as part of a more comprehensive MR evaluation. While MRE at 1.5T overall has better technical performance due to decreased artifacts,[8] both 1.5T and 3T systems offer accurate and reproducible liver stiffness measurement (LSM).

Magnetic resonance elastography technique

- Available on all major vendor platforms and as an addition to an existing MR system or part of a new MR installation.

- MRE is available for both 1.5T and 3T clinical scanners
- Uses an active driver system to produce and transmit acoustic pressure waves (60 Hz frequency) into the liver.
- A passive driver is strapped snugly to the patient's lower chest over the liver. Passive driver is connected to an active driver with a plastic tube that transmits the acoustic waves.
- The propagating shear waves are visualized using a special phase-contrast MR sequence. As shear waves have a higher velocity in more stiff tissues, they are visualized as waves with longer wavelength.[9]
- An inversion algorithm automatically converts wave information (velocity, amplitude, and wavelength) into stiffness maps.
- Typically, 4 slices are obtained and for each slice, several images are obtained, both raw data and postprocessed images.
- Magnitude images demonstrate anatomy and confirm the appropriate location of the prescribed slices.
- Phase images can be used to confirm the presence of propagating shear waves in the liver. Gray-scale and color elastograms are used for liver stiffness measurement and visual representation of degrees of fibrosis, respectively.

MRE has been shown to be highly accurate and is widely regarded as the most accurate noninvasive method for diagnosing hepatic fibrosis.[9] Studies have consistently shown high diagnostic accuracies greater than 85%, both in detecting fibrosis as well as discriminating severe fibrosis (F3-4) from mild fibrosis.[10,11,12,13,14] In addition, numerous studies have shown the results of MRE are highly reproducible with high interobserver agreement, with studies showing intraclass correlation coefficients typically greater than 0.85, and greater than 0.9 for repeatability and reproducibility.[13–16] One advantage of MRE is that it is not significantly affected by hepatic steatosis, an important issue with the high prevalence of hepatic steatosis.[17] MRE also benefits from a rather large volume of liver sampled compared with other, non-MR based, noninvasive methods. This larger sample size leads to more accurate and consistent results, particularly in patients with heterogenous fibrosis such as in primary sclerosing cholangitis.[18]

Magnetic resonance elastography liver stiffness measurement

- There are both automated and manual methods for liver stiffness measurement

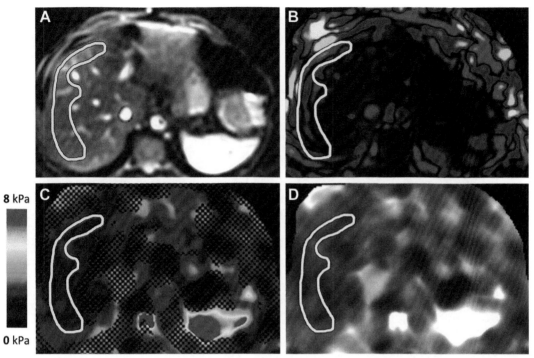

Fig. 1. MR elastogram in a patient with suspected primary sclerosing cholangitis. Magnitude (*A*), color wave (*B*), color elastogram with confidence map (*C*), and grayscale elastogram (*D*) are shown. Liver stiffness was 1.6 kPa, in the normal range.

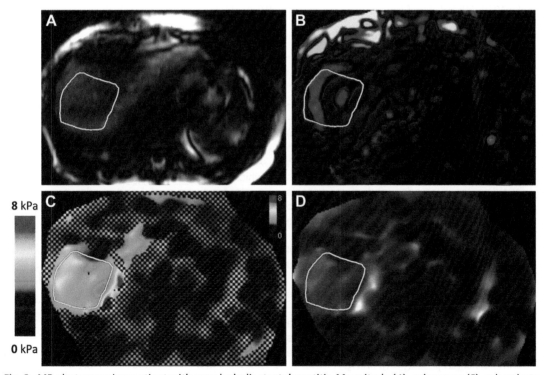

Fig. 2. MR elastogram in a patient with nonalcoholic steatohepatitis. Magnitude (*A*), color wave (*B*), color elastogram with confidence map (*C*), and grayscale elastogram (*D*) are shown. Liver stiffness was 3.8 kPa, in stage 2 to 3 fibrosis range.

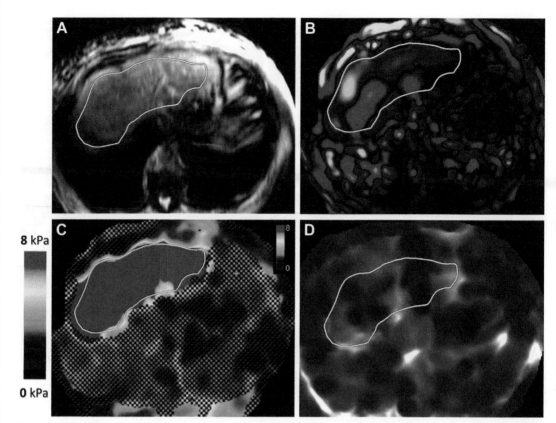

Fig. 3. MR elastogram in a patient with alcohol-related liver disease. Magnitude (*A*), color wave (*B*), color elastogram with confidence map (*C*), and grayscale elastogram (*D*) are shown. Liver stiffness was 10.3 kPa, in the stage 4 fibrosis or cirrhosis range.

(LSM) using MRE1, though currently a manual process is the widely used method clinically[19]

- The process for manual LSM varies depending on the manufacturer and sequences obtained. In the end, regions of interest (ROIs) are drawn on the gray-scale elastogram to obtain the LSM, with careful correlation with the magnitude image to ensure the ROI is avoiding the liver edge and major vessels and correlation with the wave images to ensure only good quality waves are being sampled.
- If a confidence overlay is available, the ROI should be within the available (nonhashed out) area.
- ROIs should be as large as possible to ensure the largest area of liver is sampled.[20]
- The process is repeated for all 4 slices, with a weighted arithmetical mean calculated. This mean LSM can then be used to correlate with the histologic stages of fibrosis (**Table 1**).

MRE does have a few limitations. First, any patient contraindication to MRI, such as an MR incompatible device, will preclude the use of MRE. The primary sequence obtained in MR is a gradient-recalled echo (GRE) sequence. GRE is susceptible to short T2* relaxation times with elevated hepatic iron content, especially in 3T systems, which can make a GRE MRE nondiagnostic. A spin-echo planar imaging (SE-EPI)-based MRE, which is much less affected by high hepatic iron content may be useful and studies have shown an overall greater technical success rate for

Table 1
MR elastography liver stiffness measurement (LSM) correlation with fibrosis stage

Mean LSM	Fibrosis Stage
<2.5 kPa	Normal
2.5–3.0 kPa	Normal or Inflammation
3.0–3.5 kPa	Stage 1–2 Fibrosis
3.5–4.0 kPa	Stage 2–3 Fibrosis
4.0–5.0 kPa	Stage 3–4 Fibrosis
>5.0 kPa	Stage 4 Fibrosis or Cirrhosis

SE-EPI MRE due to fewer technical failures in elevated patients with hepatic iron.[8] Another limitation of MRE are several confounding factors that can increase hepatic stiffness, unrelated to hepatic fibrosis. Examples include hepatic inflammation, hepatic congestion, biliary obstruction, portal hypertension, and infiltrative diseases such as amyloidosis.[21,22] These confounding factors should be kept in mind and the radiologist consider the clinical context when evaluating an MRE.

Diffusion-Weighted Imaging

Diffusion-weighted imaging (DWI) is a well-established MRI technique, which measures the Brownian motion of water molecules in a voxel of tissue. A fibrotic liver restricts the intravoxel motion of water, likely due to the increased connective tissue/collagen. This leads to a lower apparent diffusion coefficient (ADC), which can be measured and used to assess for and stage fibrosis. A few studies have shown an accuracy in detecting significant fibrosis with DWI,[23,24] though the technique does not perform as well as MRE.[25] A main advantage of DWI is its wide availability without additional hardware needed. However, it does have its drawbacks. ADC cutoff values can vary between studies and scanners, leading to difficulty in establishing value ranges. DWI can also be affected by noise, motion artifacts, and hepatic iron/fat content.[26,27]

Recent Advancements and Future Magnetic Resonance Techniques

Three-Dimensional Magnetic Resonance Elastography
The current predominantly used MRE technique is a 2D technique, specifically 2D GRE MRE which measures shear waves moving in a two-dimensional plane. However, as shear waves propagate in 3 dimensions in tissue, a technique measuring shear wave properties in all 3 dimensions could be more accurate. This 3D-MRE is best accomplished using an SE-EPI technique, as the large number of slices needed necessitates a fast speed of acquisition. Early studies have shown similar accuracy between 3D SE-EPI MRE and 2D GRE MRE.[28]

3D Magnetic Resonance Elastography-Derived Parameters
As discussed in the MR elastography section, there are several confounding factors in the liver that can increase liver stiffness without fibrosis. Using advanced techniques of 3D MRE, it is possible to evaluate other tissue mechanical properties with a

goal of producing a more accurate assessment of fibrosis. The technical details are out of scope for this review, though the technique uses multiple frequencies and complex inversion algorithms. Among the parameters obtained include liver viscosity, dispersion of shear wave velocity, damping ratio, and volumetric strain.[29] Of these, shear modulus has been shown to correlate with fibrosis; while others correlate more with steatosis (dispersion of shear wave velocity) or necroinflammation (damping ratio and loss modulus), for example.[29,30] More research is needed to bring these factors into clinical use, though their potential to improve MRE is promising.

Hepatocyte Function Using Hepatobiliary Contrast Agents
Hepatobiliary contrast agents (HBA) are taken up by functioning hepatocytes, with a peak hepatobiliary phase enhancement of about 20 minutes with gadoxetate disodium and about 60 to 180 minutes with gadobenate dimeglumine. As the liver becomes more fibrotic, there is a decrease in functional hepatocytes and therefore decreased HBA uptake.[31] The hepatobiliary phase enhancement can be compared with precontrast images or internal comparisons such as the spleen or muscle to detect and stage fibrosis. While the research into staging fibrosis by HBA uptake is somewhat sparse, several studies have shown the ability to accurately detect fibrosis and further research is needed.[31–33]

T1 mapping
T1 mapping is a technique that takes advantage of the prolonged T1 relaxation times in tissue with higher water content. The increased extracellular space associated with fibrosis creates this increased tissue water content that can be measured and used to correlate with stages of fibrosis.[34] As hepatic iron will shorten T1 relaxation time, this technique is often performed with a compensatory algorithm to account for the iron, referred to as corrected T1 (cT1). Early studies have shown T1/cT1 to be predominantly inferior to MRE in fibrosis evaluation, though research is ongoing.[35]

Intravoxel Incoherent Motion
Earlier, we discussed DWI assessment of hepatic fibrosis. A closely related technique also being studied for the evaluation of fibrosis is intravoxel incoherent motion (IVIM). Both DWI and IVIM use gradients to evaluate the motion of water molecules in tissue. However, DWI uses stronger gradients and assesses the diffusibility of water molecules, primarily affected by cell membranes and macromolecules. On the other hand, IVIM uses smaller gradients to assess microperfusion in the capillary network.[36] Several studies have

Table 2
Additional MR techniques for the evaluation of hepatic fibrosis

Technique	Description
Spin-Lattice Relaxation in the Rotating Frame (T1ρ)	• Measures the tissue transverse magnetization relaxation while under a constant, spin-lock radiofrequency field.[65] • Sensitive to the macromolecular components of tissue, such as collagen in a fibrotic liver. • Few studies have shown promise in the technique at detecting and staging liver fibrosis, though there have been conflicting results and further research is needed.[66,67]
T2 Mapping	• Fibrosis prolongs T2 relaxation time, likely due to increased extracellular water. • Several studies have failed to show high accuracy, though research is ongoing.[34,68]
Susceptibility-Weighted Imaging (SWI)	• Gradient-echo-based sequence which demonstrates susceptibility changes from substances such as iron, calcification, or blood products. • A few studies have shown that SWI can be effective at evaluating hepatic fibrosis, presumably due to changes in the extracellular matrix and/or increased iron within the fibrotic liver[69,70]
MR Perfusion Techniques	• Assesses different parameters related to hepatic parenchymal perfusion and associated enhancement characteristics. • Multiple studies have shown good results, though data are relatively limited.[71–73]

shown high accuracy in IVIM detecting hepatic fibrosis, though cohort sizes are relatively small and further research is needed.[36,37]

Other Techniques

A few additional MR techniques in evaluating hepatic fibrosis are described in **Table 2**.

MAGNETIC RESONANCE IMAGING OF HEPATIC STEATOSIS AND IRON
Background

Hepatic steatosis, the pathognomonic and earliest histologic feature of NAFLD, is characterized by the intracellular accumulation of triglycerides within hepatocytes. In some patients, the resultant inflammatory response can drive progression to NASH and, ultimately, cirrhosis and its associated complications, such as hepatocellular carcinoma and liver failure. Furthermore, there is mounting evidence that there is a significant interplay between the development of hepatic steatosis and pathologic processes in other organ systems. One recent study documented a strong association between hepatic steatosis on noncontrast CT and coronary artery disease,[38] which accounts

for a greater fraction of mortality in patients with NAFLD than liver disease, while several recent analyses have suggested that steatosis may be a causal factor of both the metabolic syndrome and type II diabetes.[39,40]

Excessive iron deposition within the body typically stems from conditions that result in disordered intestinal absorption, such as hereditary hemochromatosis, ineffective erythropoiesis seen with inherited anemias, or repeated transfusions in patients with profound anemia such as that seen in bone marrow suppression. These mechanisms result in the pathologic accumulation of iron in the liver, damaging hepatocytes and predisposing patients to progressive hepatic fibrosis and the development of cirrhosis,[41] and a surplus of iron may accelerate hepatic injury in patients with NASH.[42] In the heart, toxic iron accumulation can result in cardiomyopathies and fatal arrhythmias, while in the pancreas, iron overload can cause exocrine dysfunction and lead to type I diabetes; iron accumulation in the anterior pituitary gland disrupts gonadotropin synthesis, yielding gonadal dysfunction and decreased serum levels of estrogen and testosterone.[41]

Hepatic Signal Fat-fraction Calculation

$$\eta = (IP\text{-}OP)/(2IP) = F/(W + F)$$

- Where η is the signal fat fraction, IP is the signal from the fat protons (F) plus the signal from the water protons (W), and OP is the signal from the water protons minus the signal from the fat protons.
- Given that the IP and OP signals are magnitude-only signals, there is a 50% ambiguity of the fat-fraction estimate for fat concentrations greater than 50%.

Accordingly, the accurate quantification of hepatic fat and iron has long been important in the detection, prevention, and treatment of CLD. Traditional methods of diagnosing steatosis and iron overload, such as nontargeted liver biopsy, are subject to sampling error and can be complicated by pain, bleeding and high cost.[43–45] As a result, there has been increasing interest in recent years in the development of imaging biomarkers for the noninvasive identification and quantification of hepatic steatosis and iron overload.

Conventional magnetic resonance imaging techniques

In-Phase and Opposed-Phase Imaging For decades, conventional MRI imaging sequences, including in-phase and opposed-phase (IOP) imaging and fat suppression, have used the different resonance frequencies of fat and water to provide pseudoquantitative estimates of hepatic fat content.

Pseudoquantitative estimation of fat fraction
- Requires the acquisition of 2 different sets of images, with identical parameters save for one set uses fat-saturation.
- The difference in signal intensity between the sequences is assumed secondary to fat, and an approximate fat fraction can be calculated by:

$$\eta = (SNFS\text{-}SFS)/(SNFS)$$

- η is the signal fat fraction, SNFS is the liver signal intensity without fat suppression, and SFS is the signal intensity with fat suppression.
- Potential issues with this technique include the unintentional suppression of water signal and the incomplete or inhomogeneous suppression of fat, problems that would render the signal fat-fraction invalid.[46]

IOP imaging uses multiple echo times to acquire images for which the signals from water and fat are either in-phase (IP = |W + F|) or out-of-phase (OP = |W–F|), whereby the vertical bars indicated the absolute value, that is,: magnitude.

However, a number of factors confound the measurement of signal fat-fraction,[47,48] which may not accurately reflect hepatic fat content. This approach is also limited by a dynamic range of 0% to 50% hepatic fat fraction; in practice, hepatic fat fractions in excess of 50% are rare but do occur.[49]

Magnetic resonance spectroscopy Magnetic resonance spectroscopy (MRS) has also been used to quantify hepatic fat. With MRS, the resonant frequencies of water and fat protons are demonstrated on a spectral tracing and the signal intensities of the protons at their respective frequencies are quantified, yielding a signal fat fraction.[48] MRS is limited by the need for specialized expertise and time-intensive postprocessing. Furthermore, the MRS signal is usually obtained with a small voxel, meaning that sampling error is a potential problem in patients with heterogeneous hepatic fat distribution.[49]

T2 and T2* imaging The accumulation of iron in tissue impacts MRI signal by shortening the relaxation times T2*, T1, and T2. A qualitative estimate of hepatic iron overload can be obtained with either T2-or T2*-weighted images. In cases of iron overload, the liver demonstrates decreased signal intensity relative to a normal liver on T2-weighted images, which are usually acquired with fast spin-echo (FSE) sequences. IOP gradient echo (GRE) sequences have also been used to qualitatively estimate excessive iron accumulation within hepatocytes by taking advantage of T2* weighting. In IOP imaging, the second echo, given its longer echo time, is more T2* weighted than the first; hepatic parenchymal signal loss between the first echo (opposed-phase images) and the second echo (in-phase images) suggests short T2* decay and is indicative of iron deposition.[41]

Quantitative assessment of liver iron content has been performed using signal intensity ratio (SIR) techniques using either T2-or T2*-weighted imaging, MR susceptometry, and quantitative relaxometry. A comprehensive review of these methods is beyond the scope of this text but can be found elsewhere in the literature.[41]

Recent imaging techniques
Quantitative Chemical Shift-Encoded MRI Quantitative chemical shift-encoded (CSE) magnetic resonance imaging (MRI) is an imaging technique that facilitates the separation of MR signal into fat and water components by acquiring images at 3 or more echo times, although typically 6 are used. CSE MRI corrects for an assortment

of technical and biological factors—such as T1 relaxation, T2* decay, noise bias, eddy currents, and spectral complexity of fat[47,48,50,51]—that can otherwise confound accurate and reproducible measurements of signal fat-fraction within the liver. In doing so, the resultant signal fat-fraction becomes equivalent to the proton density fat-fraction, which is a fundamental property of tissue, defined as the ratio of mobile protons attributable to fat to the total number of mobile protons.[47,52]

The 2 major approaches to perform CSE MRI can be characterized as either magnitude-based or complex-based: the magnitude-based technique,[48,53,54] which is generally easier to implement, consists only of magnitude images and thus is insensitive to phase errors. The main drawbacks of magnitude-based CSE MRI are lower SNR performance and a dynamic range limited to PDFF between 0% and 50%. Complex-based technique[54–56] incorporates both phase and magnitude information, enabling the estimation of PDFF with higher SNR performance and a full dynamic range between 0% and 100%.

CSE MRI data are frequently obtained with a short breath hold and a 3D acquisition of the liver, from which a parametric map can be produced at the level of the scanner. The same acquisition used to produce an estimate of hepatic fat content in the form of PDFF can also be used to generate a confounder-corrected map of R2* (1/T2*) that is corrected for the presence of fat.[41,57,58] These maps provide a visual representation of both hepatic fat fraction, expressed as a percentage, and hepatic iron content in the form of R2*, which is directly proportional to liver iron content (LIC). Regions of interest (ROIs) can be drawn within the hepatic parenchyma on these maps to quantitate hepatic fat and iron content. Examples of PDFF and R2* images are depicted in **Figs. 4–6**.

There is no current consensus with respect to the best technique by which to analyze PDFF and R2* parametric maps, as wide variability exists with regard to the size and number of ROIs used to measure hepatic fat and iron content and the locations in which they are placed.[59–61] These differences may impede accurate comparison of PDFF and R2* values across institutions. One recent investigation[60] found that intra and interobserver variability was minimized by maximizing the volume of liver sampled through a large number of

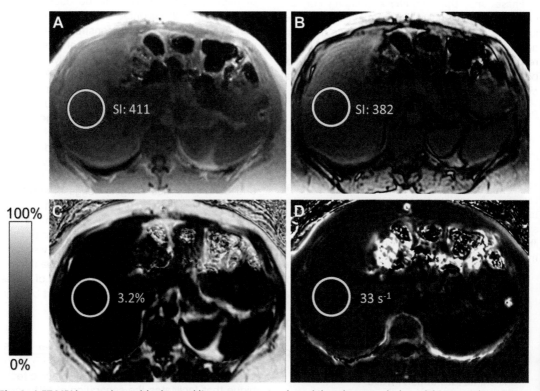

Fig. 4. 1.5T MRI in a patient with elevated liver enzymes. In-phase (*A*) and opposed-phase (*B*) images demonstrate only a small drop in signal intensity (SI) on opposed-phase images. Proton density fat fraction (*C*) images demonstrate a fat fraction (FF) of approximately 3.2%, within normal limits. R2* images (*D*) demonstrate an R2* of approximately 33 s-1, also within normal limits.

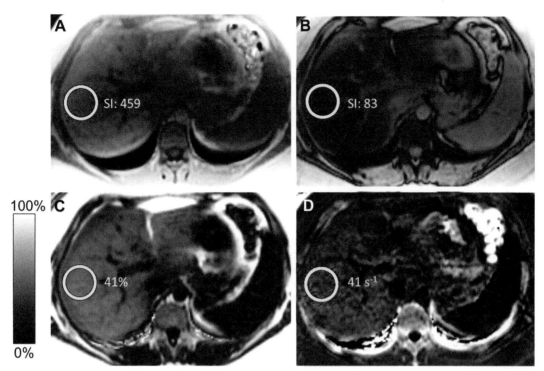

Fig. 5. 1.5T MRI in a patient with suspected hepatic steatosis. In-phase (*A*) and opposed-phase (*B*) images demonstrate a significant drop in signal intensity (SI) on opposed-phase images. Proton density fat fraction (*C*) images demonstrate a fat fraction (FF) of approximately 41% consistent with severe steatosis. R2* images (*D*) demonstrate an R2* of approximately 41 s-1, within normal limits.

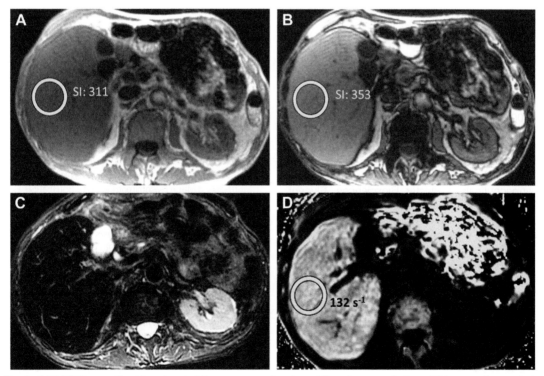

Fig. 6. 1.5T MRI in a patient for elevated liver enzymes. In-phase (*A*) and opposed-phase (*B*) images demonstrate slightly increased signal intensity (SI) on opposed-phase images. T2-weighted images (*C*) demonstrate diffusely decreased signal throughout the liver. R2* images (*D*) demonstrate an R2* of approximately 132 s-1, moderately increased.

ROIs (in either the medial, lateral, posterior, and anterior segments of the liver or in each of the 9 Couinaud segments). In the future, automated whole-liver segmentation may eliminate the need for manual ROI placement.[49]

Confounder-corrected CSE MRI techniques have demonstrated excellent correlation with PDFF as calculated by MRS,[52] have been validated in both phantoms and animals,[62,63] and, with a dynamic range of 0% to 100%, obviate challenges associated with heterogeneous hepatic fat deposition. Recently, CSE MRI techniques have been used to devise limited imaging protocols that permit the quantification of liver fat and iron in as little as 3 breath-holds and 5 total minutes of table time, at a cost similar to that of most laboratory tests,[64] highlighting the promise of this imaging method as a means of accurate, noninvasive diagnosis, and monitoring of both hepatic steatosis and iron overload.

CLINICS CARE POINTS

- MR elastography is an accurate MR technique for the diagnosing and staging hepatic fibrosis.
- Chemical shift encoded MRI provides an accurate evaluation of both hepatic fat fraction and hepatic iron content.

DISCLOSURE

This work was supported by the NIH (R01 DK100651, R41 EB025729, R01 EB031886 and R01-DK088925 and R01 EB001981) and US Department of Defense (W81XWH-19-1-0583-01). S.B. Reeder has no relevant disclosures, but wishes to disclose ownership interests in Calimetrix, Reveal Pharmaceuticals, Cellectar Biosciences, Elucent Medical, and HeartVista. S.B. Reeder also acknowledges that GE Healthcare provides research support to the University of Wisconsin-Madison. Finally, Dr S.B. Reeder is a Romnes Faculty Fellow and has received an award provided by the University of Wisconsin-Madison Office of the Vice-Chancellor for Research and Graduate Education with funding from the Wisconsin Alumni Research Foundation. Drs C.L. Welle, M.C. Olson, and S.K. Venkatesh have no relevant disclosures.

REFERENCES

1. Paik JM, Golabi P, Younossi Y, et al. Changes in the global burden of chronic liver diseases from 2012 to 2017: the growing impact of NAFLD. Hepatology 2020;72(5):1605–16.

2. Estes C, Razavi H, Loomba R, et al. Modeling the epidemic of nonalcoholic fatty liver disease demonstrates an exponential increase in burden of disease. Hepatology 2018;67(1):123–33.

3. Berger D, Desai V, Janardhan S. Con: liver biopsy remains the gold standard to evaluate fibrosis in patients with nonalcoholic fatty liver disease. Clin Liver Dis (Hoboken) 2019;13(4):114–6.

4. Dodd GD 3rd, Baron RL, Oliver JH 3rd, et al. Spectrum of imaging findings of the liver in end-stage cirrhosis: Part II, focal abnormalities. AJR Am J Roentgenol 1999;173(5):1185–92.

5. Faria SC, Ganesan K, Mwangi I, et al. MR imaging of liver fibrosis: current state of the art. Radiographics 2009;29(6):1615–35.

6. Hartleb M, Gutkowski K, Milkiewicz P. Nodular regenerative hyperplasia: evolving concepts on underdiagnosed cause of portal hypertension. World J Gastroenterol 2011;17(11):1400–9.

7. Venkatesh SK, Xu S, Tai D, et al. Correlation of MR elastography with morphometric quantification of liver fibrosis (Fibro-C-Index) in chronic hepatitis B. Magn Reson Med 2014;72(4):1123–9.

8. Kim DW, Kim SY, Yoon HM, et al. Comparison of technical failure of MR elastography for measuring liver stiffness between gradient-recalled echo and spin-echo echo-planar imaging: a systematic review and meta-analysis. J Magn Reson Imaging 2020;51(4):1086–102.

9. Tan CH, Venkatesh SK. Magnetic resonance elastography and other magnetic resonance imaging techniques in chronic liver disease: current status and future directions. Gut Liver 2016;10(5):672–86.

10. Ichikawa S, Motosugi U, Ichikawa T, et al. Magnetic resonance elastography for staging liver fibrosis in chronic hepatitis C. Magn Reson Med Sci 2012; 11(4):291–7.

11. Rustogi R, Horowitz J, Harmath C, et al. Accuracy of MR elastography and anatomic MR imaging features in the diagnosis of severe hepatic fibrosis and cirrhosis. J Magn Reson Imaging 2012;35(6):1356–64.

12. Venkatesh SK, Wang G, Lim SG, et al. Magnetic resonance elastography for the detection and staging of liver fibrosis in chronic hepatitis B. Eur Radiol 2014;24(1):70–8.

13. Lee Y, Lee JM, Lee JE, et al. MR elastography for noninvasive assessment of hepatic fibrosis: reproducibility of the examination and reproducibility and repeatability of the liver stiffness value measurement. J Magn Reson Imaging 2014;39(2):326–31.

14. Shire NJ, Yin M, Chen J, et al. Test-retest repeatability of MR elastography for noninvasive liver fibrosis assessment in hepatitis C. J Magn Reson Imaging 2011;34(4):947–55.

15. Venkatesh SK, Wang G, Teo LL, et al. Magnetic resonance elastography of liver in healthy Asians: normal

liver stiffness quantification and reproducibility assessment. J Magn Reson Imaging 2014;39(1):1–8.

16. Hoodeshenas S, Welle CL, Navin PJ, et al. Magnetic resonance elastography in primary sclerosing cholangitis: interobserver agreement for liver stiffness measurement with manual and automated methods. Acad Radiol 2019;26(12):1625–32.

17. Chen J, Allen AM, Therneau TM, et al. Liver stiffness measurement by magnetic resonance elastography is not affected by hepatic steatosis. Eur Radiol 2021.

18. Eaton JE, Dzyubak B, Venkatesh SK, et al. Performance of magnetic resonance elastography in primary sclerosing cholangitis. J Gastroenterol Hepatol 2016;31(6):1184–90.

19. Dzyubak B, Venkatesh SK, Manduca A, et al. Automated liver elasticity calculation for MR elastography. J Magn Reson Imaging 2016;43(5):1055–63.

20. Kim M, Kang BK, Jun DW, et al. MR elastography of the liver: comparison of three measurement methods. Clin Radiol 2020;75(9):715.e1–7. https://doi.org/10.1016/j.crad.2020.05.015.

21. Hoodeshenas S, Yin M, Venkatesh SK. Magnetic resonance elastography of liver: current update. Top Magn Reson Imaging 2018;27(5):319–33.

22. Venkatesh SK, Hoodeshenas S, Venkatesh SH, et al. Magnetic resonance elastography of liver in light chain amyloidosis. J Clin Med 2019;8(5):739.

23. Charatcharoenwitthaya P, Sukonrut K, Korpraphong P, et al. Diffusion-weighted magnetic resonance imaging for the assessment of liver fibrosis in chronic viral hepatitis. PLoS One 2021;16(3):e0248024.

24. Kocakoc E, Bakan AA, Poyrazoglu OK, et al. Assessment of liver fibrosis with diffusion-weighted magnetic resonance imaging using different b-values in chronic viral hepatitis. Med Princ Pract 2015;24(6):522–6.

25. Horowitz JM, Venkatesh SK, Ehman RL, et al. Evaluation of hepatic fibrosis: a review from the society of abdominal radiology disease focus panel. Abdom Radiol (NY) 2017;42(8):2037–53.

26. Bulow R, Mensel B, Meffert P, et al. Diffusion-weighted magnetic resonance imaging for staging liver fibrosis is less reliable in the presence of fat and iron. Eur Radiol 2013;23(5):1281–7.

27. Petitclerc L, Sebastiani G, Gilbert G, et al. Liver fibrosis: review of current imaging and MRI quantification techniques. J Magn Reson Imaging 2017;45(5):1276–95.

28. Morisaka H, Motosugi U, Glaser KJ, et al. Comparison of diagnostic accuracies of two- and three-dimensional MR elastography of the liver. J Magn Reson Imaging 2017;45(4):1163–70.

29. Li J, Venkatesh SK, Yin M. Advances in magnetic resonance elastography of liver. Magn Reson Imaging Clin N Am 2020;28(3):331–40.

30. Deffieux T, Gennisson JL, Bousquet L, et al. Investigating liver stiffness and viscosity for fibrosis, steatosis and activity staging using shear wave elastography. J Hepatol 2015;62(2):317–24.

31. Watanabe H, Kanematsu M, Goshima S, et al. Staging hepatic fibrosis: comparison of gadoxetate disodium-enhanced and diffusion-weighted MR imaging–preliminary observations. Radiology 2011;259(1):142–50.

32. Goshima S, Kanematsu M, Watanabe H, et al. Gd-EOB-DTPA-enhanced MR imaging: prediction of hepatic fibrosis stages using liver contrast enhancement index and liver-to-spleen volumetric ratio. J Magn Reson Imaging 2012;36(5):1148–53.

33. Kumazawa K, Edamoto Y, Yanase M, et al. Liver analysis using gadolinium-ethoxybenzyl-diethylenetriamine pentaacetic acid-enhanced magnetic resonance imaging: Correlation with histological grading and quantitative liver evaluation prior to hepatectomy. Hepatol Res 2012;42(11):1081–8.

34. Hoffman DH, Ayoola A, Nickel D, et al. T1 mapping, T2 mapping and MR elastography of the liver for detection and staging of liver fibrosis. Abdom Radiol (NY) 2020;45(3):692–700.

35. Thomaides-Brears HB, Lepe R, Banerjee R, et al. Multiparametric MR mapping in clinical decision-making for diffuse liver disease. Abdom Radiol (NY) 2020;45(11):3507–22.

36. Wang YXJ, Huang H, Zheng CJ, et al. Diffusion-weighted MRI of the liver: challenges and some solutions for the quantification of apparent diffusion coefficient and intravoxel incoherent motion. Am J Nucl Med Mol Imaging 2021;11(2):107–42.

37. Li YT, Cercueil JP, Yuan J, et al. Liver intravoxel incoherent motion (IVIM) magnetic resonance imaging: a comprehensive review of published data on normal values and applications for fibrosis and tumor evaluation. Quant Imaging Med Surg 2017;7(1):59–78.

38. Puchner SB, Lu MT, Mayrhofer T, et al. High-risk coronary plaque at coronary CT angiography is associated with nonalcoholic fatty liver disease, independent of coronary plaque and stenosis burden: results from the ROMICAT II trial. Radiology 2015;274(3):693–701.

39. Sung KC, Jeong WS, Wild SH, et al. Combined influence of insulin resistance, overweight/obesity, and fatty liver as risk factors for type 2 diabetes. Diabetes Care 2012;35(4):717–22.

40. Lonardo A, Ballestri S, Marchesini G, et al. Nonalcoholic fatty liver disease: a precursor of the metabolic syndrome. Dig Liver Dis 2015;47(3):181–90.

41. Hernando D, Levin YS, Sirlin CB, et al. Quantification of liver iron with MRI: state of the art and remaining challenges. J Magn Reson Imaging 2014;40(5):1003–21.

42. George DK, Goldwurm S, MacDonald GA, et al. Increased hepatic iron concentration in nonalcoholic steatohepatitis is associated with increased fibrosis. Gastroenterology 1998;114(2):311–8.

43. Bravo AA, Sheth SG, Chopra S. Liver biopsy. N Engl J Med 2001;344(7):495–500.

44. Rockey DC, Caldwell SH, Goodman ZD, et al. American association for the study of liver D. Liver biopsy. Hepatology 2009;49(3):1017–44.

45. Ratziu V, Charlotte F, Heurtier A, et al. Sampling variability of liver biopsy in nonalcoholic fatty liver disease. Gastroenterology 2005;128(7):1898–906.

46. Reeder SB, Cruite I, Hamilton G, et al. Quantitative assessment of liver fat with magnetic resonance imaging and spectroscopy. J Magn Reson Imaging 2011;34(4):729–49.

47. Reeder SB, Hu HH, Sirlin CB. Proton density fat-fraction: a standardized MR-based biomarker of tissue fat concentration. J Magn Reson Imaging 2012;36(5):1011–4.

48. Reeder SB, Sirlin CB. Quantification of liver fat with magnetic resonance imaging. Magn Reson Imaging Clin N Am 2010;18(3):337–57, ix.

49. Starekova J, Reeder SB. Liver fat quantification: where do we stand? Abdom Radiol (NY) 2020; 45(11):3386–99.

50. Liu CY, McKenzie CA, Yu H, et al. Fat quantification with IDEAL gradient echo imaging: correction of bias from T(1) and noise. Magn Reson Med 2007;58(2):354–64.

51. Yu H, McKenzie CA, Shimakawa A, et al. Multiecho reconstruction for simultaneous water-fat decomposition and T2* estimation. J Magn Reson Imaging 2007;26(4):1153–61.

52. Yokoo T, Serai SD, Pirasteh A, et al. Linearity, bias, and precision of hepatic proton density fat fraction measurements by using MR imaging: a meta-analysis. Radiology 2018;286(2):486–98.

53. Bydder M, Yokoo T, Hamilton G, et al. Relaxation effects in the quantification of fat using gradient echo imaging. Magn Reson Imaging 2008;26(3):347–59.

54. Yu H, Shimakawa A, Hines CD, et al. Combination of complex-based and magnitude-based multiecho water-fat separation for accurate quantification of fat-fraction. Magn Reson Med 2011;66(1):199–206.

55. Reeder SB, McKenzie CA, Pineda AR, et al. Water-fat separation with IDEAL gradient-echo imaging. J Magn Reson Imaging 2007;25(3):644–52.

56. Meisamy S, Hines CD, Hamilton G, et al. Quantification of hepatic steatosis with T1-independent, T2-corrected MR imaging with spectral modeling of fat: blinded comparison with MR spectroscopy. Radiology 2011;258(3):767–75.

57. Hernando D, Kramer JH, Reeder SB. Multipeak fat-corrected complex R2* relaxometry: theory, optimization, and clinical validation. Magn Reson Med 2013; 70(5):1319–31.

58. Kuhn JP, Hernando D, Munoz del Rio A, et al. Effect of multipeak spectral modeling of fat for liver iron and fat quantification: correlation of biopsy with MR imaging results. Radiology 2012;265(1):133–42.

59. Tang A, Tan J, Sun M, et al. Nonalcoholic fatty liver disease: MR imaging of liver proton density fat fraction to assess hepatic steatosis. Radiology 2013; 267(2):422–31.

60. Campo CA, Hernando D, Schubert T, et al. Standardized approach for roi-based measurements of proton density fat fraction and R2* in the liver. AJR Am J Roentgenol 2017;209(3):592–603.

61. Bannas P, Kramer H, Hernando D, et al. Quantitative magnetic resonance imaging of hepatic steatosis: Validation in ex vivo human livers. Hepatology 2015;62(5):1444–55.

62. Hines CD, Yu H, Shimakawa A, et al. T1 independent, T2* corrected MRI with accurate spectral modeling for quantification of fat: validation in a fat-water-SPIO phantom. J Magn Reson Imaging 2009;30(5):1215–22.

63. Hines CD, Yu H, Shimakawa A, et al. Quantification of hepatic steatosis with 3-T MR imaging: validation in ob/ob mice. Radiology 2010;254(1):119–28.

64. Pooler BD, Hernando D, Ruby JA, et al. Validation of a motion-robust 2D sequential technique for quantification of hepatic proton density fat fraction during free breathing. J Magn Reson Imaging 2018;48(6):1578–85.

65. Allkemper T, Sagmeister F, Cicinnati V, et al. Evaluation of fibrotic liver disease with whole-liver T1rho MR imaging: a feasibility study at 1.5 T. Radiology 2014;271(2):408–15.

66. Rauscher I, Eiber M, Ganter C, et al. Evaluation of T1rho as a potential MR biomarker for liver cirrhosis: comparison of healthy control subjects and patients with liver cirrhosis. Eur J Radiol 2014;83(6):900–4.

67. Takayama Y, Nishie A, Asayama Y, et al. T1 rho Relaxation of the liver: a potential biomarker of liver function. J Magn Reson Imaging 2015;42(1):188–95.

68. Lee MJ, Kim MJ, Yoon CS, et al. Evaluation of liver fibrosis with T2 relaxation time in infants with cholestasis: comparison with normal controls. Pediatr Radiol 2011;41(3):350–4.

69. Feier D, Balassy C, Bastati N, et al. The diagnostic efficacy of quantitative liver MR imaging with diffusion-weighted, SWI, and hepato-specific contrast-enhanced sequences in staging liver fibrosis–a multiparametric approach. Eur Radiol 2016;26(2):539–46.

70. Obmann VC, Marx C, Berzigotti A, et al. Liver MRI susceptibility-weighted imaging (SWI) compared to T2* mapping in the presence of steatosis and fibrosis. Eur J Radiol 2019;118:66–74.

71. Chen BB, Hsu CY, Yu CW, et al. Dynamic contrast-enhanced magnetic resonance imaging with Gd-EOB-DTPA for the evaluation of liver fibrosis in chronic hepatitis patients. Eur Radiol 2012;22(1):171–80.

72. Hagiwara M, Rusinek H, Lee VS, et al. Advanced liver fibrosis: diagnosis with 3D whole-liver perfusion MR imaging–initial experience. Radiology 2008; 246(3):926–34.

73. Xie S, Sun Y, Wang L, et al. Assessment of liver function and liver fibrosis with dynamic Gd-EOB-DTPA-enhanced MRI. Acad Radiol 2015;22(4): 460–6.

Practical Contrast Enhanced Liver Ultrasound

Judy H. Squires, MD[a,b,]*, David T. Fetzer, MD[c], Jonathan R. Dillman, MD, MSc[d,e]

KEYWORDS

- Contrast-enhanced ultrasound • Liver lesion • Adult • Child

KEY POINTS

- Ultrasound contrast agents (UCAs) used for contrast-enhanced ultrasound (CEUS) are exceedingly safe.
- Lesions with contrast retention (no washout) in the delayed phase are overwhelmingly benign.
- Lesions with contrast washout in the delayed phase are concerning for malignancy.
- The American College of Radiology CEUS Liver Imaging, Reporting, and Data System can be used to categorize liver observations, including HCC, in certain at-risk patients.

Abbreviations	
MRI	magnetic resonance imaging
GLUT-1	glucose transporter 1
CT	computed tomography
HNF-1α	hepatocyte nuclear factor - 1 alpha

INTRODUCTION

Contrast-enhanced ultrasound (CEUS) use is increasing worldwide, including in the United States, for multiple applications in patients of all ages. CEUS is most performed for focal liver lesion evaluation in adults and children because of its high safety profile and capability to yield a definitive diagnosis.[1] This often obviates multiphase CT or MRI for lesion characterization, which requires the use of ionizing radiation and potentially sedation or general anesthesia, respectively, particularly important in the pediatric population. CEUS leverages the inherent benefits of ultrasound, including portability and accessibility, using specific ultrasound contrast agents (UCAs) that are exceedingly safe, without the risk of renal or liver toxicity.[2] UCAs are cleared rapidly from the body, allowing for multiple injections during a single examination, and have no potential for deposition in the patient.[1]

The purpose of this review is to highlight the applications and technical considerations for performing CEUS for liver lesion evaluation, and to illustrate the imaging appearance of the most common liver lesions encountered in children and adults, emphasizing clinical relevance and current nomenclature.

CONTRAST-ENHANCED ULTRASOUND REQUIREMENTS

An UCA is necessary for CEUS. Current generation UCAs are composed of microbubbles of an inert insoluble fluorocarbon gas stabilized by a lipid

---

[a] Department of Radiology, UPMC Children's Hospital of Pittsburgh, 4401 Penn Avenue 2nd Fl Radiology, Pittsburgh, PA 15224, USA; [b] Department of Radiology, University of Pittsburgh School of Medicine PUH Suite E204, 200 Lothrop Street, Pittsburgh, PA 15213, USA; [c] Department of Radiology, UT Southwestern Medical Center, 5323 Harry Hines Boulevard, Dallas, TX 75390-9316, USA; [d] Department of Radiology, Cincinnati Children's Hospital Medical Center, 3333 Burnet Avenue, Cincinnati, OH 45229, USA; [e] Department of Radiology, University of Cincinnati College of Medicine, 234 Goodman Street, Cincinnati, OH 45267-0761, USA

* Corresponding author. Department of Radiology, UPMC Children's Hospital of Pittsburgh, 4401 Penn Avenue 2nd Fl Radiology, Pittsburgh, PA 15224.

E-mail address: Judy.Squires@chp.edu

Radiol Clin N Am 60 (2022) 717–730
https://doi.org/10.1016/j.rcl.2022.04.006
0033-8389/22/© 2022 Elsevier Inc. All rights reserved.

and/or protein shell, with several formulations available for clinical use. Venous access is needed, and although a peripheral intravenous line or central venous catheter may be used, intravenous contrast material injection is often a new workflow for many ultrasound departments. Additionally, 2 team members are generally needed during a CEUS examination: one to inject the UCA and another to obtain images.

Ultrasound system contrast-specific software is also necessary to perform CEUS. The contrast software automatically decreases power output and other settings to decrease mechanical index and minimize bubble destruction. Other techniques including harmonic imaging with pulse inversion are used to distinguish the bubble-specific signal, and subtract background signal from tissue, allowing for a "contrast-only" image.[3] The contrast software of most vendors' ultrasound systems uses a split-screen display, providing a grayscale image and a contrast-only image simultaneously. The grayscale image enables visualization of the soft tissues for localization. The contrast-only image provides real-time soft tissue subtraction so signal from microbubbles is relatively enhanced, and typically only very echogenic interfaces (eg, organ and vessel walls, calcifications, and bowel gas) from the grayscale image are seen.

CONTRAST-ENHANCED ULTRASOUND LIMITATIONS

Contrast-enhanced CT and/or MRI should be considered rather than CEUS for liver observation evaluation in patients with multiple different appearing liver observations, such as patients with Fontan-associated liver disease, who are at increased risk for both benign and malignant lesions. Contrast-enhanced MRI allows for characterization of the liver and all lesions simultaneously, so is preferred.[4] Portions of the liver poorly seen at grayscale ultrasound will similarly be challenging to visualize at CEUS, such as lesions near the dome of the diaphragm or in the deep right hepatic lobe in large patients or patients with hepatic steatosis. Finally, contrast-enhanced CT and/or MRI should be considered rather than CEUS for masses with high likelihood of requiring complete imaging staging, which cannot be performed at CEUS alone.[4]

CONTRAST-ENHANCED ULTRASOUND TECHNIQUE

A grayscale ultrasound examination preceding CEUS allows for a thorough survey of the hepatic parenchyma, biliary system, and vasculature, and identification of findings of hepatocellular disease

and/or portal hypertension, which may influence the differential diagnosis of focal findings in the liver. The liver lesion in question can then be precisely localized, and in a few scenarios, a definitive diagnosis can be made with grayscale ultrasound alone. These include simple hepatic cysts, classic focal fatty infiltration or sparing, and infantile hemangiomas with classic clinical features.[4] More commonly, however, the ultrasound appearance of a liver lesion is nonspecific, as many different liver lesions can seem similar at ultrasound. In addition, classic imaging findings are less commonly seen in hepatic steatosis, which is increasing in incidence.

When it is determined that CEUS may assist in making a confident diagnosis, first, an appropriate transducer should be selected. In adults, a curved array low-frequency transducer is typically ideal to best capture microbubble resonance. However, in infants and small children, a linear high-frequency transducer may allow for optimal lesion visualization, although bubble resonance (and thus perceived enhancement) may be less, and microbubble destruction rate is higher.

Second, an appropriate acoustic window should be chosen to ensure optimized and consist visualization of the observation, with the transducer placed as close as possible to the lesion. This may require placing the patient in the decubitus position, similar to routine ultrasound image optimization. An intercostal approach may be needed, with the patient's arm raised overhead to maximize the space between ribs. It is best if the lesion can be kept in the field of view during the entire respiratory cycle, so the lesion can be seen throughout the complete duration of UCA wash-in during normal respiration. The wash-in, or arterial phase, typically lasts for up to 45 seconds following UCA administration. The portal venous phase typically lasts from 30 to 120 seconds after UCA injection, which notably is earlier than CT and MRI where the portal venous phase typically begins around 45 seconds after contrast administration. The late phase lasts from 120 seconds to 4 to 6 minutes after UCA injection until clearance of the UCA.[5] Intermittent scanning should be performed during portal venous and late phases to decrease UCA destruction that can occur with continuous imaging. Artifacts at CEUS are well described and are important to minimize and consider in both performing and interpreting CEUS.[3,6,7]

BASIC INTERPRETATION PRINCIPLES

In general, CEUS interpretation predominantly relies on the appearance of the lesion in the delayed phase, with 2 possibilities: contrast material washout (hypoenhancement) or contrast material retention (no washout; isoenhancement to hyper-enhancement). Lesions without washout are over-whelmingly benign, and the specific pattern of arterial phase enhancement is important for defin-itive diagnosis.[1] Conversely, lesions that show washout, or become hypoenhancing compared with the background liver parenchyma, are much more likely to be malignant.[1] The remainder of this review details specific types of lesions, emphasizing the clinical significance and CEUS appearance. **Table 1** provides a summary of the appearance of different lesions during CEUS.

BENIGN LESIONS
Vascular Tumors

Vascular tumors in the liver are categorized using the 2018 International Society for the Study of Vascular Anomalies classification.[8] In infants and young children, the 2 most common vascular mal-formations are tumors: congenital hemangioma (also called solitary hemangioma) and infantile hem-angiomas (also called multifocal or diffuse heman-giomas). Conversely, vascular malformations such as slow or fast flow malformations (previously called "hemangiomas" and still ubiquitously called this in most adult literature) are most common after the first decade of life through adulthood.

Congenital hepatic hemangioma
A congenital hemangioma is a fast flow vascular tumor that develops in utero and is present and typically largest at birth. These generally solitary vascular tumors are typically diagnosed within 6 months of life and are commonly incidental le-sions without clinical significance. However,

Table 1
Enhancement appearance of various liver lesions at contrast-enhanced ultrasound

	Arterial Phase 10–45 s	Portal Venous Phase 30–120 s	Late Phase 120 s–6 min
Congenital hemangioma	Heterogeneous peripheral centripetal complete or incomplete fill-in	No washout of enhancing areas	No washout of enhancing areas
Infantile hemangioma	Peripheral hyperenhancement with rapid centripetal fill-in	No washout	• Hyperenhancment • Isoenhancement • Mild late washout
Hemangioma	Peripheral discontinuous nodular enhancement	Centripetal complete or partial fill-in	No washout of enhancing areas
Mesenchymal hamartoma	• Nonenhancement of cystic components • Gradual enhance-ment of septa and solid components	No washout of enhancing areas	No washout of enhancing areas
FNH	• Spoke-wheel, stellate centripetal enhancement • Possible enhancing central vessel	• No washout • Possible nonenhanc-ing central scar	• No washout • Possible nonenhanc-ing central scar
HNF-1α-inactivated adenoma	Heterogeneous hyperenhancement	No washout	No washout
Hepatoblastoma	Variable	Mild to marked washout[a]	Marked washout
HCC	Nonrim hyperenhancement	Sustained enhancement	Mild late washout
Cholangiocarcinoma	Rim hyperenhancement	Early and/or marked washout[a]	Marked washout
Metastasis	Variable	Early and/or marked washout[a]	Marked washout

[a] Early washout occurs less than 60 s. Marked washout seems nearly devoid of enhancement (punched out appearance) within 2 min.

patients with larger lesions may present with high-output congestive heart failure from vascular shunting. Most congenital hemangioma rapidly and spontaneously involute over the first year of life, termed rapidly involuting congenital hemangioma.[9] Occasionally, embolization may be necessary in infants to help cease intratumoral shunting, with resection considered when possible. No medical therapy is currently available to treat congenital hemangioma.

At ultrasound, congenital hemangioma is usually solitary and heterogeneous in echogenicity, with large vessels visible.[10] Calcifications may be seen.[11] At dynamic postcontrast imaging, there will be heterogeneous somewhat peripheral, often discontinuous and nodular enhancement that becomes more confluent at the lesion periphery over time (**Fig. 1**).[10] There may be complete fill-in with contrast material, although central portions of the tumor may not enhance, especially larger tumors, likely related to intratumoral hemorrhage, fibrosis, and/or necrosis.[9] Portions of the tumor that enhance in the arterial phase will typically remain isoenhancing to hyperenhancing in later phases without washout.[12]

Infantile hepatic hemangiomas

Infantile hepatic hemangiomas are multiple or innumerable/diffuse. These tumors develop in the first weeks or months of life and are generally not present at birth, unlike congenital hemangioma. Infantile hepatic hemangiomas are associated with cutaneous infantile hemangiomas, which are histologically identical tumors with GLUT-1 positivity. Infantile hemangiomas characteristically have rapid growth within the first year of life, followed by gradual involution during the first year of life, with small residual fibrofatty tissue. In addition to potential vascular shunting complications such as high-output heart failure, these tumors express type 3-iodothyronine deiodinase so patients may have hypothyroidism.[9] If treatment is necessary, the mainstay is propranolol.[9]

CEUS may not be necessary for diagnosis when multiple or innumerable liver lesions are encountered at grayscale ultrasound in a patient with multiple cutaneous infantile hemangiomas. At CEUS, infantile hemangiomas typically have peripheral discontinuous and nodular enhancement with very rapid homogeneous fill-in. Infantile hemangiomas are typically more homogeneous than congenital hemangiomas (**Fig. 2**).[9] There is usually sustained enhancement in the portal venous phase with hyperenhancement, isoenhancement, and mild washout all possible in the late phase.[10]

Vascular Malformations

Hemangioma

Hemangioma is a term used ubiquitously in the adult literature but is a distinct, nonneoplastic

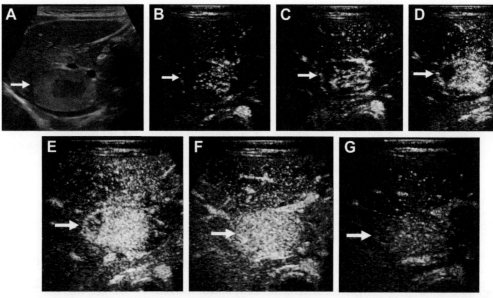

Fig. 1. A 4-month-old boy with congenital hemangioma incidentally discovered at renal ultrasound. (*A*) Transverse grayscale image demonstrates a circumscribed heterogeneous mass (*arrow*) in the inferior aspect of the right hepatic lobe. CEUS images in the transverse plane in the arterial phase at 4 (*B*), 5 (*C*), 6 (*D*), 8 (*E*), and 12 seconds (*F*) following sulfur hexafluoride lipid-type A microspheres contrast injection demonstrate heterogeneous, somewhat peripheral centripetal complete enhancement of the mass. In the late phase at 2 minutes 5 seconds following contrast injection (*G*), there is sustained enhancement of the mass without washout.

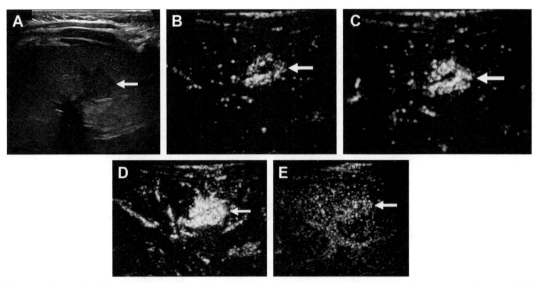

Fig. 2. A 20-month-old girl with multiple infantile hepatic hemangiomas. (*A*) Grayscale ultrasound image in the transverse plane shows a representative irregularly shaped hypoechoic lesion in the left hepatic lobe (*arrow*), with other hemangiomas not shown. CEUS images in the transverse plane in the arterial phase at 8 (*B*), 9 (*C*), and 10 seconds (*D*) after sulfur hexafluoride lipid-type A microspheres contrast injection show rapid peripheral discontinuous nodular enhancement with centripetal fill-in of the lesion. In the late phase, 2 minutes 10 seconds following contrast injection (*E*), there is sustained enhancement without washout.

lesion that is different from congenital and infantile hemangiomas. In adolescents and adults, these lesions are more appropriately called slow flow or fast flow malformations because they are not true hemangiomas.[8] Similar to their appearance at multiphase CT and MRI, at CEUS, these vascular malformations demonstrate peripheral discontinuous nodular enhancement with expanding puddles of contrast material that fill centripetally (outward to inward; **Fig. 3**). Fill-in can be complete or partial, potentially due to central clot or fibrosis. There is classically no washout, although mild late washout has been reported in some hemangiomas, which should not be a confusing finding if the characteristic arterial phase enhancement pattern is present.[6]

Mesenchymal Hamartoma

Hepatic mesenchymal hamartoma is a benign congenital lesion of uncoordinated primitive mesenchyme proliferation with pseudocysts in the periportal tracts, and no connection to bile ducts.[13,14] This lesion is usually diagnosed by 2 years of age, although patients may present prenatally.[14] Large lesions may cause abdominal distention and difficulty breathing.[14] Treatment is complete surgical resection. There is potential for local recurrence, and malignant transformation to undifferentiated embryonal sarcoma has been reported.[13,14]

Mesenchymal hamartoma is typically large (>10 cm) and unifocal, although multifocal cases have been reported.[12] At ultrasound, these lesions are typically almost completely cystic with variable amounts of internal fibrotic septations. At CEUS, the cystic components will not enhance, whereas enhancement of linear septations and any solid portions will be seen (**Fig. 4**).

Focal Nodular Hyperplasia

Focal nodular hyperplasia (FNH) is a benign tumor composed of hepatocytes, Kupffer cells, malformed blood vessels, and immature bile ducts with a vascular central scar and is thought to occur due to a congenital or acquired vascular insult.[11,13,15] FNH classically occurs in young women with normal background liver parenchyma. In patients with diffuse liver disease, such as prior chemotherapy or Fontan-associated liver disease, these are called "FNH-like" lesions although they are similar to true FNH.[11,16] FNH can slowly enlarge over time, although spontaneously resolution has been reported.[15] No treatment is necessary unless there are symptoms related to mass effect when excision may be considered.[16]

At ultrasound, spoke-wheel internal vascularity is diagnostic. At CEUS, FNH is hypervascular, with stellate, spoke-wheel centrifugal (in to out) arterial phase hyperenhancement (APHE; **Fig. 5**). A central

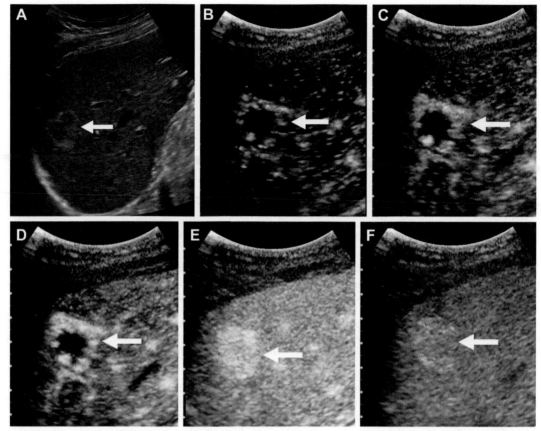

Fig. 3. A 55-year-old woman with hemangioma incidentally seen on CT (not shown) performed for abdominal pain. Grayscale ultrasound (*A*) shows an irregularly shaped mass (*arrow*) near the dome of the right lobe with echogenic rim and central hypoechogenicity. Following the intravenous administration of sulfur hexafluoride lipid-type A microspheres, at 11 seconds (*B*), peripheral discontinuous nodular enhancement is shown, with progressive puddling of contrast and centripetal enhancement at 13 seconds (*C*) and 14 seconds (*D*), with complete fill in by 48 seconds (*E*). No washout was seen at 2 minutes (*F*).

feeding vessel may be seen. Complete contrast fill-in is typical, although washout from a small central scar may be seen, as with other imaging modalities. FNH-like lesions are more commonly multiple, are usually smaller, and are less likely to have a central scar compared with FNH.[12] In the delayed phase, sustained enhancement occurs in about 90% of cases. Importantly, in cancer survivors, the lack of portal venous and late phase washout helps differentiate multiple FNH-like lesions from metastases, which typically show marked contrast agent washout by 2 minutes.[17]

Hepatocellular Adenoma

Hepatocellular adenoma is a benign hepatic neoplasm that predominantly occurs in women. Given increasing molecular and genetic information, our understanding of these lesions continues to evolve. Adenomas are now categorized into 7 distinct subtypes: inflammatory, HNF-1α-

inactivated, β-catenin-activated (also called β-catenin mutated, caused by a mutation of exon 3), weak β-catenin-activated (caused by a mutation of exon 7/8), sonic hedgehog pathway activated, unclassified hepatocellular adenoma, as well as 2 subtypes with overlapping features of the inflammatory and β-catenin-activated subtypes.[11,18] The subtypes with currently best-described appearance at CEUS are further detailed below.

Inflammatory hepatocellular adenoma

Inflammatory hepatocellular adenoma (previously called telangiectatic adenoma or telangiectatic FNH) is the most common subtype and is associated with estrogen exposure, including oral contraceptive use or obesity.[16,19] Patients may present with fever, anemia, leukocytosis, and elevated serum C-reactive protein on laboratory analysis.[16] Risk of spontaneous rupture and

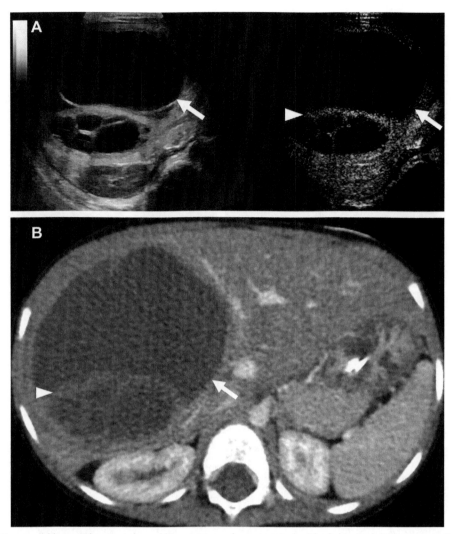

Fig. 4. A 3-year-old boy with mesenchymal hamartoma who presented with abdominal distention. At CEUS using sulfur hexafluoride lipid-type A microspheres, transverse split-screen image (*A*) with grayscale (left panel), and contrast (right panel) demonstrates a large mostly cystic mass (*arrow*) with nonenhancement of cystic areas and enhancement of internal septa and solid portions (*arrowhead*). Contrast-enhanced axial CT (*B*) at a similar level demonstrates a similar appearance with predominant cystic component (*arrow*) and a few internal enhancing components (*arrowhead*).

hemorrhage are greatest with this subtype, particularly when tumor diameter exceeds 5 cm.[11,19,20]

Background liver steatosis may make lesion visualization challenging. At CEUS in the arterial phase, inflammatory hepatocellular adenomas are hypervascular with subcapsular hyperenhancing arteries and a centripetal or heterogeneous filling pattern. Inflammatory hepatocellular adenomas will most commonly show mild washout in the portal venous phase or late phases,[20,21] with sustained enhancement less common.[21,22] Central, irregularly shaped areas of hypoenhancement are seen by the late arterial phase in up to one-third of inflammatory hepatocellular

adenomas.[20] An enhancing rim may also be seen in the late phase.[21] Given overlap in appearance with HCC, biopsy may be necessary for diagnosis.

HNF-1α-inactivated hepatocellular adenoma

HNF-1α-inactivated hepatocellular adenomas (previously called steatotic adenomas) account for 35% to 50% of adenomas and are usually seen in women with oral contraceptive use[16] as well as patients with autosomal dominant maturity onset diabetes of the young type 3 (MODY3).[19] The clinical course for this subtype is typically uncomplicated, and treatment may entail simply discontinuing oral contraceptive use.[11,16] Potential

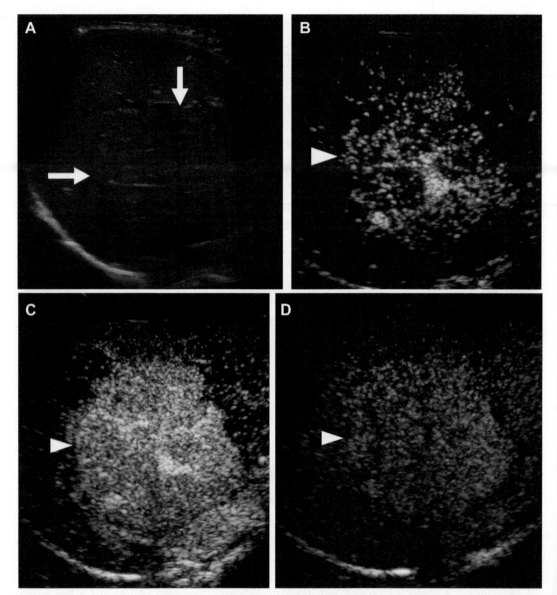

Fig. 5. A 16-year-old boy with FNH who presented with vague abdominal pain. (*A*) Transverse grayscale ultrasound demonstrates a heterogeneous somewhat circumscribed predominantly isoechoic mass (*arrows*) in the right hepatic lobe. Transverse CEUS images in the arterial phase at 26 seconds (*B*) and 32 seconds (*C*) following sulfur hexafluoride lipid-type A microspheres contrast injection demonstrate spoke-wheel centrifugal hyperenhancement of the mass (*arrowhead*) with an early enhancing central vessel. In the late phase at 6 minutes following contrast injection (*D*), there is overall contrast retention of the mass compared with the surrounding liver parenchyma (no washout).

for bleeding is lowest in this subtype, and there is also the lowest risk of malignant transformation.[18]

At CEUS, HNF-1α-inactivated hepatocellular adenomas show homogeneous hyperenhancement in the arterial phase (Fig. 6). Lesions show hyperenhancement or isoenhancement in the portal venous and late phases, with washout seen less commonly.[20–22] Sustained enhancement of HNF-1α-inactivated hepatocellular adenomas helps distinguish from the other adenoma subtypes and HCC, which often have mild late washout.

β-Catenin-activated hepatocellular adenoma

β-Catenin-activated hepatocellular adenomas account for 10% to 18% of adenomas. This subtype is the most frequent found in men, and there is an association with exogeneous androgen exposure,

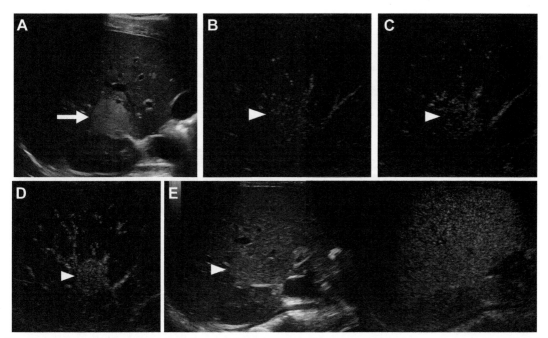

Fig. 6. A 14-year-old girl with MODY3 and HNF-1α-inactivated hepatocellular adenoma who presented with abdominal pain. Sagittal grayscale ultrasound image (*A*) demonstrates an echogenic mass in the posterior right hepatic lobe (*arrow*). Transverse CEUS images in the arterial phase at 14 seconds (*B*), 15 seconds (*C*), and 16 seconds (*D*) after sulfur hexafluoride lipid-type A microspheres contrast injection, there is heterogeneous early enhancement of the mass (*arrowhead*) with complete fill-in of contrast material. Split-screen CEUS image with grayscale (left panel) and contrast (right panel) in the late phase at 8 minutes 49 seconds after contrast injection (*E*) shows sustained enhancement of the mass (*arrowhead*), without washout.

such as for treatment of Fanconi anemia or for bodybuilding, as well as familial adenomatous polyposis and glycogen storage diseases.[11,16,19] Importantly, this subtype has the highest rate of malignant transformation at up to 50%; therefore, some authors suggest excision of any hepatic adenoma in a male patient.[11,19]

At CEUS, APHE is typically diffuse and homogeneous, with either portal venous or late phase washout in almost 90% of lesions.[20] Given overlap in appearance with HCC, biopsy may be necessary for diagnosis.

MALIGNANT LESIONS
Hepatoblastoma

Hepatoblastoma is the most common primary pediatric hepatic malignancy and 95% of cases are discovered by age 4 years.[23] Patients may present with abdominal distension or weight loss,[12] and serum alpha-fetoprotein level is elevated in 90% of patients.[11] The appearance of hepatoblastoma at CEUS has not been well studied, although a few published cases have demonstrated washout in the late phase, as expected for a primary hepatic malignancy (**Fig. 7**).[1] Hepatoblastoma staging uses PRE-Treatment EXTent of tumor,[24] which

cannot be completed with CEUS alone; contrast-enhanced MRI and/or CT are mandatory for adequate hepatoblastoma staging.

Hepatocellular Carcinoma

In adults, HCC is the most common primary liver malignancy and the fourth most common cause of cancer-related death worldwide.[25] The American College of Radiology Liver Imaging, Reporting, and Data System (LI-RADS) published CEUS LI-RADS for the diagnosis of liver observations suspicious for HCC in at-risk patients.[5,26,27] Similar to the CT/MRI LI-RADS diagnostic algorithm, CEUS LI-RADS provides the technique, interpretation, and recommended management for untreated observations in patients at-risk for HCC. The various categories convey the increasing likelihood of HCC, ranging from LR-1 (definitely benign) to LR-5 (definitely HCC), similar to the CT/MRI LI-RADS diagnostic system. Additional categories, LR-NC (not characterizable due to image omission or degradation), LR-TIV (tumor-in-vein), and LR-M (probably malignant but not HCC specific) are also included.

Major CEUS LI-RADS criteria include: 1) lesion size, 2) presence or absence of APHE (nonrim; nondiscontinuous peripheral nodular, which would

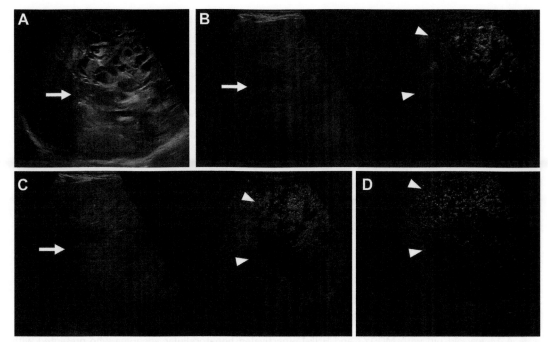

Fig. 7. A 7-month-old boy with hepatoblastoma who presented with abdominal distention. Sagittal grayscale ultrasound (*A*) demonstrates a large heterogeneous liver mass (*arrow*). Split-screen sagittal CEUS image with grayscale image (left panel) and contrast image (right panel) shows the heterogeneous mass (*arrow*), which has very heterogeneous arterial phase enhancement (*arrowheads*) at 14 seconds following sulfur hexafluoride lipid-type A microspheres contrast injection (*B*), with some fill-in of contrast material at 18 seconds (*C*). Washout of the mass (*arrowheads*) is seen at 2 minutes 9 seconds after contrast injection (*D*). In this child, CEUS was performed to better evaluate vascular involvement of the hepatoblastoma following CT and MRI.

indicate hemangioma), and 3) presence or absence of washout. Unique to CEUS LI-RADS, washout is characterized by its timing (early or late; <60 sec, or ≥ 60 sec, respectively) as well as by its degree (mild or marked). Marked washout is defined as a "punched out" appearance, nearly devoid of enhancement, within 2 minutes after contrast injection. Unlike CT/MRI LI-RADS, capsule is not a feature in CEUS. HCC classically shows nonrim APHE and mild, late washout. (Fig. 8) LR-M features include rim-APHE, early washout (<60 sec) or marked washout (punched out within 2 minute). As with LR-M observations in CT/MRI, biopsy is often needed.

Ancillary features favoring malignancy include definite growth, defined as 50% or greater size increase in 6 months or less, and those favoring HCC in particular include nodule-in-nodule architecture and mosaic architecture. Ancillary features favoring benignity include size stability in 2 years or greater and size reduction in absence of treatment.

Multiple recent publications in adult populations have shown that CEUS is highly specific for the diagnosis of HCC. For LR-5, positive predictive values of 97% to 98.5%, and specificity of 96%,

have been reported, equivalent to CT/MRI LI-RADS.[28-30] It has been noted that approximately 50% to 75% of LR-M observations are HCC, and there may be a higher incidence of HCC among CEUS LR-3 observations relative to CT/MRI LR-3.

The latest American Association for the Study of Liver Disease guidance document includes CEUS as a potential modality for the characterization of liver observations in at-risk patients.[31] However, at this time, the Organ Procurement and Transplant Network does not recognize CEUS for transplant consideration; however, it may be used in select patients as a trouble-shooting tool when CT or MRI is contraindicated or inconclusive. CEUS has shown promise in the assessment of response to treatment of HCC; however, this is not yet included in the LI-RADS system.

Cholangiocarcinoma

The most common subtype to be encountered and diagnosed by CEUS is the peripheral, mass-forming intrahepatic cholangiocarcinoma. Classic iCC may seem as a circumscribed or ill-defined heterogeneous mass, or may be indistinct and infiltrative in appearance. At CEUS, iCC classically

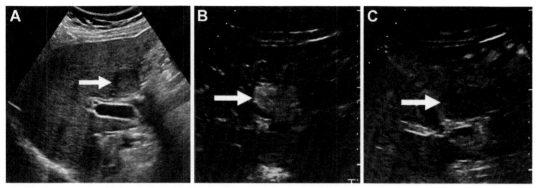

Fig. 8. A 76-year-old woman with chronic hepatitis B and a 3.6 cm hypoechoic well-differentiated HCC identified at surveillance ultrasound. Subsequent MRI was nondiagnostic due to severe motion degradation (not shown). Grayscale sagittal ultrasound image (A) shows a round, iso-to-hypoechoic nodule (arrow) in the posterior medial segment of left hepatic lobe. At CEUS using perflutren lipid microspheres, the lesion shows brisk, diffuse APHE at 17 seconds (B) with mild washout at 75 seconds (C) after contrast injection (CEUS LR-5, definitely HCC).

shows heterogeneous peripheral arterial phase hyperenhancement (rim-APHE) with washout that is rapid (<60 sec) and/or marked ("punched out" within 2 minutes) (iCC; Fig. 9).[32] The washout seen in iCC is discrepant from findings in CT and MRI, where delayed enhancement is generally seen. This discrepancy highlights one of the key differences of UCA, which are pure blood pool agents given the size of the individual microbubbles, unlike the relatively small iodinated and gadolinium-containing molecules that demonstrate an extravascular, interstitial phase allowing for delayed enhancement of otherwise nonenhancing or minimally enhancing tissue such as fibrosis/scar.

In patients at risk for HCC, rim-APHE, early and/ or marked washout are features of LR-M (probably malignant but not HCC specific), helping distinguish these masses from HCC.[33] Biopsy is generally recommended.

Metastases

In adults, there are many different types of primary malignancies that can be associated with liver metastases, although colorectal carcinoma is one of the most common.[34] The most common primary pediatric tumors with liver metastasis are neuroblastoma and Wilms tumor.[11] Identification of a primary tumor or knowledge of malignancy history is important. At CEUS, metastases are usually multiple although can be solitary. Although the arterial phase appearance is variable, metastases will nearly always demonstrate portal venous

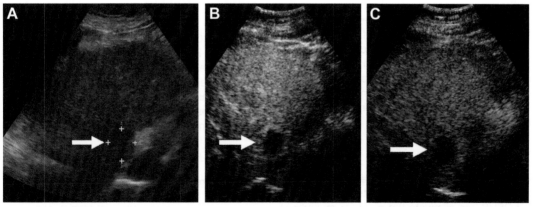

Fig. 9. A 66-year-old man with decompensated cirrhosis likely due to iron overload and alcohol abuse, presenting for transplant evaluation, was found to have a poorly differentiated adenocarcinoma at biopsy, consistent with a pancreaticobiliary primary tumor, likely representing cholangiocarcinoma. Grayscale ultrasound image (A) shows a rounded, iso-to-hypoechoic 3.3 cm nodule (arrow) high in the medial segment near the hepatic venous confluence. At CEUS performed with sulfur hexafluoride lipid-type A microspheres, the lesion demonstrates rim APHE at 20 seconds after contrast injection (B), with marked washout around 2 minutes (C).

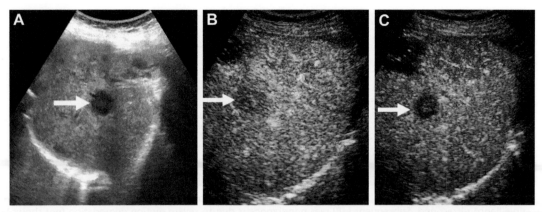

Fig. 10. A 82-year-old woman with liver metastasis due to breast cancer. Sagittal grayscale ultrasound image (*A*) demonstrates a hypoechoic nodule (*arrow*) in the right hepatic lobe. At CEUS using sulfur hexafluoride lipid-type A microspheres, there is hypoenhancement of the nodule in the arterial phase at 17 seconds following contrast injection (*B*), with early and marked washout at 42 seconds (*C*).

phase washout, typically within 1 to 2 minutes after UCA administration (**Fig. 10**)..[32,34]

INTERVENTION

Facilitated by the high safety profile of UCAs and the ability to inject multiple doses during a single encounter, CEUS has many potential uses in liver intervention.[35] CEUS may be used to improve visualization of a target lesion during biopsy or percutaneous ablation.[36–38] Microbubble contrast also helps distinguish viable (enhancing) from nonviable (nonenhancing) components of masses to help improve diagnostic yield of biopsies.[39] If multiple lesions are present, CEUS may help identify the most suspicious or accessible mass and exclude a benign cause.

CEUS is also becoming an important tool in posttreatment assessment of liver masses, particularly following transarterial chemoembolization and percutaneous ablation (radiofrequency or microwave).[40,41] The use of intraprocedural UCA immediately following an ablation procedure may help identify residual viable disease, allowing for repeat treatment during the same procedure, a benefit that has shown to improve patient outcomes.[42,43]

SUMMARY

Accurate liver lesion characterization is possible using CEUS in children and adults. UCA are safe and CEUS can eliminate the need for multiphase CT and MRI in many cases, which is particularly advantageous in children who are more susceptible to potential deleterious effects of ionizing radiation, and who may require sedation or general anesthesia to undergo diagnostic MRI.

CLINICS CARE POINTS

- Benign lesions have no washout and may have specific patterns of arterial phase enhancement that allow for definitive diagnosis.

- Hepatocellular carcinoma (HCC) demonstrate late (less than or equal to 60 seconds after contrast injection) and mild washout.

- Metastases typically demonstrate early washout (<60 seconds after contrast injection) or marked washout (nearly devoid of contrast within 2 minutes).

FUNDING SOURCES

1. Bracco Diagnostics–Unrelated to current work (bowel CEUS)
2. Philips Healthcare, GE Healthcare—Unrelated to current work (liver MRI and deep learning, free breathing body MRI)
3. Siemens Medical Solutions, Canon Medical Systems—Unrelated to current work (ultrasound markers of chronic liver disease)

DISCLOSURES

J. H. Squires: No relevant disclosures.

FUNDING SOURCES

Society for Pediatric Radiology Research & Education Foundation pilot grant (brain CEUS). D. T. Fetzer: Research agreements: GE Healthcare, Philips Healthcare, Siemens Healthineers; Advisory board, Philips Healthcare. J. R. Dillman: No relevant disclosures.

REFERENCES

1. Squires JH, McCarville MB. Contrast-enhanced ultrasound in children: implementation and key diagnostic applications. AJR Am J Roentgenol 2021. https://doi.org/10.2214/AJR.21.25713.

2. Ranganath PG, Robbin ML, Back SJ, et al. Practical advantages of contrast-enhanced ultrasound in abdominopelvic radiology. Abdom Radiol (NY) 2018; 43(4):998–1012.

3. Dietrich CF, Averkiou M, Nielsen MB, et al. How to perform Contrast-Enhanced Ultrasound (CEUS). Ultrasound Int Open 2018;4(1):E2–15.

4. Schooler GR, Squires JH, Alazraki A, et al. Pediatric Hepatoblastoma, Hepatocellular Carcinoma, and Other Hepatic Neoplasms: Consensus Imaging Recommendations from American College of Radiology Pediatric Liver Reporting and Data System (LI-RADS) Working Group. Radiology 2020;296(3): 493–7.

5. American College of Radiology. Ultrasound LI-RADS v2017. 2017. Available at: https://www.acr.org/Clinical-Resources/Reporting-and-Data-Systems/LI-RADS/Ultrasound-LI-RADS-v2017. Accessed Nov 13, 2020.

6. Fetzer DT, Kono Y, Rodgers SK. Using contrast-enhanced ultrasound to characterize focal liver lesions. Clin Liver Dis (Hoboken) 2021;17(3):119–24.

7. Fetzer DT, Rafailidis V, Peterson C, et al. Artifacts in contrast-enhanced ultrasound: a pictorial essay. Abdom Radiol (NY) 2018;43(4):977–97.

8. Anomalies ISftSoV. 2018 classification. 2020. Available at: issva.org/classification. Accessed 10/28/2020.

9. Merrow AC, Gupta A, Patel MN, et al. 2014 revised classification of vascular lesions from the international society for the study of vascular anomalies: radiologic-pathologic update. Radiographics 2016; 36(5):1494–516.

10. El-Ali AM, McCormick A, Thakrar D, et al. Contrast-enhanced ultrasound of congenital and infantile hemangiomas: preliminary results from a case series. AJR Am J Roentgenol 2020;214(3):658–64.

11. Schooler GR, Hull NC, Lee EY. Hepatobiliary MRI contrast agents: pattern recognition approach to pediatric focal hepatic lesions. AJR Am J Roentgenol 2020;214(5):976–86.

12. Pugmire BS, Towbin AJ. Magnetic resonance imaging of primary pediatric liver tumors. Pediatr Radiol 2016;46(6):764–77.

13. Chung EM, Cube R, Lewis RB, et al. From the archives of the AFIP: Pediatric liver masses: radiologic-pathologic correlation part 1. Benign tumors. Radiographics 2010;30(3):801–26.

14. Martins-Filho SN, Putra J. Hepatic mesenchymal hamartoma and undifferentiated embryonal sarcoma of the liver: a pathologic review. Hepat Oncol 2020;7(2):HEP19.

15. Masand PM. Magnetic resonance imaging features of common focal liver lesions in children. Pediatr Radiol 2018;48(9):1234–44.

16. Yoneda N, Matsui O, Kitao A, et al. Benign hepatocellular nodules: hepatobiliary phase of gadoxetic acid-enhanced MR imaging based on molecular background. Radiographics 2016; 36(7):2010–27.

17. El-Ali AM, Davis JC, Cickelli JM, et al. Contrast-enhanced ultrasound of liver lesions in children. Pediatr Radiol 2019;49(11):1422–32.

18. Nault JC, Couchy G, Balabaud C, et al. Molecular classification of hepatocellular adenoma associates with risk factors, bleeding, and malignant transformation. Gastroenterology 2017;152(4): 880–894 e6.

19. Nault JC, Paradis V, Cherqui D, et al. Molecular classification of hepatocellular adenoma in clinical practice. J Hepatol 2017;67(5):1074–83.

20. Chen K, Dong Y, Zhang W, et al. Analysis of contrast-enhanced ultrasound features of hepatocellular adenoma according to different pathological molecular classifications. Clin Hemorheol Microcirc 2020;76(3):391–403.

21. Laumonier H, Cailliez H, Balabaud C, et al. Role of contrast-enhanced sonography in differentiation of subtypes of hepatocellular adenoma: correlation with MRI findings. AJR Am J Roentgenol 2012; 199(2):341–8.

22. Manichon AF, Bancel B, Durieux-Millon M, et al. Hepatocellular adenoma: evaluation with contrast-enhanced ultrasound and MRI and correlation with pathologic and phenotypic classification in 26 lesions. HPB Surg 2012;2012:418745.

23. Chung EM, Lattin GE Jr, Cube R, et al. From the archives of the AFIP: Pediatric liver masses: radiologic-pathologic correlation. Part 2. Malignant tumors. Radiographics 2011;31(2):483–507.

24. Towbin AJ, Meyers RL, Woodley H, et al. 2017 PRETEXT: radiologic staging system for primary hepatic malignancies of childhood revised for the Paediatric Hepatic International Tumour Trial (PHITT). Pediatr Radiol 2018;48(4):536–54.

25. Moon AM, Singal AG, Tapper EB. Contemporary epidemiology of chronic liver disease and cirrhosis. Clin Gastroenterol Hepatol 2020;18(12):2650–66.

26. Lyshchik A, Kono Y, Dietrich CF, et al. Contrast-enhanced ultrasound of the liver: technical and lexicon recommendations from the ACR CEUS LI-RADS working group. Abdom Radiol (NY) 2018; 43(4):861–79.

27. Wilson SR, Lyshchik A, Piscaglia F, et al. CEUS LI-RADS: algorithm, implementation, and key

differences from CT/MRI. Abdom Radiol (NY) 2018; 43(1):127–42.

28. Terzi E, Iavarone M, Pompili M, et al. Contrast ultrasound LI-RADS LR-5 identifies hepatocellular carcinoma in cirrhosis in a multicenter restropective study of 1,006 nodules. J Hepatol 2018;68(3):485–92.

29. Zheng W, Li Q, Zou XB, et al. Evaluation of Contrast-enhanced US LI-RADS version 2017: Application on 2020 Liver Nodules in Patients with Hepatitis B Infection. Radiology 2020;294(2):299–307.

30. Huang JY, Li JW, Lu Q, et al. Diagnostic Accuracy of CEUS LI-RADS for the Characterization of Liver Nodules 20 mm or Smaller in Patients at Risk for Hepatocellular Carcinoma. Radiology 2020;294(2): 329–39.

31. Marrero JA, Kulik LM, Sirlin CB, et al. Diagnosis, staging, and management of hepatocellular carcinoma: 2018 practice guidance by the american association for the study of liver diseases. Hepatology 2018;68(2):723–50.

32. Burrowes DP, Medellin A, Harris AC, et al. Contrast-enhanced US approach to the diagnosis of focal liver masses. Radiographics 2017;37(5):1388–400.

33. Wang DC, Jang HJ, Kim TK. Characterization of Indeterminate Liver Lesions on CT and MRI With Contrast-Enhanced Ultrasound: What Is the Evidence? AJR Am J Roentgenol 2020;214(6): 1295–304.

34. Kong WT, Ji ZB, Wang WP, et al. Evaluation of liver metastases using contrast-enhanced ultrasound: enhancement patterns and influencing factors. Gut Liver 2016;10(2):283–7.

35. Malone CD, Fetzer DT, Monsky WL, et al. Contrast-enhanced US for the Interventional Radiologist: Current and Emerging Applications. Radiographics 2020;40(2):562–88.

36. Yoon SH, Lee KH, Kim SY, et al. Real-time contrast-enhanced ultrasound-guided biopsy of focal hepatic lesions not localised on B-mode ultrasound. Eur Radiol 2010;20(8):2047–56.

37. Wu W, Chen MH, Yin SS, et al. The role of contrast-enhanced sonography of focal liver lesions before percutaneous biopsy. AJR Am J Roentgenol 2006; 187(3):752–61. https://doi.org/10.2214/AJR.05. 0535.

38. Acord MR, Cahill AM, Durand R, et al. Contrast-enhanced ultrasound in pediatric interventional radiology. Pediatr Radiol 2021. https://doi.org/10.1007/ s00247-020-04853-4.

39. Grossjohann HS, Bachmann Nielsen M. Ultrasound contrast agents may help in avoiding necrotic areas at biopsy. Ultraschall Med 2006;27(1):2–3.

40. Salvaggio G, Campisi A, Lo Greco V, et al. Evaluation of posttreatment response of hepatocellular carcinoma: comparison of ultrasonography with second-generation ultrasound contrast agent and multidetector CT. Abdom Imaging 2010;35(4): 447–53.

41. Solbiati L, Ierace T, Tonolini M, et al. Guidance and monitoring of radiofrequency liver tumor ablation with contrast-enhanced ultrasound. Eur J Radiol 2004;51(Suppl):S19–23.

42. Minami Y, Kudo M, Kawasaki T, et al. Treatment of hepatocellular carcinoma with percutaneous radiofrequency ablation: usefulness of contrast harmonic sonography for lesions poorly defined with B-mode sonography. AJR Am J Roentgenol 2004;183(1): 153–6.

43. Minami Y, Kudo M, Chung H, et al. Contrast harmonic sonography-guided radiofrequency ablation therapy versus B-mode sonography in hepatocellular carcinoma: prospective randomized controlled trial. AJR Am J Roentgenol 2007;188(2):489–94.

Hepatobiliary Dual-Energy Computed Tomography

Sergio Grosu, MD[a,b], Benjamin M. Yeh, MD[a,*]

KEYWORDS

- Computed tomography • X-Ray • DECT • Humans • Abdomen • Liver • Gallstones • Bile duct

KEY POINTS

- Dual-energy computed tomography (DECT) imaging increases confidence in computed tomography evaluation of the liver, bile ducts, and gallbladder.
- Low-kiloelectronvolt (keV) virtual monoenergetic (MonoE) images and iodine density maps improve the conspicuity of liver lesions and allow more confident liver lesion characterization.
- Material decomposition algorithms enable the assessment of steatosis and hepatic iron deposition in unenhanced DECT scans and fibrosis/cirrhosis in delayed phase contrast-enhanced DECT scans.
- Virtual noncontrast images and low-keV virtual MonoE images improve the conspicuity of cholesterol gallstones.

Abbreviations	
METAVIR	meta-analysis of histological data in viral hepatitis
AUC	Area Under the Receiver Operator Characteristic Curve
UCSF	University of California–San Francisco

INTRODUCTION

The evaluation of the liver and bile ducts is a central focus of abdominal imaging. Computed tomography (CT) is often the imaging modality of choice, as it is fast, reliable, not examiner-dependent, intrinsically quantitative, and cost-effective. However, conventional single-energy CT has several well-known technical limitations. Radiodensities may be ambiguous as to whether or not they represent iodine enhancement versus calcification versus other radiodense material. Subtle liver lesions or isodense noncalcified gallstones are commonly missed. The detection and quantification of diffuse liver disease is also constrained.

Dual-energy CT (DECT) overcomes several limitations of single-energy CT, particularly for the evaluation of the liver, gallbladder, and bile ducts. In contrast to single-energy CT, which displays images derived from a single polychromatic X-ray photon energy spectrum, DECT displays results from both a high and a low X-ray photon energy spectrum that allows the differentiation of materials based on their characteristic attenuation properties of the 2 X-ray energy spectra.[1–3] Exploitation of this data allows for more accurate detection and characterization of liver lesions and gallstones and more precise assessment of diffuse liver diseases.[4–6] Furthermore, DECT allows the decrease in beam hardening artifacts from metallic

[a] Department of Radiology and Biomedical Imaging, University of California, 505 Parnassus Avenue, M391, Box 0628, San Francisco, CA 94143-0628, USA; [b] Department of Radiology, University Hospital, LMU Munich, Marchioninistr 15, 81377 Munich, Germany
* Corresponding author. UCSF Department of Radiology and Biomedical Imaging, University of California, 505 Parnassus Avenue, M391, Box 0628, San Francisco, CA 94143-0628.
E-mail address: benjamin.yeh@ucsf.edu

Radiol Clin N Am 60 (2022) 731–743
https://doi.org/10.1016/j.rcl.2022.05.006

surgical implant, which is beneficial for the evaluation of the liver and bile ducts.[7] These advantages of DECT may be achieved with similar or only slightly increased radiation dose compared with conventional scanners.[8] Future innovations in image displays, artificial intelligence, photon-counting hardware, and novel contrast agents are expected to further expand the value of DECT in everyday imaging. Our review describes the basic technical aspects of DECT image reconstructions, current clinical applications, current challenges, and future directions of DECT for the evaluation of the liver and bile ducts.

BASIC CONCEPTS OF DUAL-ENERGY COMPUTED TOMOGRAPHY

Typically, abdominal single-energy CT scans are acquired using a single X-ray source with a tube voltage of 120 kilovoltage-peak (kVp), which produces a single polychromatic X-ray beam with an energy peak of 120 kVp and an average energy of approximately 75 kiloelectronvolt (keV).[1] The X-rays that pass through the imaged object hit the detectors and are simply reconstructed into CT images where the Hounsfield Unit (HU) of each voxel reflects the attenuation of the X-ray beam.[3,9,10] In this setting, many different materials can result in the same HU values. For example, dilute iodine, moderately dense calcium, or densely packed organic material can all seem as 200 HU at 120 kVp.

However, different materials attenuate low and high X-ray energy spectra in material-specific extent. For instance, a voxel of dilute iodine that shows similar HU as a voxel of moderately dense calcium at an X-ray energy spectrum of 120 kVp will show a predictable magnitude of higher HU when imaged with an X-ray energy spectrum of 80 kVp.[3,9,10] This information is lost in single-energy CT.

DECT exploits this phenomenon of unique and predictable relative X-ray attenuation of different materials at low and high X-ray energies to allow differentiation of different materials in a given voxel.[3,11] In the following, we present current clinical implementations of DECT scan acquisition.

Different Vendor Implementations

The dual-source DECT scanner uses 2 X-ray tubes and detector arrays mounted orthogonally in the gantry. One X-ray tube produces a high-energy spectrum operating at 140 to 150 kVp, the other a low-energy spectrum operating at 70 to 100 kVp.[2,12] Generally, the X-ray tube located closer to the patient has a slightly smaller field of view of 26 to 36 cm, which limits the dual-energy evaluation to this central portion of the image.[2,3,9,12] The strength of dual-source DECT is good spectral separation, further improved with a tin filter applied to the high-energy X-ray tube which further increases the mean keV of that X-ray energy spectra.[2,9,12]

The twin-beam or split-filter DECT scanner uses a gold/tin split filter applied to a single X-ray tube operating at 120 kVp. The tin filter creates a high-energy spectrum in one-half and the gold filter a low-energy spectrum in the other half of the single X-ray beam.[2,3,12] Twin-beam DECT shows less vivid spectral separation than other dual-energy implementations.[3,9,13] It generally requires a slow table speed and large tube current to compensate for the added beam filtration.[3,9,13] The strength of twin-beam DECT is a full field of view for dual-energy imaging.[3]

The fast kV-switching or rapid kV-switching DECT scanner uses a single X-ray tube that switches as fast as 0.25 ms between a high-energy spectrum operating at 140 kVp and a low-energy spectrum operating at 80 kVp.[2,9,12] Techniques to reduce radiation exposure are limited because changes in current modulation and dual-energy scan pair are not possible.[9,13] A strength of fast kV-switching DECT is a full field of view for dual-energy imaging and excellent coregistration of the low-energy and high-energy projection data.[2,3,12]

The dual-layer spectral detector or sandwich detector DECT scanner uses a single X-ray tube that produces a conventional polychromatic X-ray beam. The spectral separation of the X-ray beam takes place at the detector level: The thin top-layer yttrium-based garnet scintillator detects the low-energy photons, and the thick bottom-layer gadolinium oxysulphide scintillator detects the remaining high-energy photons.[2,3,12] Spectral separation is decreased due to the close proximity of the 2 scintillators in the detector.[9] The strengths of dual-layer spectral detector DECT include a full field of view for dual-energy imaging, excellent coregistration of the low-energy and high-energy projection data, DECT information is retrospectively available on all scans, and tube current modulation is possible, enabling automatic exposure control techniques.[2,3,9,12]

Main Dual-Energy Computed Tomography Image Reconstructions

Regardless of which technique is used to acquire DECT data, the reconstructed DECT images show similar properties across the different DECT scanner models. The main types of image reconstructions are 120-kVp-like images, virtual monoenergetic (MonoE) images, virtual noncontrast (VNC) images (also referred to as water density maps), and iodine density maps **Table 1**.

Table 1
Clinical utility of different dual-energy computed tomography image reconstructions in hepatobiliary assessment

DECT Image Reconstructions	Clinical Utility
Conventional 120 kVp images 120-kVp-like blended images 70 keV MonoE images	General anatomic evaluation
Low-keV MonoE images	Liver lesion detection Liver lesion characterization Gallstone detection Gallstone characterization
High-keV MonoE images	Metal artifact reduction Gallstone detection Gallstone characterization
VNC images	Replacement of true unenhanced images Gallstone detection
Iodine density maps	Liver lesion detection Liver lesion characterization Liver fibrosis/cirrhosis staging Portal vein thrombus characterization Tumor response evaluation after hepatic RFA/TACE Gallbladder carcinoma detection Gallbladder carcinoma characterization Cholangiography
Specific material decomposition images	Liver iron quantification Liver fat quantification Liver fibrosis/cirrhosis staging

Abbreviations: MonoE, virtual monoenergetic; VNC, virtual noncontrast; RFA, radiofrequency ablation; TACE, transarterial chemoembolization

The 120-kVp-like images imitate conventional CT images acquired on a single-energy CT scanner operating at 120 kVp. To create 120-kVp-like images, the dual-source DECT scanner uses "mixed images" linearly combining data from both X-ray tubes.[9,14] Similarly, the twin-beam DECT combines the high-energy and low-energy spectra data in a "mixed image." The fast kV-switching DECT scanner adopts 70 to 75 keV MonoE images as 120-kVp-like images.[9,14] The dual-layer spectral detector DECT generates conventional 120 kVp images.[9,14]

MonoE images simulate how a CT image might look if it had been acquired with a specific MonoE X-ray photon energy.[3] Depending on the scanner type, the MonoE photon energy can be selected between 40 keV and 200 keV. High-KeV MonoE images generally show lower noise and are well suited for the reduction of metal artifacts because they are considerably less severe than in conventional images.[7] Different materials show characteristic relative changes in CT attenuation at different keV settings (Fig. 1). High-keV MonoE images can also be used as VNC images because the attenuation of iodine is minimized in those reconstructions.[3] High-keV MonoE images also minimize

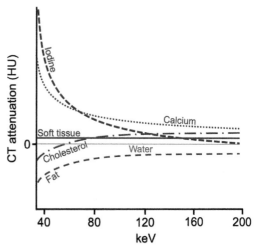

Fig. 1. HU of iodine, calcium, soft tissue, cholesterol, and fat at different X-ray photon energy levels (keV). Y-axis: CT attenuation in HU; X-axis: X-ray photon energy in keV. Note: the asymptote of iodine at high keV is the HU of the underlying tissue or blood. In the current illustration, the asymptote of iodine is chosen to be water.

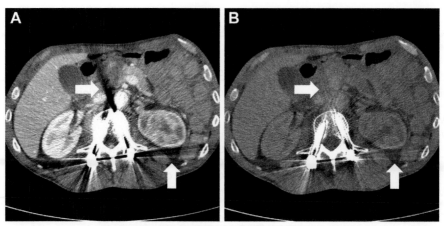

Fig. 2. Axial contrast-enhanced DECT scan of the abdomen with severe metal artifacts (*arrows*) caused by pedicle screws in the spine on a (*A*) conventional 120 kVp image and (*B*) virtual MonoE 140 keV image. Metal spray artifacts (*arrows*) are considerably less severe on (B) high-keV virtual MonoE images than on (A) conventional 120 kVp images.

streak artifact from low atomic number metals such as surgical steel (**Fig. 2**), which may otherwise degrade image quality. Low-keV MonoE images behave in the opposite way: image contrast and iodine attenuation is higher than in conventional images but also metal artifacts are more severe.[3] Low-keV monoE images are useful to emphasize iodine enhancement and have been shown to improve both hypervascular and hypovascular liver lesion detection.[15]

VNC images display materials with little or no relative decrease in HU when imaged with a low versus a high X-ray energy spectrum. This property is seen with water and most nonfatty soft tissues. Conversely, iodine density maps display materials with a relatively marked decrease in HU when imaged with a low versus a high X-ray energy spectrum. That property is particularly strong

with iodine and barium contrast agents.[3] Viewed as a pair, VNC images and iodine maps help detect and characterize iodine-enhancing lesions, bleeding, and ischemia.[16–18]

Dual-Energy Computed Tomography Protocols

Protocols specific to each DECT scanner are required due to hardware and software implementation differences between scanners. Nevertheless, some considerations apply to most DECT scanners to ensure diagnostic liver scan quality. Due to poor penetration of low-energy X-rays through thick body parts such as the upper abdomen, some institutions restrict DECT imaging only to those small-to-medium-sized patients (eg, weigh <less than 250 lbs, or abdominal diameter <43 cm). To avoid beam hardening artifacts, scans are further

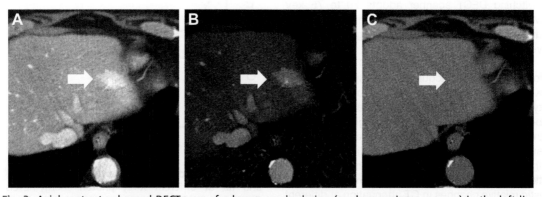

Fig. 3. Axial contrast-enhanced DECT scan of a hypervascular lesion (eg, hemangioma, *arrows*) in the left liver lobe on a (*A*) conventional 120 kVp image, (*B*) iodine density map, and (*C*) VNC image. Improved conspicuity of the hypervascular lesion on the (B) iodine density map compared with the (A) conventional 120 kVp image. Isodensity of the lesion (*arrow*) on the (C) VNC image confirms that the lesion's hyperdensity on the (A) conventional 120 kVp image is attributable to hypervascularity (increased iodine uptake).

restricted to patients where arms and other external devices can be moved well away from the imaged section of the abdomen. Although DECT may allow for marked reduction in intravenous contrast doses for many vascular and general abdominal applications, intravenous contrast dose reduction should be used with caution for DECT imaging of liver tumors where the detection and characterization of subtle lesions may depend on excellent contrast enhancement and where concern for poor contrast enhancement may outweigh the possible benefits of contrast load reduction.

FOCAL LIVER DISEASE

The benefits of DECT are readily applied to clinical evaluation of the liver. Most publications on this topic focus on improving the visualization of focal liver lesions. Other publications show the value of DECT for the assessment of diffuse liver diseases.

Hypervascular Liver Lesions

Liver lesions may be more conspicuous in low-keV (40–60 keV) MonoE image reconstructions or iodine images, which emphasize iodine attenuation[4,15,19–21] (Fig. 3). Große Hokamp and colleagues showed that the attenuation of arterially hyperenhancing liver lesions was significantly higher ($P < .001$) and subjective arterially hyperenhancing liver lesion delineation was significantly better ($P < .01$) in 40 keV MonoE images compared with conventional images.[20] In patients at high-risk for hepatocellular carcinoma (HCC), 50 keV MonoE DECT images can provide significantly better ($P < .01$) focal liver lesion conspicuity than hybrid iterative reconstruction images of standard-dose single-energy CT in nonobese patients while using lower radiation and contrast media doses.[21] Matsuda and colleagues reported

that tumor washout of HCC 2 cm or lesser was best seen on 50 keV MonoE images in the equilibrium phase.[22] However, the optimal monochromatic X-ray energy spectrum for maximizing the conspicuity of hypervascular liver lesions may be higher for larger sized abdomens.[23]

Iodine density maps may further increase the conspicuity and detection of hypervascular liver lesions.[16,24] Muenzel and colleagues showed that the liver-to-lesion contrast ratio was significantly increased ($P < .001$) and significantly more ($P < .05$) hypervascular liver lesions were correctly identified in iodine density maps compared with 65 keV MonoE images.[16] One study showed that the liver-to-lesion contrast ratio was significantly higher in DECT iodine density maps than gadolinium-enhanced breath-hold 3D T1-weighted fat-suppressed gradient-echo MR images ($P < .001$).[16] These finding were confirmed in a study of Pfeiffer and colleagues on HCC lesions.[24] Conversely, bright attenuation at virtual noncontrast DECT image reconstructions confirms that a lesion is calcified rather than enhancing with iodine (Fig. 4).

Hypovascular Liver Lesions

At portal venous phase imaging, hypovascular liver lesions can be identified more reliably at low-keV MonoE images due to an increased contrast to the higher attenuating liver parenchyma.[4,25] Caruso and colleagues demonstrated that the sensitivity for the detection of hypovascular liver lesions was higher in 50 keV MonoE images (lesion sensitivity: 95%) compared with conventional blended images (lesion sensitivity: 83%).[25] Lenga and colleagues showed that using a noise-optimization algorithm in 40 keV MonoE images could further improve hypovascular liver lesion delineation, compared with conventional

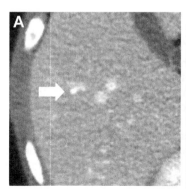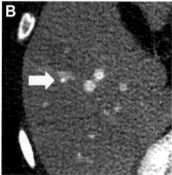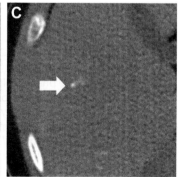

Fig. 4. Axial contrast-enhanced DECT scan of a presumably hypervascular lesion (*arrows*) in the right liver lobe on a (A) conventional 120 kVp image, (B) iodine density map, and (C) VNC image. The (C) VNC image reveals that the lesion's hyperdensity on the (A) conventional 120 kVp image is not attributable to hypervascularity (increased iodine uptake), thus unmasking the lesion as a calcified granuloma.

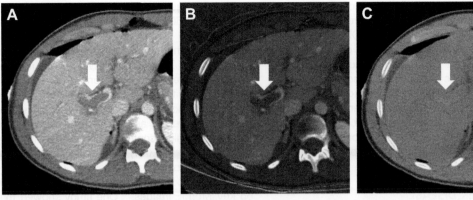

Fig. 5. Axial contrast-enhanced DECT scan of a thrombus (*arrows*) in the portal vein on a (*A*) 120-kVp-like image, (*B*) iodine density map, and (*C*) VNC image. No increased iodine uptake can be seen on the (*B*) iodine density map, indicating that the thrombus is bland and not neoplastic.

40 keV MonoE images and conventional blended images (*P* < .001).[26] However, the benefit of DECT image reconstructions for the detection of hypovascular liver lesion could be limited in patients with hepatic steatosis (liver parenchyma <40 HU at noncontrast-enhanced CT).[27]

Liver lesion characterization also benefits from DECT. Patel and colleagues showed that single-phase contrast-enhanced DECT material attenuation analysis in iodine density maps improved the characterization of small (<2.0 cm) incidental indeterminate hypovascular liver lesions compared with conventional single-energy CT evaluation.[28] Iodine quantification in iodine density maps (AUC = 0.97) performed better at differentiating benign from malignant liver lesions than HU measurements in conventional blended images (AUC = 0.81).[28] Yang and colleagues demonstrated that iodine quantification in iodine density maps (AUC = 0.87) improved the differentiation between small HCC with and without microvascular invasion, compared with 70 keV MonoE images as conventional image equivalent (AUC = 0.71).[29]

Portal Vein Thrombosis

By confirming iodine enhancement, iodine density maps in portal venous phase help differentiate neoplastic from bland macroscopic portal vein thrombi[30] (**Fig. 5**). In a pilot study by Qian and colleagues, iodine indices of neoplastic portal vein thrombi were significantly higher (*P* < .001) than those of the bland thrombi.[30] Ascenti and colleagues showed that the overall diagnostic accuracy of iodine quantification was significantly better (*P* < .001) than conventional HU measurements in distinguishing bland from neoplastic portal vein thrombosis in patients with HCC.[31]

Hepatic Tumor Response Evaluation

In a posttherapeutic setting, DECT image reconstructions could aid the identification of vital tumor burden and local recurrence.[32–34] Dai and colleagues demonstrated that volumetric iodine-uptake changes in DECT could be used to evaluate disease control in HCC patients receiving sorafenib.[32] Lee and colleagues showed that the conspicuity of ablation zones after hepatic radiofrequency ablation is improved in iodine density maps, which is helpful to assess tumor response.[33] One study showed that the rate of uncertain diagnosis of locally recurrent HCC after transarterial chemoembolization was decreased (35% vs 0%) and interobserver agreement improved (k = 0.527 vs 0.718) viewing color-coded iodine density maps, compared with conventional images.[34]

DIFFUSE LIVER DISEASE

Diffuse liver disease detection and quantification, such as for iron overload, steatosis, fibrosis, and cirrhosis, benefit from DECT.

Hepatic Iron Deposition

Because iron has a higher atomic number than the elements that compose most liver tissue, iron deposition in the liver can be quantified at DECT, with a diagnostic performance similar to MR imaging for a moderate-to-severe disease.[35–39] Liver iron quantification is among the oldest clinical applications of DECT and can be performed on any scanner simply by acquiring noncontrast images of the liver at 2 kVps[40] (**Fig. 6**). Luo and colleagues demonstrated that iron specific–based virtual iron content imaging of the liver at DECT showed strong linear correlations with MR imaging measurements of liver iron

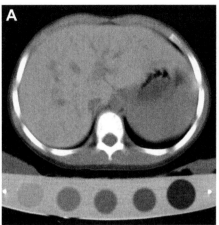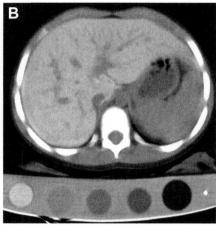

Fig. 6. Axial unenhanced CT scans of a liver with severe iron deposition acquired at (A) 120 kVp and (B) 80 kVp. In cases of hepatic iron deposition, the liver parenchyma seems brighter on (B) 80 kVp images compared with (A) 120 kVp images. Liver iron quantification at DECT is based on differences in HU of the liver parenchyma between low and high kVp images. For reference, iron-containing table phantom inserts (left 3 circles of table phantom of each image) show iron concentrations of 20, 10, and 5 mg iron/mL, from left to middle of image, respectively, show higher attenuation on the 80 kVp than the 120 kVp image.

content (r = 0.885 and 0.871).[36] In noncontrast chest-DECTs of hematologic patients intended primarily for exclusion of pulmonary infection, hepatic virtual iron content at DECT strongly correlated with serum ferritin levels (r = 0.623) and the estimated amount of transfused iron (r = 0.558).[39] Results from Abadia and colleagues showed that DECT could not only quantify liver iron content but also show the spatial distribution of iron within the liver.[41]

Liver Steatosis

The fat content in the liver can be delineated in DECT using material decomposition algorithms based on the different behavior of fat and water at low and high X-ray energy spectra[6,42–44] (Fig. 7). However, the additional value of DECT over conventional non-contrast single-energy CT for the evaluation of

hepatic steatosis is unclear, with some studies showing no additional benefit of DECT.[45,46] This can be attributed to the already good correlation of HU measurements on unenhanced single-energy CT with quantitative MR imaging methods and histologic grading of steatosis.[45–47] However, several studies indicate a promising role of DECT in the quantification of liver fat because it allows the evaluation of liver fat in iodinated contrast-enhanced CT scans where the liver steatosis delineation is less reliable, thus eliminating the need for additional unenhanced CT scans.[6,43,44,48,49] Hyodo and colleagues showed that a multimaterial decomposition algorithm in contrast-enhanced DECT was comparable to MR imaging spectroscopy in liver fat volume fraction measurements.[6] There was no significant difference (P > .05, respectively) between liver fat volume fraction measurements in unenhanced

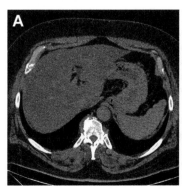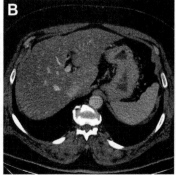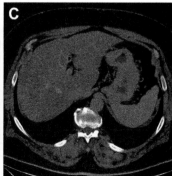

Fig. 7. (A) Axial true noncontrast CT scan and (B-C) axial contrast enhanced DECT scan of a fatty liver. (B) A 120-kVp-like reconstruction and (C) a VNC reconstruction of the contrast-enhanced DECT scan. For the evaluation of liver steatosis, (A) true noncontrast CT images may be replaced with (C) VNC DECT images to remove the need for additional unenhanced CT scans.

DECT scans and each phase of the contrast-enhanced DECT scans.[6] In a phantom study by Fischer and colleagues, DECT with the use of an iron-specific 3-material decomposition algorithm allowed for the accurate quantification of liver fat content in the presence of iodinated contrast material as well as iron.[44]

Liver Fibrosis and Cirrhosis

To understand how contrast-enhanced CT may quantify liver fibrosis, one must recognize that water within the liver parenchyma resides in 3 compartments: the intracellular space; interstitial (or extracellular extravascular) space; and intravascular space.[50,51] The combined interstitial and intravascular spaces comprise the extracellular volume fraction.[51] Liver fibrosis refers to the accumulation of collagen in the interstitial space. This expansion of the interstitial space increases the hepatic extracellular extravascular volume fraction of water.[51,52] After injection, intravenous extracellular iodinated contrast material moves freely between the intravascular and interstitial spaces of the liver and reaches an equilibrium state within roughly 3 to 5 minutes, depending on the amount of fibrosis. The extracellular volume fraction can be calculated from HU measurements of the blood pool versus the liver parenchyma at this equilibrium phase relative to the noncontrast CT HU measurements.[50,51,53,54] DECT provides semiquantitative liver fibrosis evaluation because iodine-quantification data is readily available without the need for a separate noncontrast scan.[55–59] Soufe and colleagues demonstrated that iodine density measurements from DECT scans could reliably stage liver fibrosis with an AUC ranging from 0.795 to 0.855 for assignment of each histopathologic METAVIR fibrosis stage.[55] Bak and colleagues showed that extracellular volume fraction scores derived from DECT iodine density maps could serve as an indicator of disease severity in cirrhotic patients.[56] Extracellular volume fraction scores were independently associated (odds ratio 1.27–1.32) with the presence of hepatic decompensation and could accurately predict (hazard ratio 1.40) liver-related events in the group with compensated liver cirrhosis.[56]

CLINICAL APPLICATIONS FOR GALLSTONE AND BILE DUCT EVALUATION
Gallstones

DECT considerably expands the potential of CT imaging to detect gallstones, which may otherwise be invisible or ambiguous at standard CT[5,60–66] (Fig. 8). VNC DECT images may replace true unenhanced images for gallstone identification to reduce radiation dose.[65] Interestingly, it was reported that the visibility of noncalcified gallstones was even increased on VNC DECT images compared with true unenhanced images.[62] Improved detection does not apply to calcified stones, which do not require DECT for detection and small gallstones that may be missed regardless of CT technique.[62,67] Uyeda and colleagues demonstrated that 40 keV and 190 keV MonoE images significantly increased ($P < .0001$) the contrast between noncalcified gallstones and bile compared with 70 keV MonoE images as conventional image equivalent.[5] Soesbe and colleagues used a cholesterol-bile 2-material decomposition algorithm to achieve an AUC of 0.99 for the detection of isoattenuating gallstones of all sizes in a phantom model.[61] Further study is needed to assess for accuracy in community practice.

In addition to improving gallstone detection, DECT also provides insight into gallstone composition, knowledge of which can help appropriately triage patients to nonsurgical treatment options.[68,69] Bauer and colleagues showed in a phantom model that 140 kVp and 80 kVp images allowed for reliable identification of gallstones containing a high percentage of cholesterol and no calcium component.[68] Sectors in gallstones containing more than 70% of cholesterol and no calcium could be identified with 95% sensitivity and 100% specificity on DECT.[68] Furthermore, Yin and colleagues demonstrated that DECT is helpful in differentiating between cholesterol and adenomatous gallbladder polyps 1.0 to 2.0 cm in size.[70] Mean attenuation value changes between 140 kVp and 80 kVp images as well as 100 keV and 40 keV MonoE images were significantly different ($P < .05$) between cholesterol and adenomatous polyps.[70]

Gallbladder Disease

Although in cases of suspected acute cholecystitis ultrasound is the imaging modality of choice, CT is often the first imaging examination performed in patients with uncharacteristic abdominal pain. DECT may further increase the confidence in diagnosing acute cholecystitis. Iodine density maps help visualize increased iodine uptake in the pericholecystic liver parenchyma and gallbladder wall, which is associated with acute cholecystitis.[71] Additionally, the detection and characterization of gallbladder carcinoma may be improved with DECT imaging.[71] Iodine density maps help visualize the increased iodine uptake of gallbladder carcinoma compared with benign entities such as adenomyomatosis or xanthogranulomatous cholecystitis.[71] However, these finding need further evaluation to assess for sensitivity and specificity.

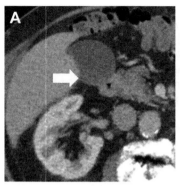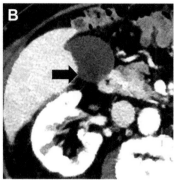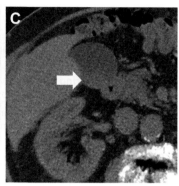

Fig. 8. Axial contrast-enhanced DECT scan of a noncalcified gallstone (*arrows*) in the gallbladder on (*A*) conventional 120 kVp image, (*B*) virtual MonoE 40 keV image, and (*C*) virtual MonoE 200 keV image. Improved conspicuity of the noncalcified gallstone on the (*B*) virtual MonoE 40 keV image where the gallstone is dark and (*C*) virtual MonoE 200 keV image where the gallstone is bright compared with the (*A*) conventional 120 kVp image.

Bile Ducts

The diagnostic value of CT cholangiography is improved with the use of DECT, but a CT cholangiographic contrast agent is no longer available in the United States. Sommer and colleagues reported that DECT imaging allowed the precise analysis of the contrast-enhanced biliary system in potential donors for living-related liver transplantation.[72] Iodine and contrast-optimized DECT images significantly increased image quality (signal-to-noise ratio: *P* < .001; contrast-to-noise ratio: < 0.01) compared with conventional images.[72] Intravenous morphine comedication could further improve bile duct visualization of DECT-cholangiography.[73] True unenhanced images may be replaced with VNC images in DECT-cholangiography to reduce radiation dose, with improved (*P* < .001) contrast-to-noise ratio for bile duct evaluation.[74]

DISCUSSION

In contrast to single-energy CT, DECT uses 2 X-ray photon energy spectra to differentiate materials that exhibit varying attenuation properties at different photon energies. In this way, additional information is gained in DECT scans that would be lost in single-energy CT scans. As a result, DECT has several advantages over single-energy CT in hepatobiliary imaging. MonoE and material decomposition DECT images have proven to be helpful in answering questions regarding disease of the liver and bile ducts for which conventional CT images reach their limits.

Recent developments may further increase the potential of DECT hepatobiliary imaging. For instance, a pilot study demonstrated that machine learning-based analysis of DECT image data using radiomics may further improve the differentiation of solid benign and malignant hepatic lesions.[75] Photon-counting CT detectors promise to improve

spectral X-ray beam separation and increase CT image resolution, which could open new opportunities for hepatobiliary CT imaging.[76] In addition, novel noniodinated contrast agents such as tantalum oxide or novel gadolinium-based agents could potentially provide application in DECT imaging of the liver and bile ducts.[77–82]

SUMMARY

DECT imaging enables improved CT diagnostic of the liver, bile ducts, and gallbladder. Low-keV MonoE images and iodine density maps improve the conspicuity of liver lesions and allow liver lesion characterization. Specific material decomposition algorithms enable the assessment of hepatic iron deposition, steatosis, and fibrosis/cirrhosis. Gallstones can be detected more securely on VNC and low-keV MonoE images as well as characterized using low and high MonoE images. In CT-cholangiography, image quality is increased in DECT iodine density maps, and unenhanced images may be replaced with VNC images to reduce radiation dose. Iodine density maps may improve the detection and characterization of gallbladder carcinoma. All these developments may be integrated in a time-effective and comparatively inexpensive way into clinical routine and could therefore lead to a rising utilization of DECT for hepatobiliary imaging.

CLINICS CARE POINTS

- Dual-energy computed tomography (CT) imaging enables more confident CT diagnoses of the liver, bile ducts, and gallbladder.
- Focal liver lesions are better detected and characterized in low-kiloelectronvolt (keV)

virtual monoenergetic (MonoE) images and iodine density maps.

- Diffuse liver disease can be quantified using specific material decomposition images.
- Disease monitoring of liver tumors is improved by iodine density maps.
- Gallstones are better detected and characterized in low-keV virtual MonoE images and virtual unenhanced images.
- Gallbladder carcinoma detection and characterization is improved by iodine density maps.

DISCLOSURE

B M. Yeh received grant funding from Philips Healthcare, General Electric Healthcare, is a consultant for Canon and General Electric Healthcare, is a speaker for Philips Healthcare and General Electric Healthcare, receives royalties for patents from UCSF and book royalties from Oxford University Press, is a shareholder in and serves on the board of directors for Nextrast, Inc.

REFERENCES

1. Coursey CA, Nelson RC, Boll DT, et al. Dual-energy multidetector CT: how does it work, what can it tell uis, and when can we use it in abdominopelvic imaging? Radiographics 2010;30(4):1037–55.
2. McCollough CH, Leng S, Yu L, et al. Dual- and multi-energy ct: principles, technical approaches, and clinical applications. Radiology 2015;276(3):637–53.
3. Yeh BM, Obmann MM, Westphalen AC, et al. Dual energy computed tomography scans of the bowel: benefits, pitfalls, and future directions. Radiol Clin North Am 2018;56(5):805–19.
4. Shuman WP, Green DE, Busey JM, et al. Dual-energy liver CT: Effect of monochromatic imaging on lesion detection, conspicuity, and contrast-to-noise ratio of hypervascular lesions on late arterial phase. AJR Am J Roentgenol 2014;203(3):601–6.
5. Uyeda JW, Richardson IJ, Sodickson AD. Making the invisible visible: improving conspicuity of noncalcified gallstones using dual-energy CT. Abdom Radiol (NY) 2017;42(12):2933–9.
6. Hyodo T, Yada N, Hori M, et al. Multimaterial decomposition algorithm for the quantification of liver fat content by using fast-kilovolt-peak switching dual-energy CT: clinical evaluation. Radiology 2017; 283(1):108–18.
7. Bamberg F, Dierks A, Nikolaou K, et al. Metal artifact reduction by dual energy computed tomography using monoenergetic extrapolation. Eur Radiol 2011; 21(7):1424–9.
8. Megibow AJ, Sahani D. Best Practice: Implementation and use of abdominal dual-energy ct in routine patient care. AJR Am J Roentgenol 2012;199(5 Suppl):S71–7.
9. Mileto A, Ananthakrishnan L, Morgan DE, et al. Clinical implementation of dual-energy CT for gastrointestinal imaging. AJR Am J Roentgenol 2020; 217(3):651–63.
10. Parakh A, Lennartz S, An C, et al. Dual-energy CT images: pearls and pitfalls. Radiographics 2021; 41(1):98–119.
11. Hounsfield GN. Computerized transverse axial scanning (tomography). 1. description of system. Br J Radiol 1973;46(552):1016–22.
12. Rajiah P, Parakh A, Kay F, et al. Update on multienergy CT: physics, principles, and applications. Radiographics 2020;40(5):1284–308.
13. McCollough CH, Boedeker K, Cody D, et al. Principles and applications of multienergy CT: report of AAPM task group 291. Med Phys 2020;47(7): e881–912.
14. Siegel MJ, Kaza RK, Bolus DN, et al. White paper of the society of computed body tomography and magnetic resonance on dual-energy CT, part 1: technology and terminology. J Comput Assist Tomogr 2016;40(6):841–5.
15. Altenbernd J, Heusner TA, Ringelstein A, et al. Dual-energy-CT of hypervascular liver lesions in patients with HCC: investigation of image quality and sensitivity. Eur Radiol 2011;21(4):738–43.
16. Muenzel D, Lo GC, Yu HS, et al. Material density iodine images in dual-energy CT: detection and characterization of hypervascular liver lesions compared to magnetic resonance imaging. Eur J Radiol 2017;95:300–6.
17. Sun H, Hou XY, Xue HD, et al. Dual-source dual-energy CT angiography with virtual non-enhanced images and iodine map for active gastrointestinal bleeding: image quality, radiation dose and diagnostic performance. Eur J Radiol 2015;84(5): 884–91.
18. Potretzke TA, Brace CL, Lubner MG, et al. Early small-bowel ischemia: dual-energy CT improves conspicuity compared with conventional CT in a swine model. Radiology 2015;275(1):119–26.
19. Marin D, Ramirez-Giraldo JC, Gupta S, et al. Effect of a noise-optimized second-generation monoenergetic algorithm on image noise and conspicuity of hypervascular liver tumors: an in vitro and in vivo study. AJR Am J Roentgenol 2016;206(6):1222–32.
20. Große Hokamp N, Höink AJ, Doerner J, et al. Assessment of arterially hyper-enhancing liver lesions using virtual monoenergetic images from spectral detector CT: phantom and patient experience. Abdom Radiol (NY) 2018;43(8):2066–74.
21. Yoon JH, Chang W, Lee ES, et al. Double low-dose dual-energy liver CT in Patients at high-risk of

HCC: a prospective, randomized, single-center study. Invest Radiol 2020;55(6):340–8.

22. Matsuda M, Tsuda T, Kido T, et al. Dual-energy computed tomography in patients with small hepatocellular carcinoma: utility of noise-reduced monoenergetic images for the evaluation of washout and image quality in the equilibrium phase. J Comput Assist Tomogr 2018;42(6):937–43.

23. Mileto A, Nelson RC, Samei E, et al. Dual-energy MDCT in hypervascular liver tumors: effect of body size on selection of the optimal monochromatic energy level. AJR Am J Roentgenol 2014;203(6): 1257–64.

24. Pfeiffer D, Parakh A, Patino M, et al. Iodine material density images in dual-energy CT: quantification of contrast uptake and washout in HCC. Abdom Radiol (NY) 2018;43(12):3317–23.

25. Caruso D, De Cecco CN, Schoepf UJ, et al. Can dual-energy computed tomography improve visualization of hypoenhancing liver lesions in portal venous phase? assessment of advanced image-based virtual monoenergetic images. Clin Imaging 2017;41:118–24.

26. Lenga L, Czwikla R, Wichmann JL, et al. Dual-energy CT In patients with colorectal cancer: improved assessment of hypoattenuating liver metastases using noise-optimized virtual monoenergetic imaging. Eur J Radiol 2018;106:184–91.

27. Nattenmüller J, Hosch W, Nguyen TT, et al. Hypodense liver lesions in patients with hepatic steatosis: do we profit from dual-energy computed tomography? Eur Radiol 2015;25(12):3567–76.

28. Patel BN, Rosenberg M, Vernuccio F, et al. Characterization of small incidental indeterminate hypoattenuating hepatic lesions: added value of single-phase contrast-enhanced dual-energy CT material attenuation analysis. AJR Am J Roentgenol 2018;211(3):571–9.

29. Yang CB, Zhang S, Jia YJ, et al. Dual energy spectral CT imaging for the evaluation of small hepatocellular carcinoma microvascular invasion. Eur J Radiol 2017;95:222–7.

30. Qian LJ, Zhu J, Zhuang ZG, et al. Differentiation of neoplastic from bland macroscopic portal vein thrombi using dual-energy spectral CT imaging: a pilot study. Eur Radiol 2012;22(10):2178–85.

31. Ascenti G, Sofia C, Mazziotti S, et al. Dual-energy CT with iodine quantification in distinguishing between bland and neoplastic portal vein thrombosis in patients with hepatocellular carcinoma. Clin Radiol 2016;71(9):938.E931–E939.

32. Dai X, Schlemmer HP, Schmidt B, et al. Quantitative therapy response assessment by volumetric iodine-uptake measurement: initial experience in patients with advanced hepatocellular carcinoma treated with sorafenib. Eur J Radiol 2013;82(2): 327–34.

33. Lee SH, Lee JM, Kim KW, et al. Dual-energy computed tomography to assess tumor response to hepatic radiofrequency ablation: potential diagnostic value of virtual noncontrast images and iodine maps. Invest Radiol 2011;46(2):77–84.

34. Lee JA, Jeong WK, Kim Y, et al. Dual-energy CT to detect recurrent HCC after TACE: initial experience of color-coded iodine CT imaging. Eur J Radiol 2013;82(4):569–76.

35. Joe E, Kim SH, Lee KB, et al. Feasibility and accuracy of dual-source dual-energy CT For noninvasive determination of hepatic iron accumulation. Radiology 2012;262(1):126–35.

36. Luo XF, Xie XQ, Cheng S, et al. Dual-energy CT for patients suspected of having liver iron overload: can virtual iron content imaging accurately quantify liver iron content? Radiology 2015;277(1):95–103.

37. Fischer MA, Reiner CS, Raptis D, et al. Quantification of liver iron content with CT-added value of dual-energy. Eur Radiol 2011;21(8):1727–32.

38. Oelckers S, Graeff W. In situ measurement of iron overload in liver tissue by dual-energy methods. Phys Med Biol 1996;41(7):1149–65.

39. Werner S, Krauss B, Haberland U, et al. Dual-energy CT for liver iron quantification in patients with haematological disorders. Eur Radiol 2019;29(6): 2868–77.

40. Chapman RW, Williams G, Bydder G, et al. Computed tomography for determining liver iron content in primary haemochromatosis. Br Med J 1980;280(6212):440–2.

41. Abadia AF, Grant KL, Carey KE, et al. Spatial distribution of iron within the normal human liver using dual-source dual-energy CT imaging. Invest Radiol 2017;52(11):693–700.

42. Elbanna KY, Mansoori B, Mileto A, et al. Dual-energy CT in diffuse liver disease: is there a role? Abdom Radiol (NY) 2020;45(11):3413–24.

43. Patel BN, Kumbla RA, Berland LL, et al. Material density hepatic steatosis quantification on intravenous contrast-enhanced rapid kilovolt (peak)-switching single-source dual-energy computed tomography. J Comput Assist Tomogr 2013;37(6): 904–10.

44. Fischer MA, Gnannt R, Raptis D, et al. Quantification of liver fat in the presence of iron and iodine: an ex-vivo dual-energy CT study. Invest Radiol 2011;46(6): 351–8.

45. Kramer H, Pickhardt PJ, Kliewer MA, et al. Accuracy of liver fat quantification with advanced CT, MRI, and ultrasound techniques: prospective comparison with MR spectroscopy. AJR Am J Roentgenol 2017; 208(1):92–100.

46. Artz NS, Hines CD, Brunner ST, et al. Quantification of hepatic steatosis with dual-energy computed tomography: comparison with tissue reference standards and quantitative magnetic resonance

imaging in the Ob/Ob mouse. Invest Radiol 2012; 47(10):603–10.

47. Guo Z, Blake GM, Li K, et al. Liver fat content measurement with quantitative CT validated against MRI proton density fat fraction: a prospective study of 400 healthy volunteers. Radiology 2020;294(1): 89–97.

48. Hur BY, Lee JM, Hyunsik W, et al. Quantification of the fat fraction in the liver using dual-energy computed tomography and multimaterial decomposition. J Comput Assist Tomogr 2014;38(6):845–52.

49. Zhang Q, Zhao Y, Wu J, et al. Quantification of hepatic fat fraction in patients with nonalcoholic fatty liver disease: comparison of multimaterial decomposition algorithm and fat (water)-based material decomposition algorithm using single-source dual-energy computed tomography. J Comput Assist Tomogr 2021;45(1):12–7.

50. Varenika V, Fu Y, Maher JJ, et al. Hepatic fibrosis: evaluation with semiquantitative contrast-enhanced CT. Radiology 2013;266(1):151–8.

51. Zissen MH, Wang ZJ, Yee J, et al. Contrast-enhanced CT quantification of the hepatic fractional extracellular space: correlation with diffuse liver disease severity. AJR Am J Roentgenol 2013;201(6): 1204–10.

52. Afdhal NH, Nunes D. Evaluation of liver fibrosis: a concise review. Am J Gastroenterol 2004;99(6): 1160–74.

53. Yoon JH, Lee JM, Klotz E, et al. Estimation of hepatic extracellular volume fraction using multiphasic liver computed tomography for hepatic fibrosis grading. Invest Radiol 2015;50(4):290–6.

54. Benedetti N, Aslam R, Wang ZJ, et al. Delayed enhancement of ascites after i.v. contrast material administration at CT: time course and clinical correlation. AJR Am J Roentgenol 2009;193(3):732–7.

55. Sofue K, Tsurusaki M, Mileto A, et al. Dual-energy computed tomography for non-invasive staging of liver fibrosis: accuracy of iodine density measurements from contrast-enhanced data. Hepatol Res 2018;48(12):1008–19.

56. Bak S, Kim JE, Bae K, et al. Quantification of liver extracellular volume using dual-energy ct: utility for prediction of liver-related events in cirrhosis. Eur Radiol 2020;30(10):5317–26.

57. Dong J, He F, Wang L, et al. Iodine density Changes in hepatic and splenic parenchyma in liver cirrhosis with dual energy CT (DECT): a preliminary study. Acad Radiol 2019;26(7):872–7.

58. Doda Khera R, Homayounieh F, Lades F, et al. Can dual-energy computed tomography quantitative analysis and radiomics differentiate normal liver from hepatic steatosis and cirrhosis? J Comput Assist Tomogr 2020;44(2):223–9.

59. Shang S, Cao Q, Han X, et al. Assessing liver hemodynamics in children with cholestatic cirrhosis by use of dual-energy spectral CT. AJR Am J Roentgenol 2020;214(3):665–70.

60. Yang CB, Zhang S, Jia YJ, et al. Clinical application of dual-energy spectral computed tomography in detecting cholesterol gallstones from surrounding bile. Acad Radiol 2017;24(4):478–82.

61. Soesbe TC, Lewis MA, Xi Y, et al. A technique to identify isoattenuating gallstones with dual-layer spectral CT: an ex vivo phantom study. Radiology 2019;292(2):400–6.

62. Lee HA, Lee YH, Yoon KH, et al. Comparison of virtual unenhanced images derived from dual-energy CT with true unenhanced images in evaluation of gallstone disease. AJR Am J Roentgenol 2016; 206(1):74–80.

63. Li H, He D, Lao Q, et al. Clinical value of spectral CT in diagnosis of negative gallstones and common bile duct stones. Abdom Imaging 2015; 40(6):1587–94.

64. Chen AL, Liu AL, Wang S, et al. Detection of gallbladder stones by dual-energy spectral computed tomography imaging. World J Gastroenterol 2015; 21(34):9993–8.

65. Bae JS, Lee DH, Joo I, et al. Utilization of virtual non-contrast images derived from dual-energy CT in evaluation of biliary stone disease: virtual non-contrast image can replace true non-contrast image regarding biliary stone detection. Eur J Radiol 2019; 116:34–40.

66. Zhang DM, Wang X, Xue HD, et al. Determinants of detection of stones and calcifications in the hepatobiliary system on virtual nonenhanced dual-energy CT. Chin Med Sci J 2016;31(2):76–82.

67. Kim JE, Lee JM, Baek JH, et al. Initial assessment of dual-energy CT in patients with gallstones or bile duct stones: can virtual nonenhanced images replace true nonenhanced images? AJR Am J Roentgenol 2012;198(4):817–24.

68. Bauer RW, Schulz JR, Zedler B, et al. Compound analysis of gallstones using dual energy computed tomography–results in a phantom model. Eur J Radiol 2010;75(1):E74–80.

69. Voit H, Krauss B, Heinrich MC, et al. [Dual-source CT: in vitro characterization of gallstones using dual energy analysis]. Rofo 2009;181(4):367–73.

70. Yin SN, Chi J, Liu L, et al. Dual-energy CT to differentiate gallbladder polyps: cholesterol versus adenomatous. Acta Radiol 2021;62(2):147–54.

71. Ratanaprasatporn L, Uyeda JW, Wortman JR, et al. Multimodality imaging, including dual-energy CT, in the evaluation of gallbladder disease. Radiographics 2018;38(1):75–89.

72. Sommer CM, Schwarzwaelder CB, Stiller W, et al. Dual-energy computed-tomography cholangiography in potential donors for living-related liver transplantation: initial experience. Invest Radiol 2010;45(7):406–12.

73. Sommer CM, Schwarzwaelder CB, Stiller W, et al. Dual-energy CT-cholangiography in potential donors for living-related liver transplantation: improved biliary visualization by intravenous morphine co-medication. Eur J Radiol 2012;81(9):2007–13.

74. Sommer CM, Schwarzwaelder CB, Stiller W, et al. Iodine removal in intravenous dual-energy CT-chol-angiography: is virtual non-enhanced imaging effective to replace true non-enhanced imaging? Eur J Radiol 2012;81(4):692–9.

75. Homayounieh F, Singh R, Nitiwarangkul C, et al. Semiautomatic segmentation and radiomics for dual-energy CT: a pilot study to differentiate benign and malignant hepatic lesions. AJR Am J Roent-genol 2020;215(2):398–405.

76. Leng S, Bruesewitz M, Tao S, et al. Photon-counting detector CT: system design and clinical applications of an emerging technology. Radiographics 2019; 39(3):729–43.

77. Lambert JW, Sun Y, Stillson C, et al. An intravascular tantalum oxide-based CT contrast agent: preclinical evaluation emulating overweight and obese patient size. Radiology 2018;289(1):103–10.

78. Rathnayake S, Mongan J, Torres AS, et al. In vivo comparison of tantalum, tungsten, and bismuth enteric contrast agents to complement intravenous iodine for double-contrast dual-energy CT of the bowel. Contrast Media Mol Imaging 2016;11(4): 254–61.

79. Dilger SKN, Nelson N, Venkatesh SK, et al. Computed tomography cholangiography using the magnetic resonance contrast agent gadoxetate disodium: a phantom study. Invest Radiol 2019; 54(9):572–9.

80. Mongan J, Rathnayake S, Fu Y, et al. In vivo differentiation of complementary contrast media at dual-energy CT. Radiology 2012;265(1):267–72.

81. Mongan J, Rathnayake S, Fu Y, et al. Extravasated contrast material in penetrating abdominopelvic trauma: dual-contrast dual-energy CT for improved diagnosis–preliminary results in an animal model. Radiology 2013;268(3):738–42.

82. Yeh BM, Fitzgerald PF, Edic PM, et al. Opportunities for new CT contrast agents to maximize the diagnostic potential of emerging spectral CT technologies. Adv Drug Deliv Rev 2017;113:201–22.

Hepatobiliary Trauma Imaging Update

Johnathon Stephens, MD, Hei Shun Yu, MD, Jennifer W. Uyeda, MD*

KEYWORDS

- Hepatobiliary • Trauma • CT • DECT

KEY POINTS

- Conservative nonsurgical management is the preferred treatment for blunt solid visceral injuries and accurate and timely diagnosis and characterization are heavily reliant on CT findings.
- The liver is one of the most common injured solid abdominal organs and treatment requires a multidisciplinary approach.
- Biliary tract traumatic injuries are rare likely due to the protective effect of the liver and are commonly associated with additional injuries in the abdomen.

Abbreviations	
CT	computed tomography
MRI	magnetic resonance imaging
IVC	Inferior vena cava
AV	arteriovenous
HU	Hounsfield units

INTRODUCTION

The morbidity and mortality from trauma are substantial, and trauma is the leading cause of death in the United States for patients under the age of 45 years.[1] It accounts for more than one-third of all visits to the emergency department and accounts for over $80 billion per year in health care costs.[1] CT examinations of the head, neck, chest, abdomen, and pelvis, the "panscan," is a critical component in the evaluation, assessment, and decision-making algorithm of hemodynamically stable trauma patients.[2] Injuries in the abdomen and pelvis are treatable if they are promptly and accurately diagnosed, and the radiologist plays an essential role in the evaluation of polytrauma patients. The liver is one of the most commonly injured abdominal organs though it is not uncommon that multiple organs are affected simultaneously.[3,4]

Conservative nonsurgical management has become the preferred treatment for most blunt solid visceral injuries, and the accurate diagnosis and characterization are heavily reliant on CT examination findings.[3,5–8] This article will review hepatobiliary trauma and associated vascular injuries as well as their associated complications.

MECHANISMS AND PATHOPHYSIOLOGY OF HEPATOBILIARY INJURY

Abdominal trauma can result from penetrating or blunt trauma. The liver is one of the most commonly injured organs in the abdomen and pelvis. Common mechanisms of blunt hepatobiliary trauma include motor vehicle collisions (MVCs), falls from height, sports accidents, and assaults,[1,3] and common mechanisms of penetrating trauma are firearm injury or stab wound.[1,9]

The authors have nothing to disclose.
Department of Radiology, Brigham and Women's Hospital, 75 Francis Street, Boston, MA 02115, USA
* Corresponding author.
E-mail address: JUYEDA@BWH.HARVARD.EDU

radiologic.theclinics.com

In blunt abdominal trauma, significant forces are needed to injure solid viscera, and the mechanisms of injury include deceleration, external compression, and crush injuries (Hughes). The specific organ injured depends on several factors including the energy delivered during the trauma, body part struck first, patient's body habitus, and use of a restraint device in MVC.[3] Understanding these patterns of injury is beneficial for the radiologists interpreting the panscan CT. This article will focus on blunt hepatic trauma.

Penetrating trauma may result from peritoneal violation from a stab wound or firearm injury.[9] Given that these traumatic injuries can have subtle or complex imaging findings, they may pose a challenge for the interpreting radiologist. Knowledge and familiarity with projectile kinetics are advantageous for the radiologist in diagnosing subtle and overt traumatic injuries.

MANAGEMENT

Hepatobiliary trauma is among the most common traumatic injuries in the abdomen and pelvis and as such, and its management is often multidisciplinary and includes emergency medicine, emergency radiology, interventional radiology, and surgery.[3] Advancements in health care have led to a preference for conservative nonoperative management (NOM), which has been shown to be effective for hemodynamically stable patients even those patients with high-grade injuries. The preferred conservative NOM highlights the emphasis of rapid and accurate diagnosis of traumatic injuries on the initial CT to decrease morbidity and mortality in patients who have sustained trauma.

The chest, abdomen, and/or pelvis are usual sources of bleeding in patients with persistent clinical findings of occult ongoing hemorrhage.[3] Compromised hemodynamic status despite adequate resuscitation with continued intraabdominal hemorrhage is an indication of emergent surgery.[3] Hemodynamic instability with evisceration and peritonitis is also an indication for surgical management.[9]

IMAGING

Contrast-enhanced CT is the standard imaging modality in diagnosing and characterizing hepatobiliary trauma due to its fast image acquisition time and superior spatial resolution. It rapidly detects parenchymal and vascular injuries and can roughly quantify the resulting volume of hemoperitoneum. Optimizing the CT technique is critical and requires consideration of various factors including the use of contrast material, acquisition of the

number of phases, and timing of the phases. All patients who have sustained trauma should receive intravenous contrast, approximately 100 to 150 mL of 350 mg of iodine per milliliter with an injection rate of 3 to 5 mL/s via a power injector through a 18 or 20 gauge cannula in a large peripheral vein.[3]

Dual-energy CT (DECT) offers improved material characterization by using different attenuation properties of different materials at low 80 to 100 kVp and high 140 kVp photon energy spectra and can be applied in hepatic trauma.[10–12] Low 80 to 100 kVp virtual monoenergetic imaging improves the contrast to noise ratio and increases the conspicuity of hepatic traumatic injuries[10] (Fig. 1). DECT iodine-selective imaging also increases the visibility of subtle lesions based on differences in iodine content and is beneficial in detecting hepatic parenchymal traumatic injuries.[10–12]

At our institution, we routinely acquire a portal venous phase through the abdomen and pelvis with a 70-s delay. An optional delayed phase is acquired 5 to 10 minutes after contrast administration to evaluate suspected or confirmed traumatic injuries on the portal venous phase.[13] A radiologist is present at the CT scanner to review all images although the patient is still in the CT scanner and determines the need for delayed phase image acquisition. The delayed phase increases the detection of urinary tract injuries and characterization of solid organ injury involving the vasculature.[13]

Recent literature shows the utility in obtaining an arterial phase of the abdomen and/or pelvis in select patients. We routinely image the abdomen in an arterial phase through the iliac crests as a continuation of the CT chest that is acquired as part of the panscan. The arterial phase of the chest and abdomen are acquired using a tracking bolus at the descending thoracic aorta. The arterial phase of the abdomen aid in detecting vascular injuries in the solid organs such as pseudoaneurysms and active bleeding and traumatic injuries to the vessels.[14,15] In the pelvis, the arterial phase facilitates characterization and detection of active arterial extravasation and aids in the differentiation from osseous or venous sources of bleeding.[16,17]

CLASSIFICATION OF HEPATIC AND EXTRAHEPATIC BILIARY TREE INJURIES

The AAST (American Association for the Surgery of Trauma) Organ Injury Scale is the most widely used traumatic organ injury classification system and was most recently updated in 2018 (Tables 1 and 2).[18] It classifies hepatic injury severity by

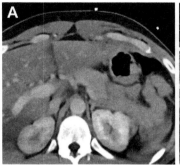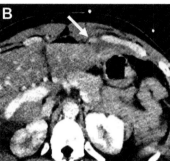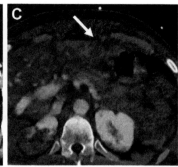

Fig. 1. Dual-energy CT abdomen and pelvis mixed image (*A*), low 100 kV image (*B*), and iodine overlay image (*C*). A 2.7 cm liver laceration in hepatic segments II/III is more conspicuous on the 100 kV and iodine overlay images (*arrows*) and is very subtle on the mixed image.

extent and location, as well as the presence of vascular injury.

A few points to remember:

- Advance one grade if multiple injuries are present, up to grade III.
- Vascular injury refers to a pseudoaneurysm or AV fistula, described below
- Grade II injuries are the most common, followed by Grade I.
- AAST grade is ultimately based on the highest grade assessed on imaging, at the time of operation, or on pathology.

ANATOMIC REVIEW

Understanding the basic hepatic anatomy and its blood supply is helpful in characterizing traumatic injuries.

The liver is functionally divided into Couinaud segments. The left hepatic lobe is composed of segments II–IVB, the right lobe is composed of segments V–VIII, and the caudate lobe is segment I. The portal veins divide the respective sections vertically, and the middle hepatic vein divides them horizontally. The liver receives blood via the hepatic arteries and portal vein, and the hepatic veins return blood to the systemic circulation. The bare area of the liver is located at the posterosuperior aspect of segment VII; its anatomic importance derives from its communication with the retroperitoneal space.

The biliary tree is composed of intrahepatic and extrahepatic divisions. The intrahepatic bile duct branches run parallel to the portal veins and drain into the common hepatic duct that then joins the cystic duct to form the common bile duct.

HEPATIC INJURIES

Contrast-enhanced CT is the imaging modality of choice in evaluating blunt liver trauma in patients

who are hemodynamically stable.[6,19–21] The major blunt hepatic traumatic injuries seen on CT include laceration, hematoma, active hemorrhage, pseudoaneurysm, and major venous injury.

Laceration

Hepatic lacerations are the most common hepatic parenchymal injury.[19] As NOM is increasingly being used in blunt hepatic injuries, early and accurate

Table 1 AAST liver injury scale	
AAST Grade	**Imaging Criteria (CT Findings)**
I	Subcapsular hematoma <10% Parenchymal laceration <1 cm depth
II	Subcapsular hematoma 10%–50% surface area; intraparenchymal hematoma <10 cm in diameter Laceration 1–3 cm in depth and ≤10 cm length
III	Subcapsular hematoma >50% surface area; ruptured subcapsular or parenchymal hematoma Intraparenchymal laceration >10 cm Laceration >3 cm depth Any injury in the presence of a liver vascular injury or active bleeding contained within liver parenchyma
IV	Parenchymal disruption involving 25%–75% of a hepatic lobe Active bleeding extending beyond the liver parenchyma into the peritoneum
V	Parenchymal disruption >75% of hepatic lobe Juxtahepatic venous injury to include retrohepatic vena cava and central major hepatic veins

Table 2
AAST extrahepatic biliary tree injury scale

AAST Grade	Description of Injury
I	Gallbladder contusion/hematoma Portal triad contusion
II	Partial gallbladder avulsion from liver bed; cystic duct intact Laceration or perforation of the gallbladder
III	Complete gallbladder avulsion from the liver bed Cystic duct laceration
IV	Partial or complete right hepatic duct laceration Partial or complete left hepatic duct laceration (<50%) Partial common hepatic duct laceration (<50%) Partial common bile duct laceration (<50%)
V	>50% transection of common hepatic duct >50% transection of common bile duct Combined right and left hepatic duct injuries Intraduodenal or intrapancreatic bile duct injuries

diagnosis is imperative in guiding clinical management. On CT, they are seen as linear or branching hypoattenuating areas in the parenchyma (**Fig. 2**). Lacerations can be classified as superficial if equal to or less than 3 cm in depth and deep if greater than 3 cm in depth (**Fig. 3**). Notably, lacerations involving the bare area of the liver that extend to the posterior and superior aspect of segment VII can lead to large retroperitoneal hematomas as it is not covered by the peritoneal reflection resulting in direct communication with the retroperitoneum.

Hematoma

Hematomas are classified as either subcapsular or intraparenchymal, representing collections of blood contained by the liver capsule or parenchyma, respectively. Intraparenchymal hematomas are rounded or elliptical in morphology, whereas subcapsular hematomas are more crescent shaped and peripherally located. Both subcapsular and intraparenchymal hematomas displace the hepatic parenchyma, differentiating them from perihepatic hemorrhage.

The AAST grade depends on the size and location of hematomas, intraparenchymal or subcapsular. Intraparenchymal hematomas appear on imaging as a hypoattenuating area in the parenchyma, and subcapsular hematomas are identified as crescentic hypoattenuating areas that compress the underlying parenchyma (**Fig. 4**).

Active Hemorrhage

Active hemorrhage after hepatic trauma is defined as blood extravasating at the time of imaging. Active extravasation appears as focal hyperattenuating areas on early/arterial phase CT that increase in size on the portal venous phase and the delayed phase, if obtained (**Fig. 5**). Active

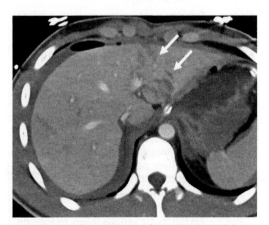

Fig. 2. Hepatic lacerations in the left hepatic lobe are seen as linear or branching hypoattenuating areas in the parenchyma.

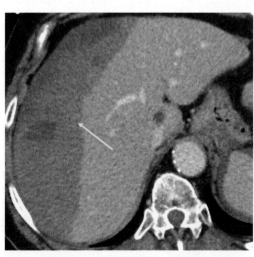

Fig. 3. Hepatic laceration seen as a large hypoattenuating area in the liver classified as AAST III hepatic laceration greater than 10 cm and greater than 3 cm in depth.

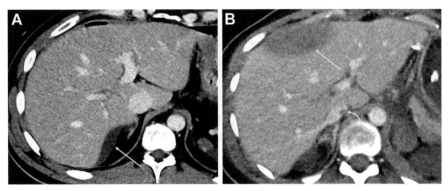

Fig. 4. Hepatic hematomas in two different patients with a AAST grade 1 subcapsular hematoma (*A*) that appears as a crescentic hypoattenuating areas (*arrow*) that compress the underlying parenchyma, whereas the intraparenchymal hematoma is rounded or elliptical in morphology (*arrow*) (*B*). Of note the patient in Fig 4B has an IVC injury seen as a contour abnormality in the intrahepatic portion of the IVC (curved *arrow*).

hemorrhage can occur in the parenchyma or around the liver and into the peritoneal space. The extravasated contrast is termed contrast blush and has similar HU as the parent vessel, which is a helpful tip when trying to determine the site of origin in ambiguous cases. The sentinel clot sign, the phenomenon where the densest clot (highest HU) is often close to the site of hemorrhage, is also useful when troubleshooting.

Detecting active hemorrhage after hepatic trauma on CT is critical for clinical management as it is a strong predictor of the need for surgical or angiographic intervention.[19,22,23] Active contrast extravasation on CT indicates ongoing bleeding, which may be life threatening and predicts failure of NOM.[19,22,23]

Active hepatic artery hemorrhage seen on CT can be effectively treated with embolization in patients who have sustained trauma to the liver.[24,25] Indications for hepatic artery embolization in blunt hepatic trauma are hemostatic control in a hemodynamically stable patient with active bleeding on CT and adjunctive hemostatic control in patients suspected uncontrolled arterial bleeding after emergency laparotomy.[26]

Pseudoaneurysm

A pseudoaneurysm is a vascular injury where damage to the arterial wall results in a contained hematoma, being contained (at least temporarily) only by adjacent structures such as adjacent fat or organ parenchyma. In the liver, pseudoaneurysms originate from branches of the hepatic artery. Most result from blunt trauma and increase in prevalence with increasing injury grade, up to 17% with AAST Grade V injuries.[27] On CT, a pseudoaneurysm will have the same attenuation as that of the aorta and adjacent major arteries on all phases of image acquisition and is a circumscribed round or oval area of contrast-enhanced blood[19,27,28] **(Fig. 6)**.

Regardless of etiology, pseudoaneurysms are often asymptomatic and are found incidentally. Patients may become symptomatic if the pseudoaneurysm ruptures and clinical manifestations include hemobilia, hematemesis, melena, or shock from life-threatening hemorrhage. Therefore, a high degree of suspicion should be applied in the setting of trauma and urgent angioembolization is recommended although some do spontaneously thrombose.

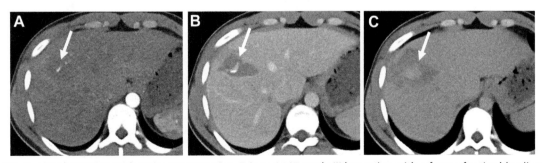

Fig. 5. Liver laceration with active extravasation. 7.0 cm AAST grade III laceration with a focus of active bleeding on the arterial phase (*A*), portal venous phase (*B*), and delayed phase (*C*) showed active arterial bleeding that increases in size and changes morphology on subsequent portal venus and delayed phases.

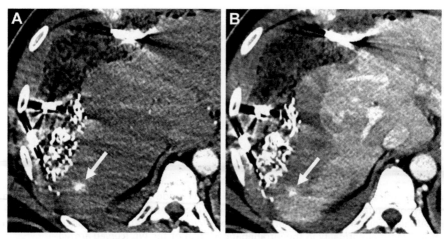

Fig. 6. Pseudoaneurysm in a patient with traumatic hepatic injury. The arterial phase (*A*) and portal venous phase (*B*) demonstrate a circumscribed round or oval area of contrast-enhanced blood in hepatic segment VII that follows the attenuation of the abdominal aorta on both phases (*arrows*).

Major Venous Injury

Major venous injuries can be life threatening with mortality rates ranging from 34% to 70% and are seen in severe hepatic traumatic injuries[19,29,30] (**Fig. 7**). On CT, major venous injuries are suspected if a hepatic laceration extends into the IVC and/or hepatic veins. Imaging findings of IVC injury in blunt hepatic trauma include extravasation, contour abnormality, and associated hepatic injury[30] (see **Fig. 4**B). The presence of major venous injury is associated with 6.5 times more likely to require operative management when the hepatic laceration extends into one or more hepatic veins.[7] Moreover, hepatic injuries involving one or more hepatic veins were 3.5 times more frequently associated with hepatic arterial bleeding.[6] The location of IVC injuries has prognostic implications where mortality rates are up to 100%, 78%, and 33% for suprahepatic, retrohepatic, and suprarenal injuries, respectively.[30,31]

SURGICAL CONSIDERATIONS

Angioembolization or surgery is reserved for actively hemorrhaging or hemodynamically unstable patients. Other warning signs are flattening of the IVC and periportal hypodensity. Hemorrhage dissecting along the periportal connective tissues can manifest as periportal hypodensity on CT; a flat IVC may indicate hypovolemia.

BILIARY TRACT INJURIES

Biliary tract traumatic injuries are rare, occurring in up to 2% to 3% of blunt trauma, likely due to the protective effect of the liver.[32–35] The gallbladder is the most common location of biliary tract injury

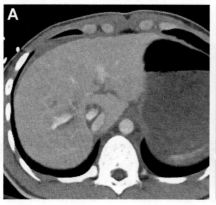
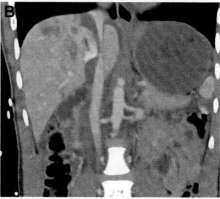

Fig. 7. Right portal vein and IVC injury with hepatic lacerations in the right lobe of the liver. The lacerations extend into the IVC and hepatic veins.

followed by the common bile duct and the intrahepatic bile ducts.[32] Biliary tract traumatic injuries are associated with additional injuries in the abdomen including hepatic, splenic, and duodenal injuries occurring in up to 91%, 54%, and 54% of cases, respectively[32] (Fig. 8).

Gallbladder injuries are classified as contusion, laceration/perforation, or avulsion[32] with contusions representing intramural hematomas and are the mildest form of injury. Gallbladder lacerations and perforations are full-thickness injuries often requiring surgical cholecystectomy[32] (see Fig. 8). Avulsion injury of the gallbladder may involve the cystic duct and cystic artery potentially leading to major blood loss.[34]

Although injuries are rare, delayed diagnosis contributes to prolonged hospital stays and higher morbidity and mortality. Injury diagnosis is often difficult due to nonspecific findings, as free bile is fluid density on CT and indistinguishable from the ascitic or postoperative fluid. For this reason, in the setting of trauma, contained intrahepatic or free perihepatic low-density fluid should raise suspicion for a biliary injury. Gallbladder wall collapse, wall thickening, or discontinuous mural enhancement are important clues. Notably, these are more evident on DECT. Gallbladder wall thickening and poor definition of the gallbladder wall are suggestive of traumatic injury.[32]

Hepatic injury extending to the gallbladder fossa should raise concern for gallbladder injury. Factors that predispose the gallbladder to injury are distention and increased sphincter of Oddi tone resulting in increased biliary pressure that predisposes the gallbladder to compression injury.

CT and MR cholangiopancreatography (MRCP) are the most used imaging studies used to diagnose gallbladder injuries. MRCP affords improved visualization of the biliary tract and assessment of injury particularly with hepatobiliary contrast agents. Active bile leaks are readily detected with hepatobiliary scintigraphy given the high sensitivity (Fig. 9). Endoscopic retrograde cholangiopancreatography (ERCP) plays a large diagnostic and therapeutic role in biliary tract injuries. It can show the site of bile duct disruption and simultaneously allows for stent placement.

IMAGING FOLLOW-UP

Follow-up imaging is generally not needed in asymptomatic, low-grade hepatic trauma.[19,36] However, it can be useful in ensuring the resolution of higher-grade injuries, and the need for repeat imaging should be based on clinical criteria including increased or new pain, fever, leukocytosis, or decreasing hemoglobin levels. As a rule of thumb, hemoperitoneum will resolve in approximately 1 week; lacerations in 3 weeks; hematomas 6 to 8 weeks; and a new baseline should be reached around 3 months after the initial injury.[19,37]

DELAYED COMPLICATIONS OF HEPATOBILIARY TRAUMATIC INJURY

With increasing use of nonsurgical management of hepatobiliary traumatic injuries particularly with complex liver lesions (AAST Grades IV–VI), the prevalence of delayed complications has increased with an overall prevalence range of 5%–23%.[38,39] Delayed complications seen on follow-up CT can occur weeks to months after the injury.[19,40] Posttraumatic complications of hepatobiliary injury include delayed hemorrhage, abscess, pseudoaneurysm, and biliary

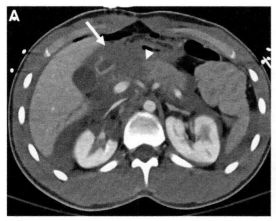 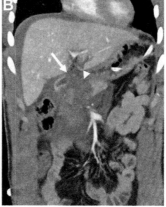

Fig. 8. Gallbladder avulsion in a patient with sustained polytrauma. Associated traumatic pancreatic laceration through the neck (*arrowhead*) and massive duodenopanceatic complex disruption with discontinuity of the proximal duodenum (*arrow*). Nonspecific gallbladder wall thickening and pericholecystic fluid render diagnosing the gallbladder avulsion injury challenging on CT, which was confirmed at the time of surgery.

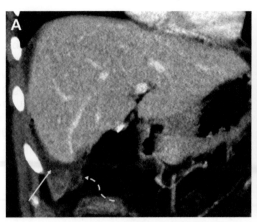
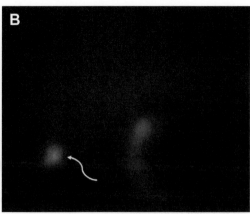

Fig. 9. Bile leak in a patient with a hepatic laceration. Coronal CT (*A*) shows a laceration through segment VI of the liver (*arrow*) with surrounding fluid containing a focus of hyperdensity (*dotted curved arrow*). HIDA scan (*B*) shows the accumulation of bile in a biloma.

complications. Early treatment relies on interventional radiology with low rates of mortality.[19]

Delayed Hemorrhage

Delayed hemorrhage is the most common complication in liver trauma, with a prevalence of up to 5.9%.[24,41] Delayed hemorrhage may be caused by an increase in initially minimal injury or rupture of a biloma-induced pseudoaneurysm.

Abscess

An abscess is a focal collection of purulent byproducts from infectious processes and resulting parenchymal destruction. On CT, these appear hypodense, spherical collections with a thick, enhancing wall surrounded by low-density edema with possible internal foci of gas. As a secondary sign, transient hepatic attenuation difference (THAD) may be seen due to local hyperemia and portal vein occlusion or compression.

In the trauma setting, abscesses often occur from hematoma or infarct superinfection.

Foci of gas may form within necrotic tissue, making differentiating necrosis from an abscess difficult. An enhancing wall favors abscess. Percutaneous drainage is therapeutic and diagnostic. The drained fluid is sent to the laboratory for culture and assessed for biliary content.

Biliary Complications

Biliary leak from a hepatic laceration is commonly seen and is usually transient and self-limiting.[19] With increased utilization of NOM of hepatic injuries, biliary leaks are a source of morbidity particularly in the setting of a delayed diagnosis.[42–45] Biliary complications resulting in bile leakage include biloma, biliary fistula, and bile

peritonitis.[19] Injury to the intrahepatic bile ducts may result in bile influx into the hematoma resulting in increased pressure within the hematoma and subsequent necrosis of the surrounding hepatic parenchyma and formation of a biloma.[46] Free intraperitoneal bile leaks are associated with prolonged hospital stays and more imaging studies and procedures compared with patients who have hepatic trauma with no bile duct injury or bile leak.[44]

The AAST liver injury grade along with the location of the liver laceration with a decreased distance of the laceration to the IVC is predictive of bile leaks.[42] On CT, an increase in the size of a well-defined low attenuation intraparenchymal or perihepatic collection in a hepatic traumatic injury suggests the presence of a biloma (see **Fig. 8**). Most bilomas resolve spontaneously, but they can enlarge and result in pain and obstructive symptoms and may also become infected requiring percutaneous drainage.[19,42]

Intraperitoneal spillage of contrast from a bile leak can result in bile peritonitis. Symptoms include fever, persistent abdominal pain, abdominal distension, and leukocytosis, however, making a diagnosis is challenging leading to the high associated morbidity and mortality.[19] On CT, bile peritonitis can be seen as persistent or increase in the amount of intraperitoneal fluid and thickening and enhancement of the peritoneum.[19] Treatment options include laparotomy or laparoscopic irrigation and drainage with endoscopic bile duct stent placement.[19]

Rarely, a posttraumatic hepatobiliary lesion can lead to a persistent pleural effusion of bile. In this setting, MRI will demonstrate contrast within the pleural space. Alternatively, thoracentesis will demonstrate intrathoracic biliary contents.

SUMMARY

Hepatobiliary trauma is best assessed by contrast-enhanced CT in hemodynamically stable patients. Early and accurate diagnosis of hepatobiliary traumatic injuries and associated vascular injuries guides management and allows for successful nonsurgical management of the traumatic injuries. CT can accurately detect and characterize hepatobiliary traumatic injuries and the associated vascular injuries in addition to evaluating delayed complications.

CLINICS CARE POINTS

- Hepatobiliary trauma is best assessed by contrast-enhanced CT provided patients are hemodynamically stable.
- Prompt and accurate diagnosis of hepatobiliary traumatic injuries and associated vascular injuries provides optimal care in trauma patients by avoiding delays in care and decreasing complications.

REFERENCES

1. NVDRS Infographic|Violence Prevention |Violence Prevention|Injury Center|CDC. 2020. Available at: https://www.cdc.gov/violenceprevention/communication resources/infographics/nvdrs-infographic.html. Accessed October 15, 2021.
2. Petrowsky H, Raeder S, Zuercher L, et al. A quarter century experience in liver trauma: a plea for early computed tomography and conservative management for all hemodynamically stable patients. World J Surg 2012;36(2):247–54.
3. Soto JA, Anderson SW. Multidetector CT of blunt abdominal trauma. Radiology 2012;265(3):678–93.
4. Cox EF. Blunt abdominal trauma. A 5-year analysis of 870 patients requiring celiotomy. Ann Surg 1984;199(4):467–74.
5. Becker CD, Gal I, Baer HU, et al. Blunt hepatic trauma in adults: correlation of CT injury grading with outcome. Radiology 1996;201(1):215–20.
6. Poletti PA, Mirvis SE, Shanmuganathan K, et al. CT criteria for management of blunt liver trauma: correlation with angiographic and surgical findings. Radiology 2000;216(2):418–27.
7. Croce MA, Fabian TC, Menke PG, et al. Nonoperative management of blunt hepatic trauma is the treatment of choice for hemodynamically stable patients. Results of a prospective trial. Ann Surg 1995; 221(6):744–53 [discussion: 753–755].
8. Stassen NA, Bhullar I, Cheng JD, et al. Eastern Association for the Surgery of Trauma. Nonoperative management of blunt hepatic injury: an Eastern Association for the Surgery of Trauma practice management guideline. J Trauma Acute Care Surg 2012; 73(5 Suppl 4):S288–93.
9. Naeem M, Hoegger MJ, Petraglia FW 3rd, et al. CT of Penetrating Abdominopelvic Trauma. Radiographics 2021;41(4):1064–81.
10. Sun EX, Wortman JR, Uyeda JW, et al. Virtual monoenergetic dual-energy CT for evaluation of hepatic and splenic lacerations. Emerg Radiol 2019;26(4): 419–25.
11. Sodickson AD, Keraliya A, Czakowski B, et al. Dual energy CT in clinical routine: how it works and how it adds value. Emerg Radiol 2021;28(1): 103–17.
12. Wortman JR, Uyeda JW, Fulwadhva UP, et al. Dual-energy CT for abdominal and pelvic trauma. Radiographics 2018;38(2):586–602.
13. Stuhlfaut JW, Lucey BC, Varghese JC, et al. Blunt abdominal trauma: utility of 5-minute delayed CT with a reduced radiation dose. Radiology 2006; 238(2):473–9.
14. Boscak AR, Shanmuganathan K, Mirvis SE, et al. Optimizing trauma multidetector CT protocol for blunt splenic injury: need for arterial and portal venous phase scans. Radiology 2013;268(1): 79–88.
15. Uyeda JW, LeBedis CA, Penn DR, et al. Active hemorrhage and vascular injuries in splenic trauma: utility of the arterial phase in multidetector CT. Radiology 2014;270(1):99–106.
16. Anderson SW, Soto JA, Lucey BC, et al. Blunt trauma: feasibility and clinical utility of pelvic CT angiography performed with 64-detector row CT. Radiology 2008;246(2):410–9.
17. Uyeda J, Anderson SW, Kertesz J, et al. Pelvic CT angiography: application to blunt trauma using 64MDCT. Emerg Radiol 2010;17(2):131–7.
18. Kozar RA, Crandall M, Shanmuganathan K, et al. AAST patient assessment committee. organ injury scaling 2018 update: spleen, liver, and kidney. J Trauma Acute Care Surg 2018;85(6):1119–22.
19. Yoon W, Jeong YY, Kim JK, et al. CT in blunt liver trauma. Radiographics 2005;25(1):87–104.
20. Shanmuganathan K, Mirvis SE. CT evaluation of the liver with acute blunt trauma. Crit Rev Diagn Imaging 1995;36:73–113.
21. Becker CD, Mentha G, Terrier F. Blunt abdominal trauma in adults: role of CT in the diagnosis and management of visceral injuries. Eur Radiol 1998; 8:553–62.
22. Fang JF, Chen RJ, Wong YC, et al. Classification and treatment of pooling of contrast material on computed tomographic scan of blunt hepatic trauma. J Trauma 2000;49:1083–8.

23. Wong YC, Wang LJ, See LC, et al. Contrast material extravasation on contrast-enhanced helical computed tomographic scan of blunt abdominal trauma: its significance on the choice, time, and outcome of treatment. J Trauma 2003;54:164–70.

24. Hagiwara A, Yukioka T, Ohta S, et al. Nonsurgical management of patients with blunt hepatic injury: efficacy of transcatheter arterial embolization. AJR Am J Roentgenol 1997;169:1151–6.

25. Wahl WL, Ahrns KS, Brandt M, et al. The need for early angiographic embolization in blunt liver injuries. J Trauma 2002;52:1097–101.

26. Letoublon C, Morra I, Chen Y, et al. Hepatic arterial embolization in the management of blunt hepatic trauma: indications and complications. J Trauma 2011;70(5):1032–6 [discussion: 1036-7].

27. Wagner ML, Streit S, Makley AT, et al. Hepatic pseudoaneurysm incidence after liver trauma. J Surg Res 2020;256:623–8.

28. Yu J, Fulcher A, Turner M, et al. Multidetector Computed Tomography of Blunt Hepatic and Splenic Trauma: Pearls and Pitfalls. Semin Roentgenol 2012;47(4):352–61.

29. Taourel P, Vernhet H, Suau A, et al. Vascular emergencies in liver trauma. Eur J Radiol 2007;64(1):73–82.

30. Tsai R, Raptis C, Schuerer D, et al. CT appearance of traumatic inferior vena cava injury. Am J Roentgenol 2016;207(4):705–11.

31. Rosengart MR, Smith DR, Melton SM, et al. Prognostic factors in patients with inferior vena cava injuries. Am Surg 1999;65:849–55 [discussion: 855–856].

32. Gupta A, Stuhlfaut J, Fleming K, et al. Blunt trauma of the pancreas and biliary tract: a multimodality imaging approach to Diagnosis. RadioGraphics 2014; 24(5):1381–95.

33. Erb RE, Mirvis SE, Shanmuganathan K. Gallbladder injury secondary to blunt trauma: CT findings. J Comput Assist Tomogr 1994;18:778–84.

34. Chen X, Talner LB, Jurkovich GJ. Gallbladder avulsion due to blunt trauma. AJR Am J Roentgenol 2001;177:822.

35. Burgess P, Fulton L. Gallbladder and extrahepatic biliary duct injury following abdominal trauma. Injury 1992;23:413–4.

36. Cuff RF, Cogbill TH, Lambert PJ. Nonoperative management of blunt liver trauma: the value of follow-up abdominal computed tomography scans. Am Surg 2000;66:332–6.

37. Delgado Millan MA, Deballon PO. Computed tomography, angiography, and endoscopic retrograde cholangiopancreatography in the nonoperative management of hepatic and splenic trauma. World J Surg 2001;25:1397–402.

38. Carrillo EH, Spain DA, Wohltmann CD, et al. Interventional techniques are useful adjuncts in nonoperative management of hepatic injuries. J Trauma 1999;46:619–22.

39. Goldman R, Zilkoski M, Mullins R, et al. Delayed celiotomy for the treatment of bile leak, compartment syndrome, and other hazards of nonoperative management of blunt liver injury. Am J Surg 2003;185:492–7.

40. Goffette PP, Laterre PF. Traumatic injuries: imaging and intervention in post-traumatic complications (delayed intervention). Eur Radiol 2002;12:994–1021.

41. Griffen M, Ochoa J, Boulanger BR. A minimally invasive approach to bile peritonitis after blunt liver injury. Am Surg 2000;66:309–12.

42. LeBedis CA, Anderson SW, Mercier G, et al. The utility of CT for predicting bile leaks in hepatic trauma. Emerg Radiol 2015;22(2):101–7.

43. Feliciano DV. Biliary injuries as a result of blunt and penetrating trauma. Surg Clin North Am 1994; 74(4):897–907 [discussion: 909-12].

44. Fleming KW, Lucey BC, Soto JA, et al. Posttraumatic bile leaks: role of diagnostic imaging and impact on patient outcome. Emerg Radiol 2006;12(3):103–7.

45. Bala M, Gazalla SA, Faroja M, et al. Complications of high grade liver injuries: management and outcome with focus on bile leaks. Scand J Trauma Resusc Emerg Med 2012;23:20.

46. Sugimoto K, Asari Y, Sakaguchi T, et al. Endoscopic retrograde cholangiography in the nonsurgical management of blunt liver injury. J Trauma 1993;35:192–9.

Focal Benign Liver Lesions and Their Diagnostic Pitfalls

Edouard Reizine, MD, Sébastien Mulé, MD, PhD*, Alain Luciani, MD, PhD

KEYWORDS

• Liver neoplasms • Focal nodular hyperplasia • Hepatocellular adenoma • Hemangioma

KEY POINTS

- A combination of MRI features – including contrast on T1/T2WI, homogeneity, dynamic enhancement profile, lack of capsule, presence of a typical central stellate area – is required for the diagnosis of focal nodular hyperplasia. These features remain specific even in male patients or in FNH lesions containing fat. However, isolated central stellate areas or hyperintensity on hepatobiliary phase acquisitions can be observed in other lesions, including malignant lesions.
- Different subtypes of hepatocellular adenomas – including inflammatory HCA, HNF1α-inactivated HCA, and ß catenin-mutated HCA – are associated with specific MRI features including native T1IP/OP, T2, dynamic enhancement profile, and various uptake patterns on hepatobiliary phase after liver-specific contrast agent injection. Nevertheless, some other features can be misleading, mimicking focal nodular hyperplasia or malignant lesions.
- Hepatic cysts and liver hemangiomas are common incidental findings in liver MRI. However, some features, such as septations or internal heterogeneous content within a cyst, should be analyzed carefully. Moreover, some atypical hemangioma presentations can be misleading, and sometimes formal diagnosis by pathology is warranted to exclude malignant lesions.
- The specific features associated with benign liver lesions can only be assessed provided that chronic liver disease or underlying primary malignant lesions have been excluded, using clinical, biological and radiological data.

INTRODUCTION

Focal hepatic lesions are frequently discovered incidentally on cross-sectional imaging or abdominal ultrasound,[1,2] and in the general population, a vast majority of those incidental findings are benign entities.[1] However, the formal diagnosis of benign liver lesions is not always straightforward and may require advanced imaging modalities, such as MRI with hepatobiliary contrast agent or contrast-enhanced ultrasound (CEUS).[3] This review presents the typical features of the main benign liver lesions, including focal nodular hyperplasia (FNH), hepatocellular adenoma (HCA), hepatic cysts, hemangioma, angiomyolipoma, and pseudotumors, such as inflammatory pseudotumors or hepatic granulomas. However, beyond the specific and classical MRI features, some lesions may present atypical patterns. Moreover, arterial phase hyperenhancement, often present in benign liver lesions, can be seen in malignant lesions such as hepatocellular carcinoma. Hence, accurate analysis of clinical and biological contexts is mandatory to optimize our diagnostic performance. The objective of this investigation was, therefore, to review the specific

Medical Imaging, Henri Mondor University Hospital, Faculté de Médecine, Universite Paris Est, INSERM Unit U 955, Equipe 18, Creteil 94010, France
* Corresponding author.
E-mail address: sebastien.mule@aphp.fr

Radiol Clin N Am 60 (2022) 755–773
https://doi.org/10.1016/j.rcl.2022.05.005

radiologic.theclinics.com

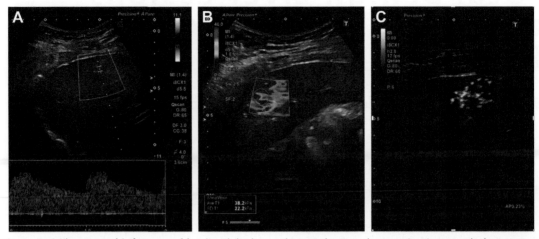

Fig. 1. Typical sonographic features of focal nodular hyperplasia. Color Doppler examination reveals the presence of a penetrating arterial vessel (*A*), and shear wave elastography shows high stiffness values (*B*). On contrast-enhanced ultrasound, after the injection of 2.4 mL of sulfur hexafluoride SonoVue, the lesion was enhanced in the arterial phase, demonstrating a typical spoke-wheel aspect with centrifugal distribution (*C*).

presentations of benign liver tumors and to illustrate their diagnostic pitfalls.

HEPATOCELLULAR LESION
Focal Nodular Hyperplasia

Focal nodular hyperplasia (FNH) is the most frequent benign hepatocellular lesion,[2] even if according to the WHO classification, FNH is not a true neoplasm but rather a mass-forming hyperplastic response of hepatocytes related to localized vascular abnormalities.[4] In 80% to 90% of cases, FNH is discovered in young women and rarely in men.[4] The background liver is usually normal, but FNH can occur in association with vascular diseases.[5,6] Usually, the lesions are incidentally found on ultrasound, where FNH shows variable nonspecific patterns of appearance on grayscale US and may sometimes only be detected because of the displacement of the surrounding vessels.[7] Typically, color Doppler examination reveals the presence of penetrating arterial vessel branching from the hepatic arterial tree directed toward the lesion. The presence of a single central artery is seen in up to 77% of FNHs, and it is not correlated with the size of the lesion.[8] Few studies have focused on shear wave elastography values for the characterization of focal liver lesions, describing high stiffness values when compared with the surrounding liver and significantly higher values than other benign lesions.[9] However, they have failed to differentiate these focal liver lesions from hepatocellular adenoma (HCA).[10]

Hence, a second imaging examination is often required to provide a formal noninvasive diagnosis. This can be achieved with contrast-enhanced ultrasound (CEUS) or MR imaging, as specific features have been associated with both techniques.[11]

With CEUS, FNH enhances at the early arterial phase (ie, 10–15 s after injection) and becomes homogeneously isoechoic after 30 s in most cases. It has been associated with two specific features:

- A spoke-wheel aspect, encountered in 20% to 25% of lesions;
- A centrifugal filling, more frequent in lesions smaller than 3 cm.[12]

A summary of typical sonographic features of FNH is presented in **Fig. 1**.

However, CEUS shows reduced sensitivity in diagnosing FNH lesions larger than 35 mm,[13,14] and MRI is usually required in that setting.

On MRI, the diagnosis of FNH is based on a combination of features, using seven major criteria to assess a proper diagnosis,[8,15,16] summarized in **Box 1** and illustrated in **Fig. 2**.

However, it is crucial to remember that an isolated feature is not sufficient for a confident diagnosis of FNH. For instance, an isolated central stellate area can be present in a wide range of liver tumors, including malignant lesions, as illustrated in **Fig. 3**.

In contrast to specificity, the sensitivity of MRI for an FNH diagnosis lags below 100%,[17–19] mainly because of the lack of a central element for lesions measuring less than 3 cm.[20] As CEUS can be misleading for lesions greater than 3.5 cm,[20] use of MRI with hepatobiliary contrast agents—i.e., gadobenate dimeglumine (Gd-BOPTA, Multihance, Bracco, Milan, Italy) or gadoxetate disodium (Gd-EOB-DTPA, Eovist or

---

Box 1
Major criteria on MRI for the diagnosis of focal nodular hyperplasia

- Native contrast close to that of the liver: Not different from the liver before contrast injection, that is, iso- or hypointense on T1-weighted images and iso- or slightly hyperintense on T2-weighted images
- Homogeneity apart from the central scar
- Central stellate area: Presence of a central hypointense area on T1-weighted images and strongly hyperintense on T2-weighted images
- Dynamic enhancement profile: Intense and transient enhancement in the arterial phase without washout
- No capsule
- Lobulated aspect
- Absence of underlying chronic liver disease or clinical history of cancer

---

Primovist, Bayer Healthcare Pharmaceuticals, Whippany, NJ, USA)—can increase the sensitivity or the diagnosis of FNH.[21] In accordance with the molecular background where FNH demonstrates increased expression of OATP,[22–24] FNH appears iso- or hyperintense on hepatobiliary-phase MRI in 94%–97% of cases,[21] with four main patterns: homogeneously hyperintense, inhomogeneously hyperintense, isointense and hypointense-with-ring.[25]

Several atypical presentations of FNH have been reported, often leading to targeted liver biopsy for final diagnosis. One common pitfall in FNH imaging is the presence of internal steatosis. Even if the presence of fat within the hepatocytes in FNH is not rare—as prior studies have found that up to 50% of FNHs contain fat on pathologic analysis[26,27]—it is less commonly seen on MRI, as only 10% of all FNHs demonstrate signal drop-out on out-of-phase imaging.[28] Although fat content can be misleading in some MRI sequences; however, it should not reduce the diagnostic confidence if all the major criteria are present,[28] as illustrated in **Fig. 4**.

More rarely, FNH can appear atypical in almost all sequences, with particularly high signal intensity on T2WI sequences and persistent enhancement in the enhanced delayed phase, suggestive of inflammatory changes, as illustrated in **Fig. 5**. Such atypical presentation is usually related to an unusually marked sinusoidal dilatation within FNH lesions.[29] This presentation should not be mistaken for inflammatory hepatocellular adenoma, and targeted liver biopsy can often be proposed in this setting if hepatobiliary phase (HBP) MRI and/or CEUS appear nonconclusive.

Finally, although FNHs are rare in men, this situation can occur, and similar to the presence of internal fat, a typical appearance on MRI should not lead to questioning the diagnosis even if particular attention to all atypical features is mandatory in that setting.[30]

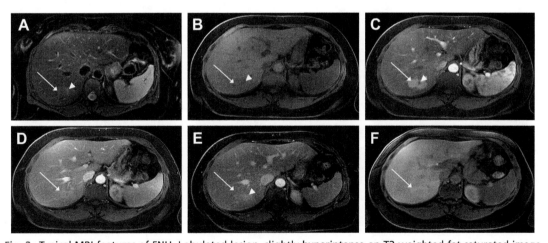

Fig. 2. Typical MRI features of FNH. Lobulated lesion, slightly hyperintense on T2-weighted fat-saturated image (*A*) and isointense on T1-weighted fat-saturated image (*B*). After injection of gadobenate dimeglumine (0.1 mL/kg), the lesion shows homogeneous arterial phase hyperenhancement (*C*) without washout in the portal venous phase (*D*) or delayed phase (*E*). There is a central element (*arrowhead*) that is hyperintense on T2-weighted fat-saturated image and hypointense on T2-weighted fat-saturated image with delayed hyperenhancement. In the hepatobiliary phase (*F*), the lesion demonstrates homogeneous hyperintensity consistent with increased uptake of the contrast agent, promoted by increased OATP expression on a molecular basis.

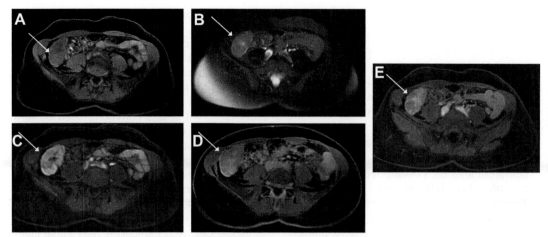

Fig. 3. Pitfall of a lesion with central element. Pedunculated lesion, hypointense on T1-weighted fat-saturated image (*A*), slightly hyperintense on T2-weighted fat-saturated image (*B*), demonstrating arterial phase hyperenhancement after injection of gadobenate dimeglumine (0.1 mL/kg) (*C*) with washout in the delayed phase (*D*), apart from delayed hyperenhancement of a central element. In the hepatobiliary phase (*E*), the lesion was hypointense with only central accumulation of gadobenate dimeglumine. The final diagnosis determined by pathology was mixed hepatocholangiocarcinoma.

HCA

Hepatocellular adenomas (HCAs) are rare benign hepatocellular tumors that mainly develop in young women.[31–33] The main risk factors are oral contraceptive use in reproductive-age women and obesity and androgen exposure in men.[34–36] The two main complications are tumor hemorrhage and malignant transformation, which can both justify liver resection in high-risk patients.[37]

A few years ago, the European Association for the Study of the Liver (EASL) issued recommendations for the management of HCA,[37] acknowledging that the risk of complications is mostly influenced by tumor size and patient sex.[38,39] Moreover, the subtyping of HCA should also be considered as different subtypes are associated with different outcomes.[34,40,41] In 2017, a new classification identified five main subgroups[34,42]:

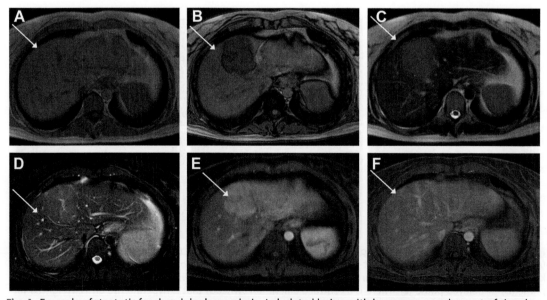

Fig. 4. Example of steatotic focal nodular hyperplasia. Lobulated lesion with homogeneous dropout of signal on the T1-opposed-phase-weighted image (A+ B), with otherwise typical features of focal nodular hyperplasia on T2-HASTE (C), T2-weighted fat-saturated image (D), arterial phase (E), and delayed phase (F).

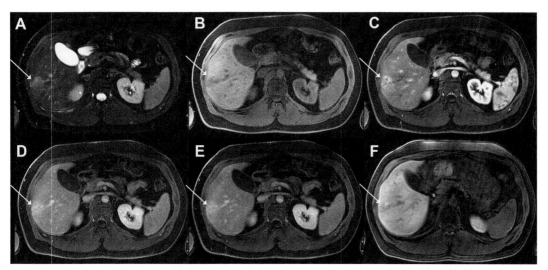

Fig. 5. Illustration of atypical FNH with sinusoidal distension. Heterogeneous lesion with irregular margins, containing area hyperintense on T2-HASTE fat-saturated image (*A*) and hypointense on T1-weighted fat-saturated image (*B*) corresponding to sinusoidal distension. The lesion showed arterial phase hyperenhancement after injection of gadobenate dimeglumine (0.1 mL/kg) (*C*), without washout in the portal venous phase (*D*) and delayed phase (*E*). The lesion exhibited peripheral uptake in the hepatobiliary phase (*F*), consistent with the final pathologic diagnosis of focal nodular hyperplasia.

- *HNF1α-inactivated HCA (HHCA)* accounts for 35%–40% of HCA and is characterized by biallelic inactivation of *hepatocyte nuclear factor 1 alpha*, thus explaining its association with maturity-onset diabetes of the young (MODY). HHCAs are usually multiple and, importantly, associated with a low risk of malignant transformation or bleeding. In pathologic analysis, HHCAs are characterized by marked steatosis, and their diagnosis is based on immunohistochemistry (IHC) to detect a downregulation of the expression of liver fatty acid-binding protein (LFABP). On MRI, a diffuse and homogeneous drop in signal intensity on out-of-phase T1-weighted MR images has a sensitivity between 87% and 91% and a specificity between 89% and 100% for the diagnosis of HHCA.[43,44] Typical HHCAs are also usually iso- or hypointense on T2-weighted images with fat suppression sequences and demonstrate faint arterial hyperenhancement.[45]

- *Inflammatory HCA (IHCA)* accounts for 35%–45% of all HCAs. IHCA is defined by activation of the IL-6/JAK/STAT pathway, leading to an inflammatory reaction. The main risk factors are estrogen exposure, obesity, alcohol use, and glycogen storage diseases. This subtype is associated with a high risk of bleeding. On IHC, there is specific overexpression of C-reactive protein (CRP) and serum amyloid A (SAA). On MRI, the combination of marked

hyperintensity on T2-weighted images and persistent enhancement in the delayed phase has a sensitivity between 85% and 88% and a specificity between 88% and 100% for the diagnosis of IHCA.[43,44] In addition, IHCA tended to appear hyperintense on T1 FS-weighted imaging (WI) precontrast, particularly when associated with underlying hepatic steatosis. Moreover, given its association with obesity, internal fat is not rare in IHCA, as illustrated in **Fig. 6**, and careful analysis of the other sequences, in particular signal intensity on T2 FS WI, is crucial to avoid mistaking IHCA for HHCA.

- *β-catenin-activated HCA (BHCA)* accounts for 15%–20% of HCAs. The main risk factors are androgen exposure, liver vascular disease, and glycogen storage diseases, which explains why it is more common in men. Approximately 50% of this subtype is associated with inflammatory changes. This subtype includes different subgroups according to the type of deletion in CTNNB1. Hence, exon 3 involvement is associated with high activation of the β-catenin pathway although exon 7 and 8 involvement is linked to low activation of the β-catenin pathway. Importantly, only high activation of the β-catenin pathway is associated with a high risk of malignant transformation.[34] In IHCA, pathologic diagnosis is based on the strong homogeneous cytoplasmic expression of glutamine synthetase with

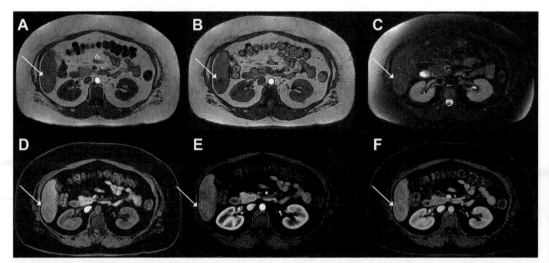

Fig. 6. IHCA-containing fat. Fat-containing lesion, with nondiffuse dropout of signal in the opposed phase (*A, B*), mildly hyperintense on T2-weighted fat-saturated image (*C*), isointense on T1-weighted fat-saturated image (*D*) with arterial phase hyperenhancement (*E*), and persistent enhancement in the delayed phase (*F*) consistent with the diagnosis of inflammatory adenoma.

nuclear positivity for β-catenin. However, those features are missing when the activation of β-catenin is lower (ie, involving exons 7 and 8), and screening for β-catenin mutations by molecular analysis is usually needed. Unfortunately, there are no validated imaging features for β-catenin-activated HCA to date, even though prior reports have shown that BHCA can demonstrate arterial phase hyperenhancement and wash out in the delayed phase, thus mimicking hepatocellular carcinoma.[43]

- *Sonic Hedgehog HCA (shHCA).* This recently described subtype remains rare, accounting for less than 5% of HCA. There is an important association with obesity, and there is a high risk of bleeding. Unfortunately, to date, the diagnosis of shHCA on imaging remains unclear.[40,46,47] As with BHCA, there are no specific MRI features, but a prior case report showed that shHCA could present peculiar intratumoral fluid cavities.[48]
- Finally, less than 5% of HCAs are still *unclassified* with no recognized molecular abnormality or IHC markers.

A summary of the main subtypes of HCA is provided in **Table 1**

Hence, using extracellular contrast agent, only the two main subtypes can be characterized with confidence on MRI, and a prior report showed that CEUS cannot be used in that setting.[49]

In the hepatobiliary phase on MRI, HCA typically appears hypointense, which can be useful for differentiation from FNH.[50,51] However, several recent studies have reported HCAs showing iso- or hyperintensity on HBP in up to 26% to 67% of cases,[52–54] especially following the injection of Gd-BOPTA. In most series, such iso- or hyperintensity was depicted in IHCA.[52–56] However, this is in contradiction to the molecular background of IHCA, as OATP expression has been shown to be lower than that of the adjacent liver.[24,57] Hence, HCA showing iso- or hyperintensity on the hepatobiliary phase could correspond to two different situations[58]:

- In lesions showing reduced contrast uptake on HBP, mainly IHCA, signal hyperintensity on HBP is not due to contrast uptake but to pre-existing signal hyperintensity on precontrast images and underlying hepatic steatosis, illustrated in **Fig. 7**.
- In lesions with true contrast uptake, specifically associated with marked activation of the β-catenin pathway,[59] which is consistent with the molecular background, prior studies have shown that OATP expression is persistent in BHCA,[24,60] as illustrated in **Fig. 8**.

Hence, HBP uptake does not always correspond to FNH but could also correspond to BHCA. Moreover, diagnosis can be challenging, as both usually develop in young patients, and both can demonstrate a central element on MRI,[61] as illustrated in **Fig. 9**.

Moreover, in addition to benign hepatocellular lesions, HBP uptake should always be analyzed carefully, and differentiated hepatocellular carcinoma or nonhepatocellular lesions with fibrotic stoma can demonstrate hyperintensity on HBP.[62]

Table 1
Summary of the main subtypes of HCA

Subtypes	HNF1α-Inactivated HCA	Inflammatory HCA	β-Catenin-activated HCA	Sonic Hedgehog HCA	Unclassified
Frequency	35%–40%	35%–45%	15%–20%	5%	<5%
Risk factors	HNF1α germline	Obesity Alcohol use Glycogen storage disease	Androgen Liver vascular disease glycogen storage disease	Obesity	
Specific staining on IHC	LFABP-	CRP++ SAA++	GS +++ β-catenin + · GS+	PTGDS + ASS1+	
Main complications		Hemorrhage	High risk of malignant transformation	Hemorrhage	
Specific MRI features	Diffuse and homogeneous drop of signal on opposed phase	Marked hyperintensity on T2 and persistent enhancement on delayed phase	No specific imaging feature associated with an uptake on the hepatobiliary phase · No specific imaging feature	No specific imaging feature	

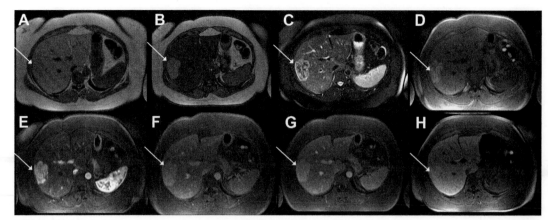

Fig. 7. Illustration of inflammatory adenoma hyperintensity in the hepatobiliary phase. Marked hepatic steatosis with homogeneous dropout of signal on the opposed-phase-weighted image (*A*, *B*), with hyperintense lesion on T2-weighted fat-saturated image (*C*), hyperintense on T1-weighted fat-saturated image (*D*), with marked arterial hyperenhancement after injection of gadobenate dimeglumine (0.1 mL/kg) (*E*) and persistent enhancement on the portal venous phase (*F*) and delayed phase (*G*). The hyperintensity on the hepatobiliary phase (*H*) seen here was related to pseudouptake in the lesion that was intrinsically hyperintense compared with the surrounding liver parenchyma due to diffuse hepatic steatosis.

There is no clear added value of metabolic imaging in HCA evaluation; however, an important pitfall is the usual avidity of HHCA on 18F-FDG PET/CT, as shown in **Fig. 10**, more so than the other HCA subtypes,[63] which mimics metastasis[64] on metabolic imaging, in particular given that this subtype is commonly associated with adenomatosis.[65]

NONHEPATOCELLULAR LESIONS
Hepatic Cysts

Hepatic cysts are the most prevalent liver lesions in the general population and can be found in 5%–18% of the general population.[66,67] On US, the characteristic imaging features are a round and completely anechoic structure, with

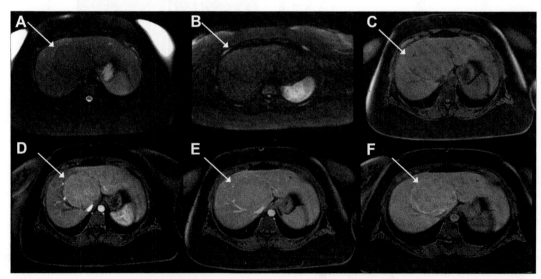

Fig. 8. β-Catenin-activated adenoma hyperintensity in the hepatobiliary phase. Large lesion hypointense on fat-saturated T2-weighted fat saturated image (*A*), without diffusion restriction (*B*), isointense on T1-weighted fat-saturated image (*C*), with arterial hyperenhancement after injection of gadobenate dimeglumine (0.1 mL/kg) (*D*) and no washout in the delayed phase (*E*). In the hepatobiliary phase (*F*), the lesion demonstrated hyperintensity consistent with a true increased uptake of gadobenate dimeglumine (0.1 mL/kg).

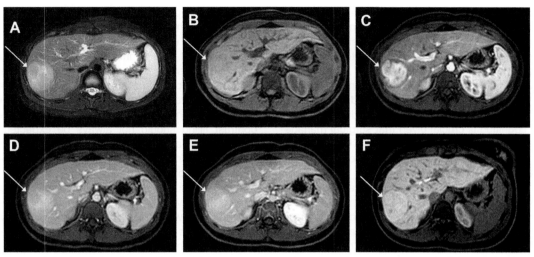

Fig. 9. Pitfall of lesion with central element hyperintensity in the hepatobiliary phase. Focal lesion slightly hyperintense on T2-weighted fat-saturated image (*A*), Isointense on T1-weighted fat-saturated image (*B*), demonstrating arterial hyperenhancement after injection of gadobenate dimeglumine (0.1 mL/kg) (*C*) without washout in the portal venous (*D*) or delayed phase (*E*) with homogeneous uptake in the hepatobiliary phase (*F*). T2 hyperintensity and minimally heterogeneous enhancement in the arterial phase were not typical for focal nodular hyperplasia. The final diagnosis made through pathology was an inflammatory β-catenin-mutated adenoma.

circumscribed margins, posterior acoustic enhancement, and no internal nodularity on color Doppler interrogation. On CT, cysts are homogeneous fluid attenuation structures, with sharp margins and no internal or mural enhancement. On MRI, they are homogenously markedly hyperintense on T2-weighted sequences, like urine, bile, and cerebrospinal fluid, with low signal on T1-weighted imaging and without any enhancement or restricted diffusion. Differential diagnosis mainly includes biliary hamartomas or von Meyenburg complexes, which are benign developmental

lesions, usually multiple and measuring less than 15 mm in diameter.[68]

Rarely, hepatic cysts can demonstrate complications such as hemorrhage.[69] In those situations, differential diagnosis between a hepatic cyst and a ciliated hepatic foregut cyst (CHFC) can be troublesome.[70] CHFC is a rare solitary benign hepatic cyst appearing histologically similar to bronchogenic and esophageal duplication cysts. The majority of CHFCs are incidentally found either on imaging or intraoperatively.[71] Typically, a CHFC is a solitary lesion measuring less than 3 cm and

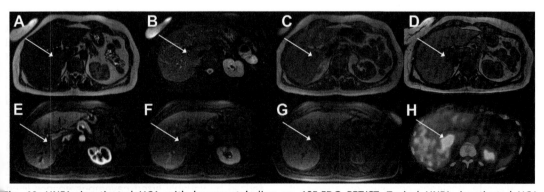

Fig. 10. HNF1α-inactivated HCA with hypermetabolism on 18F-FDG PET/CT. Typical HNF1α-inactivated HCA, slightly hyperintense on T2 HASTE (*A*) but hypointense on T2-weighted fat-saturated image (*B*), related to the diffuse and homogeneous fat content on the lesion as demonstrated by signal dropout in the T1-opposed-phase-weighted image (*C*, *D*). On postcontrast sequences after injection of gadobenate dimeglumine (0.1 mL/kg), the lesion demonstrated faint arterial hyperenhancement (*E*), with hypointensity in the delayed phase (*F*) and in the hepatobiliary phase (*G*). This lesion demonstrated marked hypermetabolism on 18F-FDG PET/CT (*H*).

is most commonly located in the subcapsular aspect of segment IV.[71] Diagnosis may be difficult on CT, as the fluid may be of greater density than simple fluid.[72,73] On MRI, signal intensity on T1-weighted images is also variable, ranging from hypointense to hyperintense,[74–76] and rarely, they may be associated with a fluid–fluid level.[77] Even if preoperative diagnosis may be difficult, CHFC recognition is crucial given that surgical management should be considered for all CHFCs.[71]

In addition to infectious lesions, one major differential diagnosis of liver cysts is mucinous cystic neoplasms, accounting for approximately 5% of all hepatic cystic lesions.[78] The previous terms "biliary cystadenoma" and "cystadenocarcinoma" should no longer be used, and according to the WHO classification, those tumors should be classified either as biliary mucinous cystic neoplasms (MCNs) of the liver and bile ducts (noninvasive for biliary cystadenoma and invasive for biliary cystadenocarcinoma) when ovarian-type stroma is present or as intraductal papillary neoplasms of the liver and bile duct (IPNB) when there is communication with bile ducts.[4] MCNs occur most commonly in Caucasian, middle-aged women.[79] A prior study found that the presence of upstream bile duct dilatation, perilesional perfusional changes, location in the left lobe, and the coexistence of fewer than three other cysts can help differentiate biliary cystic neoplasms from simple hepatic cysts.[80] In addition, a recent study found that the features most predictive of MCNs rather than simple cysts were thick septations, internal nodularity, or solid enhancing components, with advantages of MRI over CT for the detection of upstream biliary dilatation, thin septation, and internal hemorrhage or debris.[79]

Hemangioma

Hepatic hemangiomas are the most common solid benign tumors of the liver, with a prevalence between 1% and 20%.[81,82] They are frequently discovered incidentally, as most patients with hemangioma are asymptomatic and require no treatment.[82] There is a female predilection (ratio of 5:1),[82] and multiple hemangiomas may be present in 9%–22% of patients.

On ultrasound, the most common appearance consists of a homogeneous hyperechoic nodule, with discrete posterior acoustic enhancement, and without signal on Doppler evaluation.[83] On CEUS, there is peripheral discontinuous globular enhancement in the arterial phase with centripetal filling in the portal and late phases.[84] Hence, a combination of peripheral nodular arterial enhancement

and complete portal venous fill-in may have 98% sensitivity for the diagnosis of hemangioma.[85]

CT features usually include a hypodense well-defined lesion, with an internal density similar to that of the vessels. After injection, slow nodular discontinuous peripheral and centripetal enhancement is observed, with typically persistent filling in the delayed phase. However, delayed complete contrast filling should not always be expected, especially for large tumors. MRI has been shown to be the best imaging modality for diagnosing hepatic hemangiomas with high sensitivity and specificity.[86] In addition to similar enhancement as described above, typical hemangiomas are hypointense on T1-weighted MR images and markedly hyperintense on T2-weighted images. On diffusion, hepatic hemangiomas typically show suppression of high signal intensity at high b values; however, a significant rate of otherwise typical hemangiomas may demonstrate residual high signal intensity on high b-value images related to the T2 shine-through effect.[86]

There are several forms of atypical hemangiomas,[81,87,88] some of which are well known and usually have a straightforward diagnosis, such as rapidly filling hemangioma, characterized by immediate homogenous enhancement in the arterial phase of contrast administration with persistent enhancement in later phases of contrast administration on CT and MR. Perilesional hepatic parenchymal transient hyperenhancement in the arterial phase is commonly associated with these hemangiomas,[89] as illustrated in **Fig. 11**.

Another classic form of atypical hemangioma is a large hemangioma, defined as giant hemangioma when the size exceeds 4 cm,[87] even if some suggest reserving the term "giant" for hemangiomas larger than 10 cm.[90] They are characterized by heterogeneous but high hyperintensity on T2, associated with areas of different T2 intensities with internal septation.[81,87,88] The enhancement kinetics are slow but identical to those of typical hemangiomas, apart from incomplete filling of the delayed phase. An example of a giant hemangioma is shown in **Fig. 12**.

In contrast, features of sclerosed hemangioma can be misleading. On pathology, there is a difference between true sclerosed hemangiomas, characterized by extensive fibrosis with marked narrowing or obliteration of the vascular spaces, and sclerosing cavernous hemangiomas, characterized by variably sized cavernous spaces lined with flattened endothelial cells with varying degrees of stromal sclerosis.[91] However, both forms usually demonstrate atypical features, in particular slight hyperintensity on T2WI with capsular retraction and calcification.[92] After injection, most

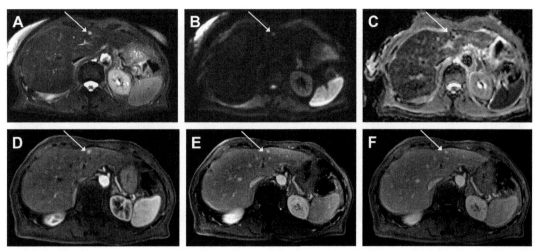

Fig. 11. Rapidly filling hemangioma. As a typical hemangioma, the lesion demonstrated marked hyperintensity on T2-weighted fat-saturated images (A), with slight hyperintensity on diffusion (B) without restriction (C). On the postcontrast sequences, enhancement was similar to that of the aorta in the arterial (D), portal venous (E), and delayed (F) phases, with perilesional transient hyperenhancement in the arterial phase.

sclerosing cavernous hemangiomas tend to demonstrate centripetal enhancement characteristics, in contrast to sclerosed hemangiomas, which usually exhibit little or no enhancement during the arterial phase and only marginal enhancement during the delayed phase.[92] Most of the time, sclerosed hemangiomas do not demonstrate diffusion restriction, which can help to differentiate them from malignant lesions,[93] as illustrated in Fig. 13.

Calcifications may occur in 20% of hemangiomas and are usually large and coarse and located centrally.[94] Rarely, calcifications may occur in almost all the lesions, as illustrated in Fig. 14.

Rare Tumors and Pseudotumors

Hepatic angiomyolipoma (HAML) is a rare mesenchymal tumor with marked female predominance and peak incidence in middle-aged adults.[4,95–97] Most of them are sporadic, and 5% to 10% of patients have tuberous sclerosis.[98]

In general, HAML is suggested when its fatty component is identified on imaging[99]; however, in addition to hepatocellular tumors that can also

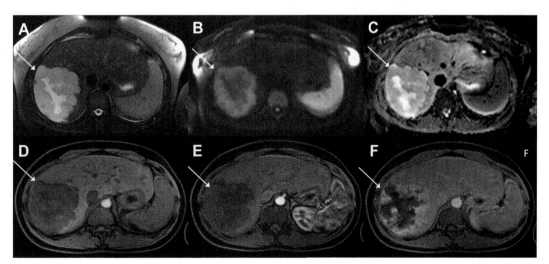

Fig. 12. Giant hemangioma. Large liver lesion with heterogeneous hyperintensity on T2-weighted fat-saturated image (A), hyperintensity on diffusion (B) without restriction (C). The lesion was hypointense on T1-weighted fat-saturated image (D) with almost no enhancement in the arterial phase I and incomplete filling in the delayed phase (F).

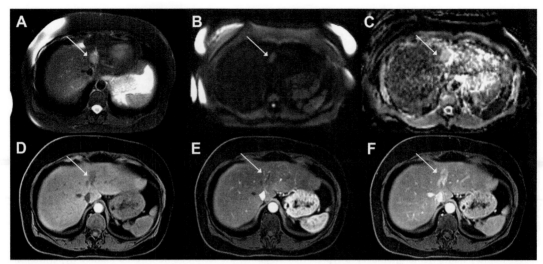

Fig. 13. Pitfalls of sclerosed hemangioma. Lesion with faint hyperintensity on fat-saturated T2-weighted image (*A*), hyperintensity on diffusion (*B*) without restriction (*C*), hypointensity on fat-saturated T1-weighted image (*D*) with faint peripheral hyperenhancement in the arterial phal(*E*) and heterogeneous rim hyperenhancement in the delayed phase (*F*). Despite the reassuring lack of diffusion restriction, a biopsy was performed to exclude fibrotic malignant lesions, and the diagnosis of sclerosed hemangioma was confirmed.

have a fat component, as seen previously, the fat content of HAML can also vary, or events sometimes cannot be recognized on MRI.[97] After contrast media injection, HAMLs demonstrate arterial hyperenhancement with typical washout on portal venous and delayed imaging,[100,101] thus mimicking hepatocellular carcinoma. In those situations, CEUS could be useful, as HAML may demonstrate specific findings such as a centripetal filling pattern or a prolonged enhancement pattern with a higher peak intensity.[102] A formal diagnosis is provided by pathology. An example of HAML is provided in **Fig. 15.**

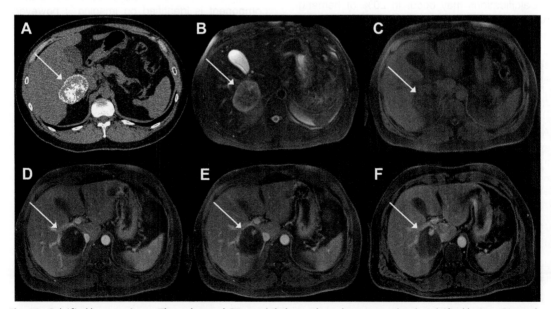

Fig. 14. Calcified hemangioma. The enhanced CT scan (*A*) showed an almost completely calcified lesion. Given the calcification, the lesion showed a heterogeneous signal intensity on fat-saturated T2-weighted imaging (*B*) and fat-saturated T1-weighted imaging (*C*). After injection of contrast, the single nodular peripheral discontinuous hyperenhancement (*D–F*) was consistent with the diagnosis of calcified hemangioma.

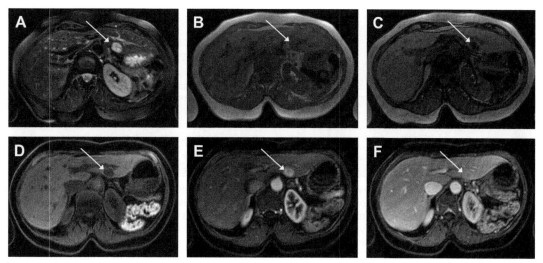

Fig. 15. Example of hepatic angiomyolipoma. Rounded lesion demonstrating faint hyperintensity on fat-suppressed T2-weighted image (*A*), with dropout of signal in the opposed phase (*B*, *C*) in keeping with the internal fat. The lesion was hypointense on fat-suppressed T1-weighted imaging (*D*), with marked arterial hyperenhancement after injection of gadobenate dimeglumine (0.1 mlg) (*E*) and no washout in the delayed phase (*F*). The diagnosis of hepatic angiomyolipoma was confirmed through biopsy.

Granulomatous hepatitis, defined as an inflammatory liver disease with the formation of granulomas in the liver, is associated with a large variety of conditions, most commonly with sarcoidosis, tuberculosis, and histoplasmosis.[103,104] According to prior reports, hepatic granulomas are present in 2.4%–10% of liver tissue specimens examined.[105,106] There is no specific imaging pattern for hepatic granulomas; however, they are often associated with diffusion restriction[107] and can mimic liver metastases,[108] as shown in **Fig. 16**.

Inflammatory pseudotumor (IPT) of the liver is a rare benign neoplasm that was first described in 1953[109] and is histologically characterized by fibroblastic and myofibroblastic proliferation with inflammatory infiltrate.[110] IPTs are now classified into two types based on IgG4 staining: IgG4-related and non-IgG4-related.[111] Usually, IPT will regress spontaneously or with conservative

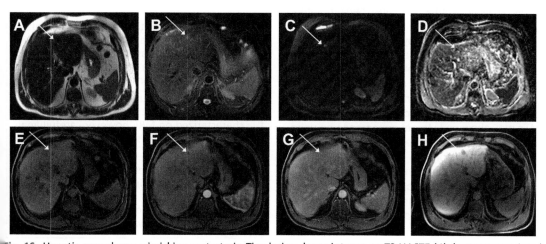

Fig. 16. Hepatic granuloma mimicking metastasis. Tiny lesion, hyperintense on T2 HASTE (*A*), better appreciated on fat-saturated T2-weighted images (*B*), hyperintense on diffusion (*C*) with restriction (*D*), hypointense on fat-saturated T1-weightelmages (*E*), with rim hyperenhancement in the arterial phase (*F*), progressive peripheral filling in the delayed phase (*G*) and no uptake in the hepatobiliary phase (*H*). Given that the patient had several similar lesions within the liver, it was mistaken for metastasis, with a final diagnosis of hepatic granuloma based on the pathologic findings.

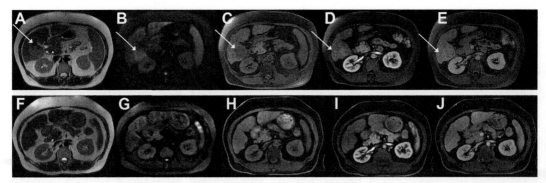

Fig. 17. Illustration of an inflammatory pseudotumor. Large lesion developed on a cirrhotic liver, hyperintense on T2 HASTE (*A*), hyperintense on diffusion (*B*), hypointense on T1 fat-suppressed WI (*C*) with arterial hyperenhancement (*D*) and no washout in the deled phase (*E*). The pathologic result was in favor of an inflammatory pseudotumor. Follow-up 3 months later showed complete resolution of the tumor on T2-weighted images (*F*), diffusion (*G*), T1 (*H*), arterial (*I*), and delayed phases (*J*).

treatment.[112] Rarely, IPT can also cause complications such as portal thrombophlebitis, portal hypertension, and biliary obstruction.[113,114] On ultrasound images, these lesions usually appear as hypoechoic masses but may also show hyperechogenicity or complex echogenicity.[115,116] On CEUS, IPTs may also display various enhancement patterns.[116] On MRI, imaging features are usually nonspecific, mostly T1 hypointense and moderately T2 hyperintense with a highly variable enhancement pattern,[117] which was the case for the example provided in **Fig. 17.** A recent study showed that IPTs may demonstrate central hypointensity with a relatively hyperintense periphery on HBP, which could be helpful to differentiate IPT from malignant lesions such as metastases.[118]

One rare differential of IPT is the inflammatory myofibroblastic tumor, a rare benign tumor, possibly representing the neoplastic counterpart of IPT,[110] characterized by fibroblastic or myofibroblastic spindle cells, admixed with lymphocytes and plasma cells, and ALK gene translocation, resulting in aberrant expression of ALK protein in the myofibroblast.[110] IMTs usually occur in children and young adults. On MRI, IMTs may show early target appearance on unenhanced T1WI, characterized by a central isointensity and a peripheral hypointense rim on unenhanced T1WI, and on early dynamic phases of gadoxetic acid-enhanced MRI, characterized by central enhancement and a peripheral hypointense rim in the arterial and portal venous phases.[119]

SUMMARY

Benign focal liver lesions include numerous tumors ranging from common incidental findings with no specific management to rare tumors with potential malignant transformation. Moreover, benign lesions can be mistaken for malignant lesions. Hence, optimal instrumentation using MRI, often performed using a hepatobiliary contrast agent, and contrast-enhanced ultrasound is the cornerstone for optimized diagnostic pathways. Multidisciplinary tumor boards, bringing together hepatologists, pathologists, radiologists, and surgeons, should address difficult cases of benign liver tumors to allow improved patient management.

CLINICS CARE POINTS

- Optimal instrumentation using MRI, often performed using a hepatobiliary contrast agent, and contrast-enhanced ultrasound are the cornerstone for optimized diagnosis in benign liver lesions.

- Typical Focal Nodular Hyperplasia and main Hepatocellular Adenoma subtypes can be characterized on MRI, however carefull analysis of MRI features is mandatory to avoid potential pitfalls.

- Hepatic cysts and liver hemangiomas are common incidental findings in liver MRI. However, some features, such as septations or internal heterogeneous content within a cyst, should be analyzed carefully.

DISCLOSURE

The authors have nothing to disclose.

REFERENCES

1. Gore RM, Pickhardt PJ, Mortele KJ, et al. Management of Incidental Liver Lesions on CT: A White Paper of the ACR Incidental Findings Committee. J Am Coll Radiol 2017;14(11):1429–37.

2. Kaltenbach TE-M, Engler P, Kratzer W, et al. Prevalence of benign focal liver lesions: ultrasound investigation of 45,319 hospital patients. Abdom Radiol 2016;41:25–32.

3. Nault J-C, Blanc J-F, Moga L, et al. Non-invasive diagnosis and follow-up of benign liver tumours. Clin Res Hepatol Gastroenterol 2021;101765. https://doi.org/10.1016/j.clinre.2021.101765.

4. Nagtegaal ID, Odze RD, Klimstra D, et al. The 2019 WHO classification of tumours of the digestive system. Histopathology 2020;76(2):182–8.

5. Sempoux C, Balabaud C, Paradis V, et al. Hepatocellular nodules in vascular liver diseases. Virchows Arch Int J Pathol 2018;473(1):33–44.

6. Vilgrain V, Paradis V, Van Wettere M, et al. Benign and malignant hepatocellular lesions in patients with vascular liver diseases. Abdom Radiol N Y 2018;43(8):1968–77.

7. Bartolotta TV, Midiri M, Scialpi M, et al. Focal nodular hyperplasia in normal and fatty liver: a qualitative and quantitative evaluation with contrast-enhanced ultrasound. Eur Radiol 2004; 14(4):583–91.

8. Ronot M, Vilgrain V. Imaging of benign hepatocellular lesions: current concepts and recent updates. Clin Res Hepatol Gastroenterol 2014;38(6):681–8.

9. Ronot M, Di Renzo S, Gregoli B, et al. Characterization of fortuitously discovered focal liver lesions: additional information provided by shearwave elastography. Eur Radiol 2015;25(2):346–58.

10. Taimr P, Klompenhouwer AJ, Thomeer MGJ, et al. Can point shear wave elastography differentiate focal nodular hyperplasia from hepatocellular adenoma. J Clin Ultrasound 2018;46(6):380–5.

11. Soussan M, Aubé C, Bahrami S, et al. Incidental focal solid liver lesions: diagnostic performance of contrast-enhanced ultrasound and MR imaging. Eur Radiol 2010;20(7):1715–25.

12. Wang W, Chen L-D, Lu M-D, et al. Contrast-enhanced ultrasound features of histologically proven focal nodular hyperplasia: diagnostic performance compared with contrast-enhanced CT. Eur Radiol 2013;23(9):2546–54.

13. Roche V, Pigneur F, Tselikas L, et al. Differentiation of focal nodular hyperplasia from hepatocellular adenomas with low-mechanical-index contrast-enhanced sonography (CEUS): effect of size on diagnostic confidence. Eur Radiol 2015;25(1):186–95.

14. Bertin C, Egels S, Wagner M, et al. Contrast-enhanced ultrasound of focal nodular hyperplasia: a matter of size. Eur Radiol 2014;24(10):2561–71.

15. Mathieu D, Rahmouni A, Anglade MC, et al. Focal nodular hyperplasia of the liver: assessment with contrast-enhanced TurboFLASH MR imaging. Radiology 1991;180(1):25–30.

16. Dioguardi Burgio M, Ronot M, Salvaggio G, et al. Imaging of Hepatic Focal Nodular Hyperplasia: Pictorial Review and Diagnostic Strategy. Semin Ultrasound CT MR 2016;37(6):511–24.

17. Bieze M, van den Esschert JW, Nio CY, et al. Diagnostic accuracy of MRI in differentiating hepatocellular adenoma from focal nodular hyperplasia: prospective study of the additional value of gadoxetate disodium. AJR Am J Roentgenol 2012;199(1): 26–34.

18. Ferlicot S, Kobeiter H, Tran Van Nhieu J, et al. MRI of atypical focal nodular hyperplasia of the liver: radiology-pathology correlation. AJR Am J Roentgenol 2004;182(5):1227–31.

19. Grazioli L, Morana G, Federle MP, et al. Focal nodular hyperplasia: morphologic and functional information from MR imaging with gadobenate dimeglumine. Radiology 2001;221(3):731–9.

20. Tselikas L, Pigneur F, Roux M, et al. Impact of hepatobiliary phase liver MRI versus Contrast-Enhanced Ultrasound after an inconclusive extracellular gadolinium-based contrast-enhanced MRI for the diagnosis of benign hepatocellular tumors. Abdom Radiol N Y 2017;42(3):825–32.

21. Suh CH, Kim KW, Kim GY, et al. The diagnostic value of Gd-EOB-DTPA-MRI for the diagnosis of focal nodular hyperplasia: a systematic review and meta-analysis. Eur Radiol 2015;25(4):950–60.

22. Yoneda N, Matsui O, Kitao A, et al. Hepatocyte transporter expression in FNH and FNH-like nodule: correlation with signal intensity on gadoxetic acid enhanced magnetic resonance images. Jpn J Radiol 2012;30(6):499–508.

23. Fujiwara H, Sekine S, Onaya H, et al. Ring-like enhancement of focal nodular hyperplasia with hepatobiliary-phase Gd-EOB-DTPA-enhanced magnetic resonance imaging: radiological-pathological correlation. Jpn J Radiol 2011; 29(10):739–43.

24. Reizine E, Amaddeo G, Pigneur F, et al. Quantitative correlation between uptake of Gd-BOPTA on hepatobiliary phase and tumor molecular features in patients with benign hepatocellular lesions. Eur Radiol 2018. https://doi.org/10.1007/s00330-018-5438-7.

25. van Kessel CS, de Boer E, ten Kate FJW, et al. Focal nodular hyperplasia: hepatobiliary enhancement patterns on gadoxetic-acid contrast-enhanced MRI. Abdom Imaging 2013;38(3): 490–501.

26. Nguyen BN, Fléjou JF, Terris B, et al. Focal nodular hyperplasia of the liver: a comprehensive pathologic study of 305 lesions and recognition of new

histologic forms. Am J Surg Pathol 1999;23(12): 1441–54.

27. Hussain SM, Semelka RC, Mitchell DG. MR imaging of hepatocellular carcinoma. Magn Reson Imaging Clin N Am 2002;10(1):31–52, v.

28. Ronot M, Paradis V, Duran R, et al. MR findings of steatotic focal nodular hyperplasia and comparison with other fatty tumours. Eur Radiol 2013; 23(4):914–23.

29. Laumonier H, Frulio N, Laurent C, et al. Focal nodular hyperplasia with major sinusoidal dilatation: a misleading entity. BMJ Case Rep 2010; 2010. bcr0920103311.

30. Luciani A, Kobeiter H, Maison P, et al. Focal nodular hyperplasia of the liver in men: is presentation the same in men and women? Gut 2002;50(6): 877–80.

31. Edmondson HA, Henderson B, Benton B. Liver-cell adenomas associated with use of oral contraceptives. N Engl J Med 1976;294(9):470–2.

32. Nault J-C, Bioulac-Sage P, Zucman-Rossi J. Hepatocellular benign tumors-from molecular classification to personalized clinical care. Gastroenterology 2013;144(5):888–902.

33. Belghiti J, Cauchy F, Paradis V, et al. Diagnosis and management of solid benign liver lesions. Nat Rev Gastroenterol Hepatol 2014;11(12):737–49.

34. Nault J-C, Couchy G, Balabaud C, et al. Molecular Classification of Hepatocellular Adenoma Associates With Risk Factors, Bleeding, and Malignant Transformation. Gastroenterology 2017;152(4): 880–94.e6.

35. Chang CY, Hernandez-Prera JC, Roayaie S, et al. Changing epidemiology of hepatocellular adenoma in the United States: review of the literature. Int J Hepatol 2013;2013:604860.

36. Brunt EM, Sempoux C, Bioulac-Sage P. Hepatocellular adenomas: the expanding epidemiology. Histopathology 2021;79(1):20–2.

37. European Association for the Study of the Liver (EASL). EASL Clinical Practice Guidelines on the management of benign liver tumours. J Hepatol 2016;65(2):386–98.

38. Dokmak S, Paradis V, Vilgrain V, et al. A single-center surgical experience of 122 patients with single and multiple hepatocellular adenomas. Gastroenterology 2009;137(5):1698–705.

39. Farges O, Ferreira N, Dokmak S, et al. Changing trends in malignant transformation of hepatocellular adenoma. Gut 2011;60(1):85–9.

40. Védie A-L, Sutter O, Ziol M, et al. Molecular classification of hepatocellular adenomas: impact on clinical practice. Hepatic Oncol 2018;5(1). https://doi.org/10.2217/hep-2017-0023.

41. Julien C, Le-Bail B, Touhami KO, et al. Hepatocellular Adenoma Risk Factors of Hemorrhage: Size is not the only Concern! Single Center Retrospective

Experience of 261 Patients. Ann Surg 2021. https://doi.org/10.1097/SLA.0000000000005108.

42. Beaufrère A, Paradis V. Hepatocellular adenomas: review of pathological and molecular features. Hum Pathol 2021;112:128–37.

43. Laumonier H, Bioulac-Sage P, Laurent C, et al. Hepatocellular adenomas: magnetic resonance imaging features as a function of molecular pathological classification. Hepatol Baltim Md 2008;48(3):808–18.

44. Ronot M, Bahrami S, Calderaro J, et al. Hepatocellular adenomas: accuracy of magnetic resonance imaging and liver biopsy in subtype classification. Hepatol Baltim Md 2011;53(4):1182–91.

45. Bise S, Frulio N, Hocquelet A, et al. New MRI features improve subtype classification of hepatocellular adenoma. Eur Radiol 2018. https://doi.org/10.1007/s00330-018-5784-5.

46. Nault J-C, Couchy G, Caruso S, et al. ASS1 and peri-portal gene expression in sonic hedgehog hepatocellular adenomas. Hepatol Baltim Md 2018. https://doi.org/10.1002/hep.29884.

47. Sala M, Gonzales D, Leste-Lasserre T, et al. ASS1 Overexpression: A Hallmark of Sonic Hedgehog Hepatocellular Adenomas; Recommendations for Clinical Practice. Hepatol Commun 2020;4(6): 809–24.

48. Frulio N, Balabaud C, Laurent C, et al. Unclassified hepatocellular adenoma expressing ASS1 associated with inflammatory hepatocellular adenomas. Clin Res Hepatol Gastroenterol 2019. https://doi.org/10.1016/j.clinre.2019.03.012.

49. Gregory J, Paisant A, Paulatto L, et al. Limited added value of contrast-enhanced ultrasound over B-mode for the subtyping of hepatocellular adenomas. Eur J Radiol 2020;128:109027.

50. Grazioli L, Morana G, Kirchin MA, et al. Accurate differentiation of focal nodular hyperplasia from hepatic adenoma at gadobenate dimeglumine-enhanced MR imaging: prospective study. Radiology 2005;236(1):166–77.

51. Grazioli L, Bondioni MP, Haradome H, et al. Hepatocellular adenoma and focal nodular hyperplasia: value of gadoxetic acid-enhanced MR imaging in differential diagnosis. Radiology 2012;262(2): 520–9.

52. Ba-Ssalamah A, Antunes C, Feier D, et al. Morphologic and Molecular Features of Hepatocellular Adenoma with Gadoxetic Acid-enhanced MR Imaging. Radiology 2015;277(1):104–13.

53. Agarwal S, Fuentes-Orrego JM, Arnason T, et al. Inflammatory hepatocellular adenomas can mimic focal nodular hyperplasia on gadoxetic acid-enhanced MRI. AJR Am J Roentgenol 2014; 203(4):W408–14.

54. Thomeer MG, Willemssen FE, Biermann KK, et al. MRI features of inflammatory hepatocellular adenomas on hepatocyte phase imaging with liver-

specific contrast agents. J Magn Reson Imaging 2014;39(5):1259–64.

55. Tse JR, Naini BV, Lu DSK, et al. Qualitative and Quantitative Gadoxetic Acid-enhanced MR Imaging Helps Subtype Hepatocellular Adenomas. Radiology 2016;279(1):118–27.

56. Glockner JF, Lee CU, Mounajjed T. Inflammatory hepatic adenomas: Characterization with hepatobiliary MRI contrast agents. Magn Reson Imaging 2017;47:103–10.

57. Yoneda N, Matsui O, Kitao A, et al. Benign Hepatocellular Nodules: Hepatobiliary Phase of Gadoxetic Acid-enhanced MR Imaging Based on Molecular Background. Radiogr Rev Publ Radiol Soc N Am Inc 2016;36(7):2010–27.

58. Reizine E, Ronot M, Pigneur F, et al. Iso- or hyperintensity of hepatocellular adenomas on hepatobiliary phase does not always correspond to hepatospecific contrast-agent uptake: importance for tumor subtyping. Eur Radiol 2019. https://doi.org/10.1007/s00330-019-06150-7.

59. Reizine E, Ronot M, Ghosn M, et al. Hepatospecific MR contrast agent uptake on hepatobiliary phase can be used as a biomarker of marked β-catenin activation in hepatocellular adenoma. Eur Radiol 2021;31(5):3417–26.

60. Yoneda N, Matsui O, Kitao A, et al. Beta-catenin-activated hepatocellular adenoma showing hyperintensity on hepatobiliary-phase gadoxetic-enhanced magnetic resonance imaging and overexpression of OATP8. Jpn J Radiol 2012;30(9):777–82.

61. Rousseau C, Ronot M, Sibileau E, et al. Central element in liver masses, helpful, or pitfall? Abdom Imaging 2015;40(6):1904–25.

62. Vernuccio F, Gagliano DS, Cannella R, et al. Spectrum of liver lesions hyperintense on hepatobiliary phase: an approach by clinical setting. Insights Imaging 2021;12(1):8.

63. Young JR, Graham RP, Venkatesh SK, et al. 18F-FDG PET/CT of hepatocellular adenoma subtypes and review of literature. Abdom Radiol N Y 2021;46(6):2604–9.

64. Lim D, Lee SY, Lim KH, et al. Hepatic adenoma mimicking a metastatic lesion on computed tomography-positron emission tomography scan. World J Gastroenterol 2013;19(27):4432–6.

65. Barbier L, Nault J-C, Dujardin F, et al. Natural history of liver adenomatosis: a long-term observational study. J Hepatol 2019. https://doi.org/10.1016/j.jhep.2019.08.004.

66. Larssen TB, Rørvik J, Hoff SR, et al. The occurrence of asymptomatic and symptomatic simple hepatic cysts. A prospective, hospital-based study. Clin Radiol 2005;60(9):1026–9.

67. Tran Cao HS, Marcal LP, Mason MC, et al. Benign hepatic incidentalomas. Curr Probl Surg 2019;56(9):100642.

68. Lev-Toaff AS, Bach AM, Wechsler RJ, et al. The radiologic and pathologic spectrum of biliary hamartomas. AJR Am J Roentgenol 1995;165(2):309–13.

69. Borhani AA, Wiant A, Heller MT. Cystic hepatic lesions: a review and an algorithmic approach. AJR Am J Roentgenol 2014;203(6):1192–204.

70. Wilson JM, Groeschl R, George B, et al. Ciliated hepatic cyst leading to squamous cell carcinoma of the liver - A case report and review of the literature. Int J Surg Case Rep 2013;4(11):972–5.

71. Ziogas IA, van der Windt DJ, Wilson GC, et al. Surgical Management of Ciliated Hepatic Foregut Cyst. Hepatol Baltim Md 2020;71(1):386–8.

72. Kimura A, Makuuchi M, Takayasu K, et al. Ciliated hepatic foregut cyst with solid tumor appearance on CT. J Comput Assist Tomogr 1990;14(6):1016–8.

73. Shoenut JP, Semelka RC, Levi C, et al. Ciliated hepatic foregut cysts: US, CT, and contrast-enhanced MR imaging. Abdom Imaging 1994;19(2):150–2.

74. Kadoya M, Matsui O, Nakanuma Y, et al. Ciliated hepatic foregut cyst: radiologic features. Radiology 1990;175(2):475–7.

75. Fang S-H, Dong D-J, Zhang S-Z. Imaging features of ciliated hepatic foregut cyst. World J Gastroenterol 2005;11(27):4287–9.

76. Ansari-Gilani K, Modaresi Esfeh J. Ciliated hepatic foregut cyst: report of three cases and review of imaging features. Gastroenterol Rep 2017;5(1):75–8.

77. Rodriguez E, Soler R, Fernandez P. MR imagings of ciliated hepatic foregut cyst: an unusual cause of fluid-fluid level within a focal hepatic lesion (2005.4b). Eur Radiol 2005;15(7):1499–501.

78. Soares KC, Arnaoutakis DJ, Kamel I, et al. Cystic neoplasms of the liver: biliary cystadenoma and cystadenocarcinoma. J Am Coll Surg 2014;218(1):119–28.

79. Anderson MA, Dhami RS, Fadzen CM, et al. CT and MRI features differentiating mucinous cystic neoplasms of the liver from pathologically simple cysts. Clin Imaging 2021;76:46–52.

80. Kim JY, Kim SH, Eun HW, et al. Differentiation between biliary cystic neoplasms and simple cysts of the liver: accuracy of CT. AJR Am J Roentgenol 2010;195(5):1142–8.

81. Caseiro-Alves F, Brito J, Araujo AE, et al. Liver haemangioma: common and uncommon findings and how to improve the differential diagnosis. Eur Radiol 2007;17(6):1544–54.

82. Gore RM, Newmark GM, Thakrar KH, et al. Hepatic incidentalomas. Radiol Clin North Am 2011;49(2):291–322.

83. Harvey CJ, Albrecht T. Ultrasound of focal liver lesions. Eur Radiol 2001;11(9):1578–93.

84. Zarzour JG, Porter KK, Tchelepi H, et al. Contrast-enhanced ultrasound of benign liver lesions. Abdom Radiol N Y 2018;43(4):848–60.

85. Dietrich CF, Mertens JC, Braden B, et al. Contrast-enhanced ultrasound of histologically proven liver hemangiomas. Hepatol Baltim Md 2007;45(5): 1139–45.

86. Duran R, Ronot M, Kerbaol A, et al. Hepatic hemangiomas: factors associated with T2 shine-through effect on diffusion-weighted MR sequences. Eur J Radiol 2014;83(3):468–78.

87. Vilgrain V, Boulos L, Vullierme MP, et al. Imaging of atypical hemangiomas of the liver with pathologic correlation. Radiogr Rev Publ Radiol Soc N Am Inc 2000;20(2):379–97.

88. Klotz T, Montoriol P-F, Da Ines D, et al. Hepatic haemangioma: common and uncommon imaging features. Diagn Interv Imaging 2013;94(9):849–59.

89. Byun JH, Kim TK, Lee CW, et al. Arterioportal shunt: prevalence in small hemangiomas versus that in hepatocellular carcinomas 3 cm or smaller at two-phase helical CT. Radiology 2004;232(2): 354–60.

90. Di Carlo I, Koshy R, Al Mudares S, et al. Giant cavernous liver hemangiomas: is it the time to change the size categories? Hepatobiliary Pancreat Dis Int 2016;15(1):21–9.

91. Makhlouf HR, Ishak KG. Sclerosed hemangioma and sclerosing cavernous hemangioma of the liver: a comparative clinicopathologic and immunohisto-chemical study with emphasis on the role of mast cells in their histogenesis. Liver 2002;22(1):70–8.

92. Jia C, Liu G, Wang X, et al. Hepatic sclerosed hemangioma and sclerosing cavernous hemangioma: a radiological study. Jpn J Radiol 2021. https://doi.org/10.1007/s11604-021-01139-z.

93. Kim Y-Y, Kang TW, Cha DI, et al. Gadoxetic acid-enhanced MRI for differentiating hepatic sclerosing hemangioma from malignant tumor. Eur J Radiol 2021;135:109474.

94. Stoupis C, Taylor HM, Paley MR, et al. The Rocky liver: radiologic-pathologic correlation of calcified hepatic masses. Radiogr Rev Publ Radiol Soc N Am Inc 1998;18(3):675–85 [quiz: 726].

95. Goodman ZD, Ishak KG. Angiomyolipomas of the liver. Am J Surg Pathol 1984;8(10):745–50.

96. Tsui WM, Colombari R, Portmann BC, et al. Hepatic angiomyolipoma: a clinicopathologic study of 30 cases and delineation of unusual morphologic variants. Am J Surg Pathol 1999;23(1):34–48.

97. Lee SJ, Kim SY, Kim KW, et al. Hepatic Angiomyolipoma Versus Hepatocellular Carcinoma in the Noncirrhotic Liver on Gadoxetic Acid-Enhanced MRI: A Diagnostic Challenge. AJR Am J Roentgenol 2016;207(3):562–70.

98. Black ME, Hedgire SS, Camposano S, et al. Hepatic manifestations of tuberous sclerosis complex: a genotypic and phenotypic analysis. Clin Genet 2012;82(6):552–7.

99. Prasad SR, Wang H, Rosas H, et al. Fat-containing lesions of the liver: radiologic-pathologic correlation. Radiogr Rev Publ Radiol Soc N Am Inc 2005;25(2):321–31.

100. Ji J, Lu C, Wang Z, et al. Epithelioid angiomyolipoma of the liver: CT and MRI features. Abdom Imaging 2013;38(2):309–14.

101. O'Malley ME, Chawla TP, Lavelle LP, et al. Primary perivascular epithelioid cell tumors of the liver: CT/MRI findings and clinical outcomes. Abdom Radiol N Y 2017;42(6):1705–12.

102. Huang Z, Wu X, Li S, et al. Contrast-Enhanced Ultrasound Findings and Differential Diagnosis of Hepatic Epithelioid Angiomyolipoma Compared with Hepatocellular Carcinoma. Ultrasound Med Biol 2020;46(6):1403–11.

103. Balci NC, Tunaci A, Akinci A, et al. Granulomatous hepatitis: MRI findings. Magn Reson Imaging 2001; 19(8):1107–11.

104. Mortelé KJ, Segatto E, Ros PR. The infected liver: radiologic-pathologic correlation. Radiogr Rev Publ Radiol Soc N Am Inc 2004;24(4):937–55.

105. Harrington PT, Gutiérrez JJ, Ramirez-Ronda CH, et al. Granulomatous hepatitis. Rev Infect Dis 1982;4(3):638–55.

106. Drebber U, Kasper H-U, Ratering J, et al. Hepatic granulomas: histological and molecular pathological approach to differential diagnosis–a study of 442 cases. Liver Int 2008;28(6):828–34.

107. Lee NK, Kim S, Kim DU, et al. Diffusion-weighted magnetic resonance imaging for non-neoplastic conditions in the hepatobiliary and pancreatic regions: pearls and potential pitfalls in imaging interpretation. Abdom Imaging 2015;40(3):643–62.

108. Zhang L, Lin WM, Li H, et al. Hepatic nontuberculous mycobacterial granulomas in patients with cancer mimicking metastases: an analysis of three cases. Quant Imaging Med Surg 2019;9(6): 1126–31.

109. Pack GT, Baker HW. Total right hepatic lobectomy; report of a case. Ann Surg 1953;138(2):253–8.

110. Yamamoto H, Yamaguchi H, Aishima S, et al. Inflammatory myofibroblastic tumor versus IgG4-related sclerosing disease and inflammatory pseudotumor: a comparative clinicopathologic study. Am J Surg Pathol 2009;33(9):1330–40.

111. Zen Y, Fujii T, Sato Y, et al. Pathological classification of hepatic inflammatory pseudotumor with respect to IgG4-related disease. Mod Pathol 2007;20(8):884–94.

112. Park JY, Choi MS, Lim Y-S, et al. Clinical features, image findings, and prognosis of inflammatory

pseudotumor of the liver: a multicenter experience of 45 cases. Gut Liver 2014;8(1):58–63.

113. Someren A. Inflammatory pseudotumor" of liver with occlusive phlebitis: report of a case in a child and review of the literature. Am J Clin Pathol 1978; 69(2):176–81.

114. Lee SL, DuBois JJ. Hepatic inflammatory pseudotumor: case report, review of the literature, and a proposal for morphologic classification. Pediatr Surg Int 2001;17(7):555–9.

115. Nam KJ, Kang HK, Lim JH. Inflammatory pseudotumor of the liver: CT and sonographic findings. AJR Am J Roentgenol 1996;167(2):485–7.

116. Kong W-T, Wang W-P, Cai H, et al. The analysis of enhancement pattern of hepatic inflammatory pseudotumor on contrast-enhanced ultrasound. Abdom Imaging 2014;39(1):168–74.

117. Patnana M, Sevrukov AB, Elsayes KM, et al. Inflammatory pseudotumor: the great mimicker. AJR Am J Roentgenol 2012;198(3):W217–27.

118. Ichikawa S, Motosugi U, Suzuki T, et al. Imaging features of hepatic inflammatory pseudotumor: distinction from colorectal liver metastasis using gadoxetate disodium-enhanced magnetic resonance imaging. Abdom Radiol N Y 2020;45(8): 2400–8.

119. Chang AI, Kim YK, Min JH, et al. Differentiation between inflammatory myofibroblastic tumor and cholangiocarcinoma manifesting as target appearance on gadoxetic acid-enhanced MRI. Abdom Radiol N Y 2019;44(4):1395–406.

Cross-Sectional Imaging Findings of Atypical Liver Malignancies and Diagnostic Pitfalls

Emphasis on Computed Tomography, and Magnetic Resonance Imaging

Michael J. King, MD[a], Indira Laothamatas, MD[a], Arthi Reddy, MD[a], Rebecca Wax, MD[a], Sara Lewis, MD[a,b,*]

KEYWORDS

- Liver malignancy • Hepatocellular carcinoma • Metastases • Sarcoma • Computed tomography
- Magnetic resonance imaging

KEY POINTS

- Atypical liver malignancies, which may be defined as either an atypical appearance of commonly encountered lesions or lesions that are encountered rarely, pose diagnostic challenges at cross-sectional imaging.
- Knowledge of key imaging findings and differential diagnostic considerations can aid in making an accurate diagnosis.

INTRODUCTION

Advances in cross-sectional imaging methods with computed tomography (CT) and magnetic resonance imaging (MRI) have improved the radiologist's ability to noninvasively characterize many liver malignancies with high accuracy. Recent developments include improvements in imaging technique, sequences, protocols, use of newer liver-specific contrast agents (ie, gadoxetic acid for MRI), as well as the incorporation of functional and/or quantitative methods (ie, diffusion-weighted MRI) into routine imaging protocols.

Malignant liver lesions include lesions that originate in the liver (primary) and lesions that are metastatic from other organs (secondary). Often, patients are either asymptomatic or have nonspecific symptoms, and thus present with advanced disease at the time of diagnosis. Apart from hepatocellular carcinoma (HCC), intrahepatic cholangiocarcinoma (ICC), and hepatic metastases, other types of malignant liver lesions are quite rare.[1] As such, despite improvements in imaging methods, atypical liver malignancies, which may be defined as either an atypical appearance of commonly encountered lesions or lesions that are encountered rarely, remain challenging to characterize on imaging. While primary liver malignancies such as HCC, and to a lesser extent ICC, have characteristic and well-described imaging appearances, atypical presentations exist, such as infiltrative, cystic, or intraductal HCC or

---

a Department of Diagnostic, Molecular and Interventional Radiology, Icahn School of Medicine at Mount Sinai, Box 1234. New York, NY 10029, USA; b BioMedical Engineering and Imaging Institute, Icahn School of Medicine Mount Sinai, 1470 Madison Avenue, New York, NY 10029, USA
* Corresponding author. One Gustave Levy Place, Department of Diagnostic, Molecular and Interventional Radiology, Icahn School of Medicine at Mount Sinai, Box 1234. New York, NY 10029.
E-mail address: sara.lewis@mountsinai.org

Radiol Clin N Am 60 (2022) 775–794
https://doi.org/10.1016/j.rcl.2022.05.003

mucinous ICC.[2] The increasingly recognized entity combined hepatocellular-intrahepatic cholangiocarcinoma (cHCC-ICC) is notoriously difficult to diagnose preoperatively or without histologic confirmation.[3] Clearly, accurate diagnosis is essential, as the management and prognosis of these lesions differ drastically. On the other hand, certain hepatic malignancies, such as primary neuroendocrine malignancy, mesenchymal sarcomas, and hematologic malignancy, occur so rarely and are highly variable in appearance, contributing to the challenge of making an accurate diagnosis. Furthermore, certain benign lesions and pseudotumors, such as inflammatory pseudotumor, vascular shunting, focal or confluent hepatic fibrosis, and focal fat deposition can mimic malignancy, especially in oncologic patients or patients at risk for HCC.[4]

Diagnostic radiologists are playing an increasingly important role in the interdisciplinary care of patients. Knowledge of the epidemiologic factors, certain cross-sectional imaging appearances, and key technical and imaging pitfalls can contribute significantly to accurate diagnosis and subsequent patient management. In this article, we review certain technical considerations and focus on atypical appearances of common primary and secondary malignant liver lesions, as well as uncommon malignant liver lesions, with emphasis on CT and MRI.

TECHNICAL PITFALLS
Imaging Technique Considerations

Careful attention to imaging protocol and acquisition technique is essential to enabling accurate liver lesion characterization. Dedicated imaging protocols have been developed and optimized for both CT and MRI, details of which are reported elsewhere.[5,6] Pre/postcontrast imaging is the cornerstone of focal liver lesion detection and characterization, and liver scanning protocols routinely include noncontrast, late arterial phase (AP), portal venous phase (PVP), and equilibrium (EP) or transitional phase (TP) or delayed phase (DP) using either extra-cellular contrast agents (CT and MRI) or liver-specific contrast agents (MRI; gadoxetic acid).

Late arterial phase is defined as hepatic artery enhancement as well as early enhancement of the portal vein, with no or minimal liver parenchymal enhancement, and is essential for the determination of arterial phase hyperenhancement (APHE) that is characteristic of certain hepatic malignancies.[5,7] Special attention to technique, timing, and image quality of late arterial phase MRI with gadoxetic acid is warranted, given the

risk of transient severe motion (TSM) and that the small volume of agent administered may result in a shortened, less avid enhancement duration.[8,9] Finally, while CT scanning is less impacted by patient motion due to rapid acquisition time, voluntary and physiologic involuntary motion during longer-acquisition MRI can result in significant image degradation and artifacts—such as blurring and ghosting which cause image duplicates from misplaced signal—all of which may impede image interpretation.[10]

Image Interpretation Pearls

Uncommonly, HCC or hepatic metastases may contain hemorrhage (ie, RCC, neuroendocrine tumor, lung cancer, or choriocarcinoma) or melanin (ie, melanoma) resulting in T1 hyperintensity or hyperdensity on noncontrast MRI and CT, respectively.[4] Scrutiny of postcontrast subtraction MRI is then recommended to better define the lesion's enhancement characteristics. Registration between pre and postcontrast imaging is needed to avoid artifacts on subtraction imaging, which can be minimized by instructing patients on breath-holding technique. Unlike CT, breath-holding for MRI may be best performed on end-expiration to ensure a more consistent location of the diaphragm. For CT, careful manual region of interest (ROI) measurement or the use of dual-energy CT may be of value to determine enhancement within such lesions.[11]

The presence of moderate to severe steatosis or iron deposition in the background liver can potentially confound the characterization of focal liver lesions as the signal intensity of a lesion is evaluated and compared relative to the background parenchyma. It has also been reported that hepatic steatosis may potentially either mask or mimic liver metastases on CT in oncology patients.[12] Scrutiny of fat sensitive sequences, such as T1 in and opposed phase imaging or dedicated fat and iron quantification sequences on MRI, is recommended to recognize the presence of steatosis or iron deposition to ensure accurate characterization of liver lesions (Fig. 1).[4]

PRIMARY LIVER CANCER
Hepatocyte Origin

Atypical hepatocellular carcinoma
According to international guidelines published by the American Association for the Study of Liver Diseases (AASLD), European Association for the Study of Liver (EASL) and Liver Reporting and Data System (LI-RADS), a liver lesion in the setting of cirrhosis with APHE followed by washout in the PVP or DP on CT or MRI is diagnostic for HCC without the need for pathologic confirmation.[13]

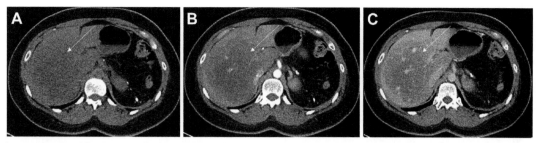

Fig. 1. 36-year-old woman with elevated liver function tests and mass-like hepatic steatosis. Axial noncontrast CT (*A*) demonstrates an ill-defined, mass-like region of decreased attenuation in the right hepatic lobe (*arrow*). The region of decreased attenuation in the right lobe measured 12 HU, compared with 57 HU in the left hepatic lobe. Postcontrast arterial phase (*B*) and portal venous phase (*C*) axial CTs demonstrate an ill-defined region of decreased attenuation in the right hepatic lobe without discrete mass (*arrows*), and otherwise normal background liver. Normal hepatic vessels are seen coursing through the hypoattenuating region without the evidence of mass effect.

However, these imaging criteria have reduced sensitivity (as low as 30%) for HCCs with atypical enhancement.[13] Atypical enhancement patterns are often seen in small and well-differentiated HCCs, and includes iso/hypovascular HCC (ie, without APHE), hypervascular HCC without PVP washout, and HCC that is hyperintense on the hepatobiliary phase (HBP) for MRI performed with liver-specific contrast agents (**Figs. 2** and **3**).[13] Isovascular or hypovascular lesions can be the first sign of early HCC, with a reported prevalence of 14% to 19.5%.[14] Choi and colleagues reported that 96.6% of hypovascular HCCs were also hypointense on the HBP, which, therefore, may be a hallmark of iso/hypovascular HCC.[15] Some HCCs are hypervascular on the AP without washout on the PVP, and there are conflicting studies on whether T2 hyperintensity can be seen as an indicator of HCC in these lesions.[13] Hypointensity on the HBP is a helpful finding but does not differentiate HCC from other lesions such as hepatic hemangiomas which also lack functioning hepatocytes.[16] Approximately 10% of HCCs are hyperintense on the HBP phase, while demonstrating the typical vascular enhancement profile on the dynamic phases of postcontrast imaging[13] However, 3% of HCCs that are hyperintense on the HBP phase may lack PVP or DP washout.[17] This can make it very difficult to distinguish atypical HCC from large regenerative nodules and other benign lesions, although scrutiny of the ancillary findings of T2 hyperintensity or restricted diffusion on diffusion weighted imaging (DWI) may be helpful for diagnosis.

Infiltrative hepatocellular carcinoma

Infiltrative HCC accounts for 7% to 20% of HCC cases and is almost always associated with cirrhosis.[18] The ill-defined appearance poses diagnostic challenges and can also mimic other liver diseases such as hepatic fat deposition, hepatic microabscesses, ICC, and diffuse metastatic disease.[18] Infiltrative HCC usually involves multiple hepatic segments, an entire hepatic lobe, or both lobes. Portal vein thrombosis is a very common finding with a frequency ranging from 68% to 100% and may often be the primary imaging feature.[18] On contrast-enhanced imaging, infiltrative HCC often has a permeative appearance, minimal and inconsistent arterial enhancement, and heterogeneous washout on the PVP. On MRI, the tumor is often heterogeneously T2 hyperintense, homogenously or heterogeneously T1 hypointense, and hyperintense on DWI compared with surrounding liver parenchyma (**Fig. 4**).[18]

Intraductal hepatocellular carcinoma

HCC will occasionally invade the bile ducts and cause bile duct tumor thrombus (BDTT) with a reported incidence of 0.53% to 12.9%.[19] The initial presentation may be obstructive jaundice and can mimic cholangiocarcinoma. Cholangiocarcinoma has a different surgical management from HCC with BDTT, and therefore, preoperative distinction is important, although is very challenging in the absence of liver parenchymal involvement. A retrospective study by Zhou and colleagues of pathologically proven HCC with hilar bile duct tumor thrombus (HBDTT) found that liver parenchymal involvement with an associated intraductal lesion, absence of hilar bile duct wall thickening, and washout in PVP were all found to have high sensitivity and high specificity for HCC with HBDTT.[19] Other imaging features with high specificity for HCC with HBDTT are vascular tumor emboli and splenomegaly. Clinical history of viral hepatitis and elevations of serum alpha-fetoprotein (AFP) level may also aid in the diagnosis.[19]

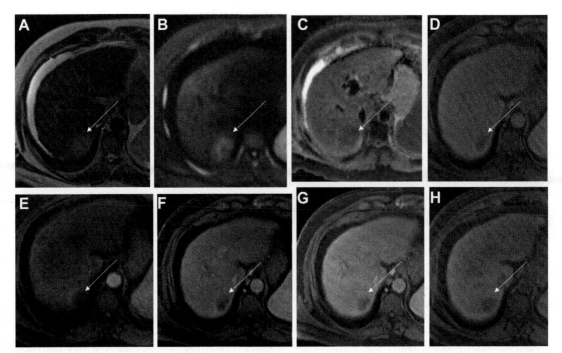

Fig. 2. 58-year-old man with nonalcoholic steatohepatitis undergoing HCC screening presenting with an atypical (hypovascular) HCC. Axial SS FSE T2WI (*A*) demonstrates a mildly T2 hyperintense, well-defined, ovoid mass in subcapsular segment 7 posteriorly (*arrow*). SS EPI DWI (b 800 s/mm2) (*B*) and corresponding ADC map (*C*) demonstrate intralesional restricted diffusion. Axial noncontrast GRE T1WI (*D*), and arterial (*E*), portal venous (*F*), and transitional (*G*) postcontrast phases demonstrate a hypointense mass in segment 7 (*arrows*) with subtle rim arterial phase hyperenhancement and progressive delayed internal enhancement. The lesion is hypointense in the hepatobiliary phase (*H*). Pathology at percutaneous biopsy was consistent with hepatocellular carcinoma.

Cystic hepatocellular carcinoma

HCC that undergoes internal necrosis, cystic degeneration, or hemorrhage can present as a multilocular cystic mass.[20] Cystic HCC is a rare entity generally seen in rapidly growing tumors.[21] Cross-sectional imaging findings that help differentiate cystic HCC from other cystic neoplasms (ie, mucinous cystic neoplasm and metastases) or benign cystic lesions (ie, hepatic abscess, echinococcal cyst, intrahepatic hematoma, and biloma) include the presence of liver cirrhosis, typical imaging characteristics of HCC within the solid components, and vascular invasion.[19,20] Compared with simple fluid, the attenuation of the cystic component of HCC is similar or slightly higher density on CT and has slightly hypointense signal intensity on T2-weighted MRI.[20] Clinical history can help distinguish cystic HCC from HCC treated with locoregional therapies with subsequent liquefactive necrosis, which can appear cystic on cross-sectional imaging.[22]

Fibrolamellar hepatocellular carcinoma

Fibrolamellar HCC mainly occurs in young adults (average age 25 years) without underlying liver disease.[23] These are classically large, well-defined (80%–100%), lobulated tumors with internal heterogeneity that can lead to a variable cross-sectional imaging appearance.[23] Fibrolamellar HCC is typically hypodense on noncontrast CT, and most (approximately 90%) demonstrate heterogeneous APHE. The lesion has a widely variable appearance on PVP CT: 48% of lesions are isodense, 16% are hyperdense, and 36% are hypodense relative to the liver. A central stellate scar is observed in 71% of the lesions. 68% of the scars contain calcifications and 95% of the scars are associated with radial septa.[23] Delayed enhancement of the scar is reported in 25% to 65% of lesions, however, should not be used as a distinguishing feature on CT as focal nodular hyperplasia (FNH) may also demonstrate delayed enhancement of the scar.[23,24]

On MRI, fibrolamellar HCC is typically T1 hypointense and T2 hyperintense, with heterogeneous enhancement on the arterial phase that becomes isointense or hypointense on the PVP and DP following contrast administration.[24] MRI may have an advantage for the characterization of the central scar, as the central scar within fibrolamellar HCC is typically T1 and T2 hypointense, compared

ic neoplasms with invasive

erred to as biliary cystadenomas, c neoplasms (MCN) are biliary neo-osed of mucin-producing epithe-re is a reported 20% risk of sformation to invasive MCN(form-o as biliary cystadenocarcinoma).[53] ely reported as occurring almost emales—theorized to be secondary l feature of ovarian-like subepithelial l has been reported in a small subset nts, typically in the fifth decade of al presentation is widely variable, either being asymptomatic or pre-ight upper quadrant/epigastric pain, lness, and/or a palpable abdominal

very rare entity, with most published nsisting of limited single-center ase reports. There are currently no ed imaging features that differentiate MCN from invasive MCN, and MCNs sected to reliably identify their degree cy.[55–57] The typical appearance of CT and MRI is a large unilocular or cystic mass with enhancement and/ on of the septa, with or without visible es (**Fig. 7**). MCNs typically do not e with an adjacent bile duct, a key g factor from cyst-forming IPN-B.[58] uctal dilatation is, therefore, less ssociated with MCN than IPN-B, and ductal dilatation to the tumor is rarely Recent studies have demonstrated ncement and septations arising from ll without an overlying indentation as itive features of MCN on CT and a subset comparison of noninvasive e MCNs, a mural nodule, calcification, lation, and intra-cystic debris were all tics of invasive MCNs.[60]

cholangiocarcinoma

cholangiocarcinoma (mCCA) is an rare variant of ICC, with nearly all pub-ature on this entity consisting of case Given the lesion's abundant mucin , differentiation from other mucin-lesions (such as invasive IPN-B, inva-, or mucinous metastasis) is prudent s extremely difficult.[61]

generally appears as a large, irregular, mass that may be almost entirely cystic solid/cystic, depending on the degree production (**Fig. 8**). Intra-tumoral calcifi-d portal vein tumor thrombus have been

described. On CT, mCCA is generally hypode and solid components are hypovascular with ripheral enhancement following contrast admini tration, lending to possible confusion with hemangioma. On MRI, it is generally T1 hypoin-tense and T2 hyperintense, and luminal communi-cation between the tumor and bile duct on MRCP sequences may be observed.[61–63] Like the more common mass-forming ICC, upstream biliary obstruction, satellite nodules, adjacent hepatic perfusion anomaly, and parenchymal atrophy may be observed in mCCA.[64]

Neuroendocrine origin

Although mainly occurring in organs of the bron-chopulmonary or gastrointestinal tract, primary neuroendocrine tumors (NETs) can occur in almost any organ.[65] Primary hepatic neuroendocrine tu-mor (PHNET), representing approximately 0.3% of all neuroendocrine tumors, is an extremely rare entity that is difficult to distinguish from the much more common metastatic hepatic NET, with fewer than 200 cases of PHNET reported in the literature.[66,67]

The clinical presentation of PHNET is nonspe-cific and may include vague abdominal pain, jaun-dice, palpable right upper quadrant mass, weight loss, and diarrhea.[67] It has been reported that less than 20% of patients with PHNET present with classic carcinoid syndrome (described as skin flushing, abdominal pain, and episodic diar-rhea).[68–70] Surgical resection is considered the mainstay of treatment, supplemented by systemic chemotherapy, radiation, and targeted locore-gional and molecular therapies.[71]

The imaging appearance of PHNET is similar to metastatic hepatic NET. On CT, the lesion is typi-cally a round, well-circumscribed, hypodense mass that demonstrates heterogeneous APHE following contrast administration. Calcification and/or internal heterogeneity/necrosis are rare yet may become more frequent as tumors grow larger.[71] On MRI, the lesion is generally a round, well-circumscribed, T1 hypointense, T2 hyperin-tense mass with APHE, DP capsule, HBP hypoin-tensity, and diffusion restriction.[67,72] They can demonstrate radiotracer avidity on both FDG and somatostatin receptor analog (eg, gallium-68 DOTATATE) PET.[73]

PRIMARY HEPATIC SARCOMAS
Angiosarcoma

Although primary hepatic angiosarcoma accounts for only 2% of primary hepatic tumors, it is the most common hepatic malignancy of mesen-chymal origin. This tumor demonstrates a strong

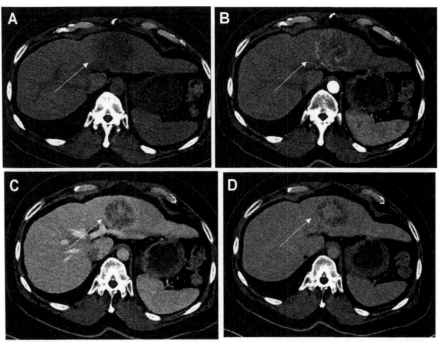

Fig. 3. 69-year-old woman with cirrhosis and incidental liver mass. Axial noncontrast CT (*A*) demonstrates a well-defined hypoattenuating mass in segment 2 (*arrow*). Postcontrast arterial phase (*B*), portal venous phase (*C*), and transitional phase (*D*) axial CTs demonstrate rim arterial phase hyperenhancement, central progressive enhance-ment, and delayed peripheral washout. Pathology at percutaneous biopsy demonstrated poorly differentiated carcinoma, with hepatocellular carcinoma favored over cholangiocarcinoma.

with the scar in FNH which is typically T2 hyperin-tense. Additionally, fibrolamellar HCC does not typically retain hepatobiliary specific contrast agents, which helps to differentiate it from FNH (**Fig. 5**).[24]

Combined hepatocellular carcinoma/intrahepatic cholangiocarcinoma

Combined hepatocellular carcinoma-cholangiocarcinoma (cHCC-ICC) is a rare primary liver tumor that demonstrates imaging and histo-logic features of both HCC and ICC.[25] Given the rarity of this entity, many of its clinical and demo-graphic features, prognostic factors and optimal treatment options remain poorly understood.[26] The preoperative diagnosis of cHCC-ICC is important as patients can proceed to transplant without histology; however, significant overlap of HCC and ICC imaging features and inherent tu-mor heterogeneity make this quite difficult.[27] Pre-vious studies have reported that imaging features of cHCC-ICC more closely resemble ICC and metastasis rather than HCC; however, a recent study of 61 cHCC-ICCs demonstrated that 54.1% of the lesions met LI-RADS criteria for

HCC, and therefore might have originally been misclassified.[28–34]

cHCC-ICC generally appears as a hypodense or isodense mass on noncontrast CT and as a T1 hypointense, T2 intermediate or hyperintense mass on MRI.[35] Diffusion restriction, intralesional fat, hemorrhage, biliary obstruction, tumor thrombus, and/or overlying capsular retraction may be visualized, lending to its individual HCC and ICC components.[27] The enhancement pattern on CT and MRI can also be quite variable, with most cHCC-ICC lesions demonstrating whole-lesion or rim APHE, either with progressive central enhancement, central or peripheral washout, or washout and progression on more delayed phases (**Fig. 6**).[27,31] The presence of washout, washout and progression, intralesional fat, and hemorrhage were all strongly associated with cHCC-ICC when directly compared with ICC.[27]

Biliary Duct Origin

Intraductal papillary neoplasm of the bile duct
Intraductal papillary neoplasm of the bile duct (IPN-B) is analogous to the intraductal

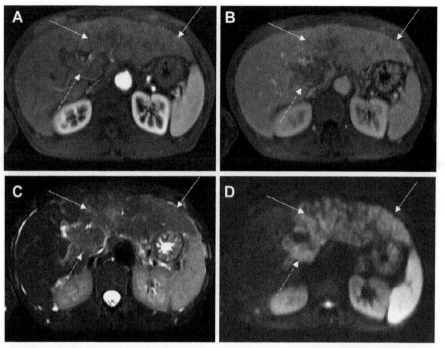

Fig. 4. 57-year-old man with elevated alpha-fetoprotein (AFP) of 544.9 ng/mL and infiltrative HCC. Axial postcontrast GRE T1WI during the arterial phase (*A*) demonstrates heterogenous enhancement in the left lobe, with ill-defined discrete and confluent hypointense nodules on portal venous phase (*arrows*) (*B*). Axial T2 FSE with fat saturation (*C*) and SS EPI DWI (b 800 s/mm2) demonstrate corresponding diffuse and heterogeneous signal hyperintensity in the left lobe, consistent with infiltrative HCC (*arrows*). Expansion of the portal vein with heterogeneous enhancement and T2/DWI hyperintensity are also present, consistent with tumor thrombus (*dashed arrows*).

papillary mucinous neoplasm of the pancreas (IPMN) given that they share similar embryologic, clinical, and histopathologic features.[36,37] Typical clinical presentation involves symptoms

related to biliary obstruction by tumor and/or thick intraductal mucin, including abdominal pain, jaundice, elevated liver enzymes, and cholangitis.[38]

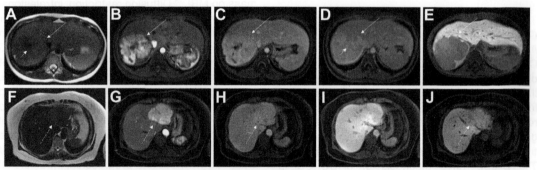

Fig. 5. Similar and contrasting imaging characteristics of fibrolamellar hepatocellular carcinoma (HCC) compared with focal nodular hyperplasia (FNH). Contrast-enhanced MRI using an extracellular contrast agent in a 15-year-old woman with an incidental liver mass reveals a 10.0 cm mildly T2 hyperintense solid mass in segments 7 and 8 (*arrow*) (*A*) with arterial phase hyperenhancement (APHE) (*B*) and no portal venous or equilibrium phase washout (*C, D*). Delayed enhancement of the T2 hypointense central scar is present (short *arrow*). Subsequent MRI with gadoxetic acid-enhanced MRI demonstrates delayed hepatobiliary phase (HBP) hypointensity (*E*). Pathology revealed fibrolamellar HCC. Similar mild T2 hyperintensity and dynamic postcontrast imaging findings are noted in an 8.3 cm solid mass in segments 2 and 3 in a 65-year-old woman (*dashed arrow*) (F through I) on gadoxetic acid-enhanced MRI. Delayed HBP (*J*) in this patient reveals hyperintensity in the lesion, diagnostic for FNH. No central scar was identified in the FNH.

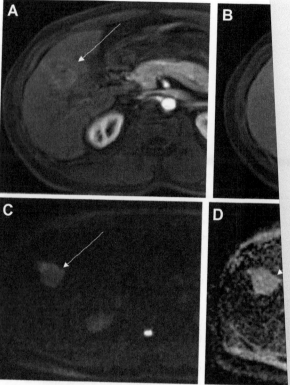

Fig. 6. 46-year-old man with chronic hepatitis B, elevated AFP (44.8 ng/mL~~ ultrasound. Axial GRE T1WI demonstrates a peripherally enhancing mass with progressive whole-lesion enhancement in the portal venous phase (*L~~ responding ADC map (*D*) demonstrate intralesional restricted diffusion, i trahepatic cholangiocarcinoma (ICC). This patient had a normal CA demonstrated cHCC-ICC.

Macroscopically, IPN-B appears as a papillary lesion within a bile duct lumen, with varying degrees of associated mucin production (mucin is detected macroscopically in approximately 1/3 of cases of IPN-B).[39] As the lesion spreads along the bile duct mucosa, multiple lesions can be seen in up to 50% of cases.[40] Surgical resection is considered the treatment of choice as the lesion may demonstrate an invasive component; accurate preoperative diagnosis is, therefore, critical as the lesion is approached surgically similar to a cholangiocarcinoma.[41–43]

Four different imaging manifestations have been described, primarily related to the balance between papillary proliferation and mucin production: (1) mass with proximal duct dilatation; (2) disproportionate duct dilatation without mass; (3) mass with proximal and distal duct dilatation (most common subtype); and (4) cyst forming.[44] When IPN-B is associated with abundant mucin production, it may cause dilatation of the bile duct distal to the lesion, which is considered a characteristic feature.[45] In the cystic subtype,

internal papilla
communication
duct is often a
cystic hepatic I

On CT, the
mass that is g
to surrounding
hypointense to
a papillary filling
on T2-weighted
administration, t
mild hyperintens
does not remain
DP, unlike intradu
shows progressiv
Diffusion restricti
solid components
filling defects on
MRCP.[49,50] Malign
in 31% to 83% of
tion to the above-c
show avidity on FD
biliary enhancemer

Mucinous cys
features
Previously ref
mucinous cyst
plasms comp
lium.[52,53] The
malignant trar
erly referred t
Although wid
exclusively in
to the essentia
stroma—MCN
of male patie
life.[54,55] Clini
with patients
senting with
abdominal fu
mass.[56]

MCN is a
literature co
studies or c
well-establis
noninvasive
are usually re
of malignan
MCN on bot
multilocular
or calcificati
mural nodu
communica
differentiatir
Adjacent d
commonly a
downstrean
observed.[58]
septal enha
the cyst wa
highly sen
MRI.[53,59] I
and invasiv
bile duct d
characteris

Mucinous
Mucinous
extremely
lished liter
reports.
productio
producing
sive MCN
but remai

mCCA
lobulated
or mixed
of mucin
cation an

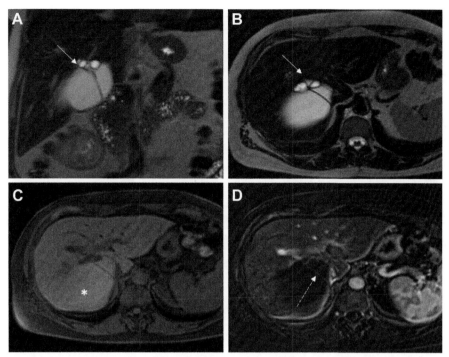

Fig. 7. 51-year-old woman with a multiloculated mucinous cystic neoplasm of the liver. Coronal (*A*) and axial (*B*) SS FSE T2WI demonstrate an 11.0 cm multiloculated cystic mass containing thin septations (*arrows*). On axial noncontrast GRE T1WI (*C*), the largest cystic component contains T1 hyperintense material, consistent with mucin (*asterisk*). Thin perceptible septal enhancement is present in the portal venous phase subtracted GRE T1WI (*dashed arrow*) (*D*). Pathologic diagnosis of multiloculated mucinous cystic neoplasm was confirmed given the presence of simple cuboidal epithelium with underlying "ovarian-like" cellular stroma that was positive for estrogen and progesterone receptors by immunohistochemistry stains following partial hepatectomy.

male predominance, and most commonly presents in the clinical setting of hematologic abnormalities, such as anemia and thrombocytopenia. Exposure to environmental carcinogens, including thorium dioxide (Thorotrast), arsenic, and vinyl chloride has previously been associated with hepatic angiosarcoma; however, exposure to these substances is now uncommon. Moreover, many cases now are reported in the absence of known risk factors.[74]

The diagnosis of hepatic angiosarcoma is often challenging due to the known vascularity and pleomorphic histopathology of this tumor, which result in both an increased risk of hemorrhage with biopsy and a varied spectrum of imaging appearances, respectively.[75] Reported CT findings include multiple small nodules, a large dominant mass, a mixed presentation with a dominant mass and multiple nodules, or diffusely infiltrating tumor.[74] Furthermore, on CT, many of these small nodular lesions are hypodense compared with the normal hepatic parenchyma on both noncontrast and AP, with some cases demonstrating mild hyperenhancement on AP.[74,75] Though often confused with benign hepatic hemangioma,

multiple recent reports have shown the enhancement pattern of hepatic angiosarcoma to vary from hemangioma in multiple ways.[16,74,75] In contrast to the characteristic progressive, nodular, discontinuous centripetal enhancement of hemangiomas, angiosarcomas demonstrate irregular central and rim enhancement of a lower attenuation than that of the aorta.[74] On MRI, larger dominant masses are typically heterogeneous and T2 hyperintense, with or without T1 hyperintense hemorrhagic components and/or fluid-fluid levels representing intra-tumoral necrosis. Postcontrast MRI demonstrates heterogeneous AP and PVP enhancement with progressive enhancement on DP, barring regions of internal necrosis, fibrosis, or hemorrhage (**Fig. 9**).[74,75]

Given the highly variable appearance of angiosarcoma, including overall lesion appearance and enhancement pattern, differential diagnostic considerations include HCC, ICC, and hypovascular and hypervascular metastases. Apart from distinguishing clinical and laboratory features, the progressive enhancement on delayed imaging of angiosarcoma is significant, as it would be atypical of HCC. In addition, periductal enhancement and

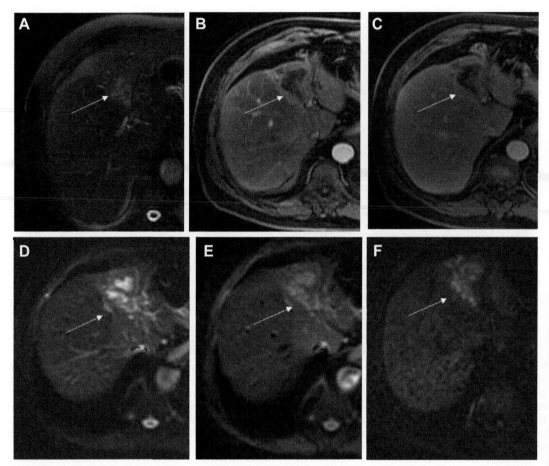

Fig. 8. 73-year-old man with new liver mass. Axial T2 FSE with fat saturation (*A*) axial GRE T1WI with arterial (*B*) and portal venous phases (*C*) and SS EPI DWI with b values of 10 s/mm2 (*D*) 500 s/mm2 (*E*) and 800 s/mm2 (*F*) demonstrate a 5.6 cm lobulated mass in segment 4A (*arrows*) with central areas of marked T2 hyperintensity. The lesion demonstrates minimal peripheral enhancement, surrounding biliary distention, and diffusion restriction. There is severe atrophy of the left lateral segment and perfusion anomaly surrounding the mass. Pathology at resection was consistent with mucinous cholangiocarcinoma.

intrahepatic biliary dilatation are findings that would favor cholangiocarcinoma.[74,76,77]

Hepatic Epithelioid Hemangioendothelioma

Hepatic epithelioid hemangioendothelioma (HEHE) is a rare and low-grade malignant tumor of vascular origin with an increased female predominance. Approximately 36% of patients demonstrate extra-hepatic lesions at diagnosis, most commonly within the lungs, lymph nodes, and peritoneum. Accurate diagnosis is essential as HEHE can often be treated with surgical resection or transplantation regardless of the presence of metastatic disease. However, diagnosis remains challenging due to the variable clinical presentation and the range of potential imaging appearances.[76,78]

Most cases of HEHE demonstrate multifocal and peripherally distributed or subcapsular lesions, which ultimately increase in size and coalesce to form larger confluent masses.[76,78] Capsular retraction and hypertrophy of the normal hepatic parenchyma have been reported. The most common cross-sectional imaging appearance is multifocal low-density hepatic nodules of varying sizes (**Fig. 10**). Earlier stage disease, as mentioned above, demonstrates a multifocal and peripheral nodular pattern, while more progressed forms have confluent masses. Associated calcification or central hypodensity on nonenhanced CT images, possibly reflecting central necrosis, are also described. Postcontrast CT images demonstrated mild peripheral enhancement in some cases.[79] On MRI, lesions typically demonstrate T1 hypointensity with heterogeneous or

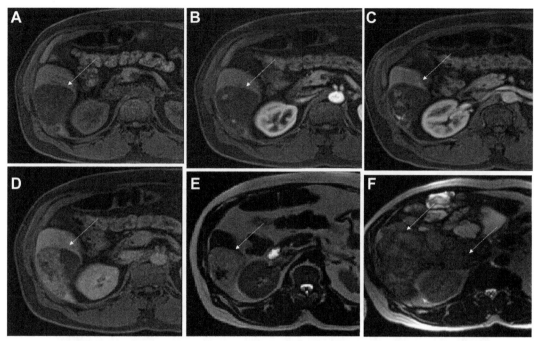

Fig. 9. 57-year-old man with hepatic epitheloid angiosarcoma. Axial noncontrast GRE T1WI (*A*) and arterial (*B*) portal venous (*C*) and transitional (*D*) postcontrast phases demonstrate a dominant hypointense mass in segment 6 (*arrows*) with progressive heterogeneous internal enhancement. No significant hemorrhage or necrosis was identified in the lesion. Three-month follow-up axial SS FSE T2WI (*E-F*) demonstrates significant tumor progression.

targetoid T2 hyperintensity. Most lesions also demonstrate immediate peripheral enhancement on postcontrast sequences. Delayed postcontrast sequences showed progressive central filling in some cases. The differential diagnosis is quite extensive, including hemangiomas, abscesses, FNH, HCC, and metastases.

The lollipop sign is an imaging sign that has been reported to increase the specificity and recognition of HEHE on cross-sectional imaging.[78,79] The lollipop sign has two components, the first being the round, well-circumscribed hypodense tumor, most commonly with an avascular core (the candy), and the second being an adjacent histologically occluded vein (the stick). Additional reported but uncommon imaging characteristics include cavitating or complex exophytic tumor, the presence of a central enhancing scar, or hyperenhancement of the lesion.[79,80]

Fibrosarcoma

Fibrosarcoma is a malignant tumor derived from fibroblasts and usually occurs in the limbs, head and neck, and the trunk, while rarely occurring in the viscera. According to Ito and colleagues from 1924 to 1990, only 33 cases of hepatic fibrosarcoma were reported in the literature.[81] Currently,

diagnosis is made at pathology as there is no imaging finding characteristic for hepatic fibrosarcoma. Case reports have described lesions containing cystic degeneration and hemorrhage, portal vein involvement, or heterogeneous AP enhancement at CT.[82,83]

Leiomyosarcoma

Primary hepatic leiomyosarcoma is extremely rare, with probable origin from the smooth muscle cells of the hepatic veins or bile ducts. Most cases generally reflect metastases from extra-hepatic sites, including the gastrointestinal system, uterus, retroperitoneum, or lung. The tumor is most commonly found in middle-aged or older patients without a gender predisposition or a clear association with chronic hepatic disease or cirrhosis.[84] Interestingly, an increased number of cases of primary hepatic leiomyosarcoma in a younger population with human immunodeficiency virus (HIV) and in immunosuppressed transplant patients have recently been reported.[85]

The most frequently described finding is a large, well-circumscribed, and heterogeneously hypodense mass with internal enhancement on postcontrast CT. An appropriate clinical history is essential as additional studies have reported an

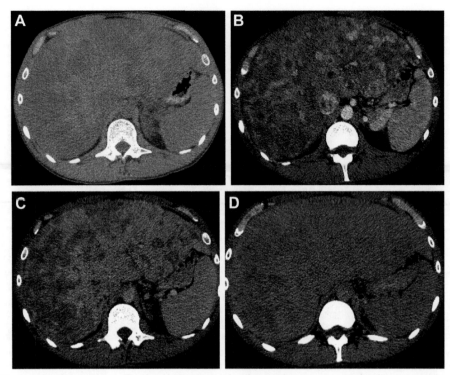

Fig. 10. 32-year-old man with epigastric pain and hepatic epithelioid hemangioendothelioma. Axial noncontrast CT (*A*) demonstrates extensive, confluent hypodense masses throughout both hepatic lobes. Postcontrast arterial phase (*B*) portal venous phase (*C*) and delayed phase (*D*) axial CTs demonstrate innumerable predominantly rim-enhancing lesions on the arterial phase with progressive central filling.

enhancing, thickened wall, which may mimic the findings of an abscess or hydatid cyst.[86] On MRI, these lesions generally demonstrate homogenous or heterogenous T1 signal, which may reflect internal hemorrhage, with associated high signal on T2-weighted sequences. Marked enhancement on the delayed postcontrast sequences is also generally noted without significant enhancement on arterial or venous phase.[83,87]

Kaposi Sarcoma

Kaposi sarcoma is a low-grade malignancy associated with human herpesvirus-8 (HHV-8) and is the most common intrahepatic neoplasm in patients with acquired immunodeficiency syndrome (AIDS). Less commonly, Kaposi sarcoma has also been reported in immunocompromised solid organ transplant recipients.[76]

Hepatic Kaposi sarcoma most commonly presents as multifocal parenchymal nodules, usually originating from the perivascular regions of the peripheral portal venous branches. Multiple hypoattenuating nodules in a perivascular and periportal distribution are noted on noncontrast CT. No significant associated enhancement is generally noted on AP or PVP, although there may be diffuse

enhancement on DP.[76,88,89] Other differential diagnoses include metastatic lesions, fungal microabscesses, and multiple hemangiomas, for which associated Kaposi cutaneous involvement would be most helpful in narrowing the diagnosis.

Malignant Fibrous Histiocytosarcoma/ Histiocytoma

Although malignant fibrous histiocytosarcoma (MFH) is the most common soft tissue sarcoma in the adult population, involvement of the visceral organs, including the liver, is very rare.[90] Most cases occur in adults over the age of fifty with a slight male predominance. The complex internal architecture of these tumors, including hemorrhage, necrosis, myxoid degeneration, and/or fibrosis results in a large, heterogenous, and predominantly hypodense mass on noncontrast CT images with occasional involvement of the adjacent liver capsule. A spectrum of postenhancement appearances has been noted including a large heterogeneously enhancing mass with internal necrosis, a large mass with an enhancing peripheral pseudo-capsule, as well as a multiloculated cystic mass with progressively enhancing fibrotic internal septations. Despite

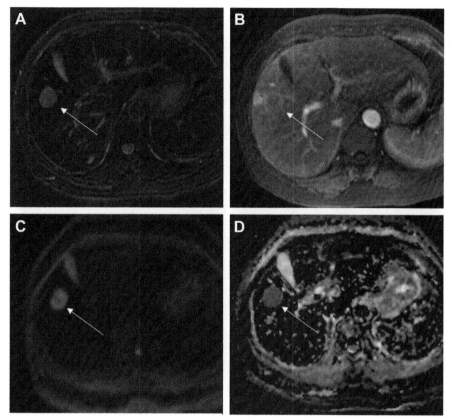

Fig. 11. 58-year-old woman with a history of allogeneic stem cell transplant for acute myeloid leukemia (AML) presenting with multiple liver lesions. Axial T2 FSE with fat saturation (*A*) demonstrates a 2.7 cm well-defined, T2 hyperintense mass in segment 5 (*arrow*). There is peripheral and mild central enhancement with surrounding shunting on portal venous phase GRE T1WI (*B*). Axial SS EPI DWI (b 800 s/mm2) (*C*) and corresponding ADC map (*D*) demonstrate intralesional diffusion restriction. Diffuse iron deposition is noted in the background liver, as evidenced by marked T2, DWI, and ADC hypointensity. Subsequent biopsy of this lesion revealed posttransplant lymphoproliferative disease (PTLD).

the rather aggressive appearance of hepatic MFH, there has been no report of bile duct obstruction, portal vein occlusion, or lymph node metastasis.[1]

Similarly, the few reported cases with MRI demonstrated a large, predominantly T1 hypointense and T2 hyperintense, lobulated mass with well-circumscribed margins and associated heterogenous and progressive enhancement. Although there is no distinctive imaging feature, hepatic MFH should be considered in a patient with an aggressive-appearing and large necrotic/cystic lesion of unknown etiology.[1,87,90]

HEMATOLOGIC ORIGIN
Primary Hepatic Lymphoma

Primary hepatic lymphoma (PHL) is a subset of non-Hodgkin lymphoma that is confined to the liver and perihepatic lymph nodes without distant involvement for at least 6 months after disease

onset.[91] Although liver involvement is common in systemic lymphoma, PHL is exceedingly rare, accounting for less than 0.4% of extranodal lymphoma and is rising in incidence.[92] As the treatment of PHL consists primarily of combination chemotherapy, correct diagnosis is crucial and may spare the patient from surgical resection.

PHL is variable in appearance and most frequently presents as a solitary mass or multiple masses. A diffuse or infiltrative pattern is rare and confers a worse prognosis.[85] On CT, PHL presents as a solitary or multiple hypoattenuating masses, and may appear heterogeneous due to internal hemorrhage or necrosis. Calcification in untreated lesions is rare.[93] Following contrast administration, PHL may demonstrate minimal to no enhancement, patchy enhancement, or rim enhancement.[94] On MRI with liver-specific contrast agents, PHL is typically T1 hypointense, T2 hyperintense, and demonstrates hypointense

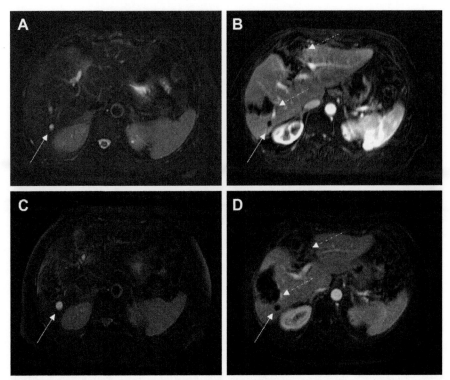

Fig. 12. 62-year-old woman with a history of cystic neuroendocrine liver metastases. Axial T2 FSE with fat satu-ration (*A*) demonstrates a 6 mm T2 hyperintense cyst in segment 6 (*arrow*) without enhancement on portal venous phase postcontrast GRE T1WI (*B*). The patient had previously undergone surgical wedge resection and ablation of other hepatic metastatic lesions in segments 4 and 6 (dashed *arrows*). Follow-up MRI 6 months later demonstrates interval enlargement of the segment 6 cystic lesion on axial T2 FSE with fat saturation (*C*) and sub-tracted portal venous phase postcontrast GRE T1WI (*D*), now measuring 12 mm.

signal on HBP.[95] Like other lymphomas, PHL dem-onstrates hyperintense signal on DWI with corre-sponding low ADC values reflective of their hypercellularity. Whole-body DWI has been shown to be comparable to FDG-PET/CT for the staging of lymphoma.[96]

Posttransplant Lymphoproliferative Disease

Posttransplant lymphoproliferative disease (PTLD) describes a spectrum of disease ranging from benign lymphoid hyperplasia to frank lymphoma following solid organ or hematopoietic stem cell transplant. It is associated with Epstein–Barr virus reactivation in the setting of immunosuppres-sion.[97] The first-line treatment is a reduction in immunosuppression, while other treatment modal-ities include rituximab, chemotherapy, radiation, and/or antiviral therapy.[97] Extranodal disease is more common than nodal disease in PTLD, with the liver being the most involved abdominal solid organ.[98]

Hepatic involvement of PTLD may manifest (in descending order of frequency) as focal liver mass or masses, ill-defined infiltrative lesions, or

as a porta hepatis mass, potentially causing hepa-tomegaly and biliary obstruction.[99] While vascular encasement may occur in PTLD, vessel invasion, thrombosis or occlusion is rare.[100] PTLD lesions are typically hypoattenuating with minimal to ab-sent contrast enhancement on CT. On MRI, PTLD typically demonstrates hypointense signal on T1, mildly hyperintense signal on T2, with min-imal to absent enhancement on postcontrast se-quences (**Fig. 11**).[99] Similar to other lymphomas, PTLD demonstrates hyperintense signal on DWI with corresponding low ADC values, making whole-body DWI a potentially viable alternative to FDG-PET-CT for the diagnosis, staging, and assessment of treatment response in patients with PTLD.[96,101]

METASTATIC DISEASE

Due in part to its dual vascular supply, the liver is one of the most frequent sites of metastasis. A study by Horn and colleagues using data from the Surveillance, Epidemiology, and End Results (SEER) database found that 5.1% of patients

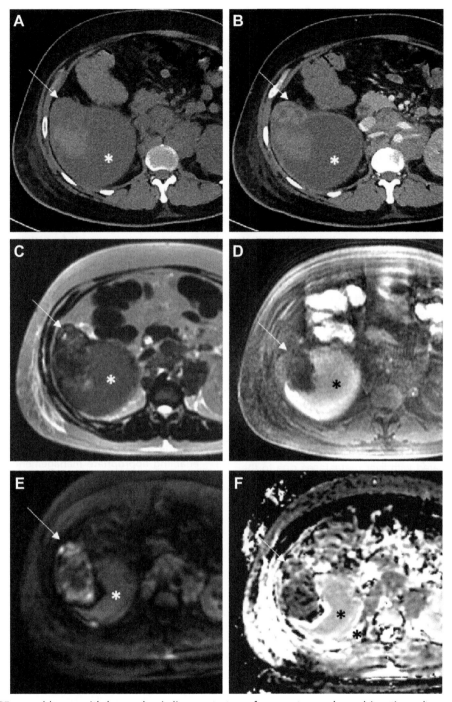

Fig. 13. 35-year-old man with hemorrhagic liver metastases from gastroesophageal junction adenocarcinoma. Pre (*A*) and postcontrast (*B*) axial CTs demonstrate a complex cystic-solid mass in hepatic segments 5/6, with a 4.0 cm enhancing component along the anterior margin (*arrows*) and a complex predominantly low attenuation cystic component posteriorly (*asterisk*). MRI was then performed for further characterization, revealing T2 intermediate (*C*) and T1 hyperintense (*D*) material in the posterior component, most consistent with hemorrhage (*asterisk*). Axial SS EPI DWI (b 800 s/mm2) (*E*) and corresponding ADC map (*F*) demonstrate intralesional restricted diffusion. Metastatic retroperitoneal lymphadenopathy is also noted.

have synchronous liver metastasis at the time of primary cancer diagnosis and that survival for patients with liver metastasis was significantly decreased compared with patients without liver metastasis.[102] The imaging features of hepatic metastases are highly variable and often depend on histology of the primary malignancy; however, atypical features include cystic components and hemorrhage, which are discussed herein.

Cystic Hepatic Metastases

Liver metastases may be cystic due to high mucin content reflective of the primary tumor, such as in ovarian cystadenocarcinoma or colorectal adenocarcinoma. Alternatively, the cystic component may be secondary to necrosis in metastasis that has been treated or has outgrown its blood supply. In general, cystic metastases have ill-defined borders, irregular walls, and demonstrate early arterial rim enhancement on CT and MRI.[103] On occasion, these metastases may be purely cystic (**Fig. 12**). The differential diagnosis includes polycystic liver disease, biliary hamartomas, abscesses, cystic HCC, and MCN or invasive MCN.[104]

Hemorrhagic Hepatic Metastases

Both hypervascular and hypovascular liver metastases have been reported to cause hepatic hemorrhage. However, hemoperitoneum is more frequently seen in association with primary liver tumors compared with liver metastases due to the higher degree of vascularity in primary liver tumors.[105] The hemorrhage may be contained or may rupture into the peritoneal space and potentially cause hemorrhagic shock and intraperitoneal tumor spillage. In the acute phase, hemorrhagic hepatic metastases are typically hyperattenuating on noncontrast CT and gradually decrease in attenuation over time. The MRI appearance of hemorrhagic hepatic metastases is highly variable depending on the age of the blood products (**Fig. 13**). The differential diagnosis includes hemorrhage into benign lesions (ie, hepatocellular adenoma) or primary liver malignancy (ie, HCC), rupture of a hepatic artery aneurysm, and spontaneous hepatic rupture in patients at risk for bleeding complications.[106]

SUMMARY

Atypical liver malignancies, which may be defined as either an atypical appearance of commonly encountered lesions or lesions that are encountered rarely, may present with a myriad of imaging appearances. Such variability at imaging poses a diagnostic challenge for the radiologist. Ultimately,

knowledge of the patient's clinical history, laboratory values, pertinent imaging findings, as well as discussion in a multi-disciplinary setting, may enable an accurate diagnosis noninvasively. In this review, we sought to summarize the key CT and MRI findings in the context of clinical information for such liver lesions. The radiologist's enhanced knowledge of atypical liver malignancies will help achieve accurate diagnosis, and thus improved clinical treatment planning and patient care.

CLINICS CARE POINTS

- Liver malignancies result from the development of tumor from variety of cells in the liver (hepatocytes, biliary epithelium, hepatocytes, lymphocytes, neuroendocrine cells, et cetera) and secondarily from spread to the liver from other sites (metastatic disease).

- Certain tumors may have a characteristic appearance on cross sectional imaging, while certain tumors can be highly variable in appearance.

- The diagnostic radiologist's knowledge of atypical liver malignancies and unusual presentations of more common liver malignancies can aid the multidisciplinary clinical team in reaching the correct diagnosis and enabling appropriate management for the patient.

- Careful attention to imaging protocols and awareness of certain technical pitfalls can help in avoiding imaging misinterpretation.

DISCLOSURE

The authors have nothing to disclose.

REFERENCES

1. Tan Y, Xiao EH. Rare hepatic malignant tumors: dynamic CT, MRI, and clinicopathologic features: with analysis of 54 cases and review of the literature. Abdom Imaging 2013;38(3):511–26.
2. Kim JH, Joo I, Lee JM. Atypical appearance of hepatocellular carcinoma and its mimickers: how to solve challenging cases using gadoxetic acid-enhanced liver magnetic resonance imaging. Korean J Radiol 2019;20(7):1019–41.
3. Lewis S, et al. Volumetric quantitative histogram analysis using diffusion-weighted magnetic resonance imaging to differentiate HCC from other primary liver cancers. Abdom Radiol (NY) 2019;44(3):912–22.

4. Siegelman ES, Chauhan A. MR characterization of focal liver lesions: pearls and pitfalls. Magn Reson Imaging Clin N Am 2014;22(3):295–313.

5. Donato H, et al. Liver MRI: From basic protocol to advanced techniques. Eur J Radiol 2017;93:30–9.

6. Kartalis N, Brehmer K, Loizou L. Multi-detector CT: Liver protocol and recent developments. Eur J Radiol 2017;97:101–9.

7. Erkan B, et al. Non-invasive diagnostic criteria of hepatocellular carcinoma: Comparison of diagnostic accuracy of updated LI-RADS with clinical practice guidelines of OPTN-UNOS, AASLD, NCCN, EASL-EORTC, and KLSCG-NCC. PLoS One 2019;14(12):e0226291.

8. Chernyak V, et al. Use of gadoxetate disodium in patients with chronic liver disease and its implications for liver imaging reporting and data system (LI-RADS). J Magn Reson Imaging 2019;49(5):1236–52.

9. Aslam A, et al. Assessing locoregional treatment response to Hepatocellular Carcinoma: comparison of hepatobiliary contrast agents to extracellular contrast agents. Abdom Radiol (NY) 2021;46(8):3565–78.

10. Wile GE, Leyendecker JR. Magnetic resonance imaging of the liver: sequence optimization and artifacts. Magn Reson Imaging Clin N Am 2010;18(3):525–547, xi.

11. Marin D, et al. State of the art: dual-energy CT of the abdomen. Radiology 2014;271(2):327–42.

12. Karcaaltincaba M, Akhan O. Imaging of hepatic steatosis and fatty sparing. Eur J Radiol 2007;61(1):33–43.

13. Kovac JD, et al. An overview of hepatocellular carcinoma with atypical enhancement pattern: spectrum of magnetic resonance imaging findings with pathologic correlation. Radiol Oncol 2021;55(2):130–43.

14. Leoni S, et al. The impact of vascular and nonvascular findings on the noninvasive diagnosis of small hepatocellular carcinoma based on the EASL and AASLD criteria. Am J Gastroenterol 2010;105(3):599–609.

15. Choi JW, et al. Hepatocellular carcinoma: imaging patterns on gadoxetic acid-enhanced MR Images and their value as an imaging biomarker. Radiology 2013;267(3):776–86.

16. White PG, Adams H, Smith PM. The computed tomographic appearances of angiosarcoma of the liver. Clin Radiol 1993;48(5):321–5.

17. Renzulli M, Golfieri R, Bologna Liver Oncology Group. Proposal of a new diagnostic algorithm for hepatocellular carcinoma based on the Japanese guidelines but adapted to the Western world for patients under surveillance for chronic liver disease. J Gastroenterol Hepatol 2016;31(1):69–80.

18. Reynolds AR, et al. Infiltrative hepatocellular carcinoma: what radiologists need to know. Radiographics 2015;35(2):371–86.

19. Zhou X, et al. Hepatocellular carcinoma with hilar bile duct tumor thrombus versus hilar Cholangiocarcinoma on enhanced computed tomography: a diagnostic challenge. BMC Cancer 2020;20(1):54.

20. Qian LJ, et al. Spectrum of multilocular cystic hepatic lesions: CT and MR imaging findings with pathologic correlation. Radiographics 2013;33(5):1419–33.

21. Vachha B, et al. Cystic lesions of the liver. AJR Am J Roentgenol 2011;196(4):W355–66.

22. Abraham SC, et al. Histologic abnormalities are common in protocol liver allograft biopsies from patients with normal liver function tests. Am J Surg Pathol 2008;32(7):965–73.

23. Ichikawa T, et al. Fibrolamellar hepatocellular carcinoma: imaging and pathologic findings in 31 recent cases. Radiology 1999;213(2):352–61.

24. Ganeshan D, et al. Imaging features of fibrolamellar hepatocellular carcinoma. AJR Am J Roentgenol 2014;202(3):544–52.

25. Yin X, et al. Combined hepatocellular carcinoma and cholangiocarcinoma: clinical features, treatment modalities, and prognosis. Ann Surg Oncol 2012;19(9):2869–76.

26. Jarnagin WR, et al. Combined hepatocellular and cholangiocarcinoma: demographic, clinical, and prognostic factors. Cancer 2002;94(7):2040–6.

27. Sammon J, et al. MRI features of combined hepatocellular- cholangiocarcinoma versus mass forming intrahepatic cholangiocarcinoma. Cancer Imaging 2018;18(1):8.

28. de Campos RO, et al. Combined hepatocellular carcinoma-cholangiocarcinoma: report of MR appearance in eleven patients. J Magn Reson Imaging 2012;36(5):1139–47.

29. Hwang J, et al. Differentiating combined hepatocellular and cholangiocarcinoma from mass-forming intrahepatic cholangiocarcinoma using gadoxetic acid-enhanced MRI. J Magn Reson Imaging 2012;36(4):881–9.

30. Fowler KJ, et al. Combined hepatocellular and cholangiocarcinoma (biphenotypic) tumors: imaging features and diagnostic accuracy of contrast-enhanced CT and MRI. AJR Am J Roentgenol 2013;201(2):332–9.

31. Potretzke TA, et al. imaging features of biphenotypic primary liver carcinoma (hepatocholangiocarcinoma) and the potential to mimic hepatocellular carcinoma: LI-RADS analysis of CT and MRI features in 61 cases. AJR Am J Roentgenol 2016;207(1):25–31.

32. Aoki K, et al. Combined hepatocellular carcinoma and cholangiocarcinoma: clinical features and

computed tomographic findings. Hepatology 1993; 18(5):1090–5.

33. Jeon TY, et al. The value of gadobenate dimeglumine-enhanced hepatobiliary-phase MR imaging for the differentiation of scirrhous hepatocellular carcinoma and cholangiocarcinoma with or without hepatocellular carcinoma. Abdom Imaging 2010;35(3):337–45.

34. Wells ML, et al. Biphenotypic hepatic tumors: imaging findings and review of literature. Abdom Imaging 2015;40(7):2293–305.

35. Maximin S, et al. Current update on combined hepatocellular-cholangiocarcinoma. Eur J Radiol Open 2014;1:40–8.

36. Ohtsuka M, et al. Similarities and differences between intraductal papillary tumors of the bile duct with and without macroscopically visible mucin secretion. Am J Surg Pathol 2011;35(4):512–21.

37. Kloek JJ, et al. A comparative study of intraductal papillary neoplasia of the biliary tract and pancreas. Hum Pathol 2011;42(6):824–32.

38. Egri C, et al. intraductal papillary neoplasm of the bile duct: multimodality imaging appearances and pathological correlation. Can Assoc Radiol J 2017;68(1):77–83.

39. Katabathina VS, et al. Biliary diseases with pancreatic counterparts": cross-sectional imaging findings. Radiographics 2016;36(2):374–92.

40. Kang MJ, et al. Impact of macroscopic morphology, multifocality, and mucin secretion on survival outcome of intraductal papillary neoplasm of the bile duct. J Gastrointest Surg 2013;17(5):931–8.

41. Fuente I, et al. intraductal papillary neoplasm of the bile duct (IPNB): case report and literature review of a challenging disease to diagnose. J Gastrointest Cancer 2019;50(3):578–82.

42. Luvira V, et al. Long-term outcome of surgical resection for intraductal papillary neoplasm of the bile duct. J Gastroenterol Hepatol 2017;32(2):527–33.

43. Ohtsuka M, et al. Intraductal papillary neoplasms of the bile duct. Int J Hepatol 2014;2014:459091.

44. Park HJ, et al. Intraductal papillary neoplasm of the bile duct: clinical, imaging, and pathologic features. AJR Am J Roentgenol 2018;211(1):67–75.

45. Wu CH, et al. Comparative radiological pathological study of biliary intraductal tubulopapillary neoplasm and biliary intraductal papillary mucinous neoplasm. Abdom Radiol (NY) 2017; 42(10):2460–9.

46. Lim JH, et al. Cyst-forming intraductal papillary neoplasm of the bile ducts: description of imaging and pathologic aspects. AJR Am J Roentgenol 2011;197(5):1111–20.

47. Ogawa H, et al. CT findings of intraductal papillary neoplasm of the bile duct: assessment with multiphase contrast-enhanced examination using multi-detector CT. Clin Radiol 2012;67(3):224–31.

48. Wan XS, et al. Intraductal papillary neoplasm of the bile duct. World J Gastroenterol 2013;19(46): 8595–604.

49. Hong GS, et al. Thread sign in biliary intraductal papillary mucinous neoplasm: a novel specific finding for MRI. Eur Radiol 2016;26(9):3112–20.

50. Lim JH, Jang KT, Choi D. Biliary intraductal papillary-mucinous neoplasm manifesting only as dilatation of the hepatic lobar or segmental bile ducts: imaging features in six patients. AJR Am J Roentgenol 2008;191(3):778–82.

51. Schlitter AM, et al. Intraductal papillary neoplasms of the bile duct: stepwise progression to carcinoma involves common molecular pathways. Mod Pathol 2014;27(1):73–86.

52. Bosman FT, World Health Organization., International Agency for Research on Cancer. WHO classification of tumours of the digestive system. In: World Health Organization classification of tumours. 4th edition. Lyon: International Agency for Research on Cancer; 2010. p. 417.

53. Boyum JH, et al. Hepatic mucinous cystic neoplasm versus simple biliary cyst: assessment of distinguishing imaging features using CT and MRI. AJR Am J Roentgenol 2021;216(2):403–11.

54. Choi HK, et al. Differential diagnosis for intrahepatic biliary cystadenoma and hepatic simple cyst: significance of cystic fluid analysis and radiologic findings. J Clin Gastroenterol 2010;44(4): 289–93.

55. Arnaoutakis DJ, et al. Management of biliary cystic tumors: a multi-institutional analysis of a rare liver tumor. Ann Surg 2015;261(2):361–7.

56. Simo KA, et al. Invasive biliary mucinous cystic neoplasm: a review. HPB (Oxford) 2012;14(11): 725–40.

57. Sang X, et al. Hepatobiliary cystadenomas and cystadenocarcinomas: a report of 33 cases. Liver Int 2011;31(9):1337–44.

58. Kim HJ, et al. CT differentiation of mucin-producing cystic neoplasms of the liver from solitary bile duct cysts. AJR Am J Roentgenol 2014;202(1):83–91.

59. Kovacs MD, et al. Differentiating biliary cystadenomas from benign hepatic cysts: Preliminary analysis of new predictive imaging features. Clin Imaging 2018;49:44–7.

60. Seo JK, et al. Appropriate diagnosis of biliary cystic tumors: comparison with atypical hepatic simple cysts. Eur J Gastroenterol Hepatol 2010; 22(8):989–96.

61. Hagiwara K, et al. Resected primary mucinous cholangiocarcinoma of the liver. Surg Case Rep 2018;4(1):41.

62. Sumiyoshi T, et al. Mucinous cholangiocarcinoma: clinicopathological features of the rarest type of cholangiocarcinoma. Ann Gastroenterol Surg 2017;1(2):114–21.

63. Hayashi M, et al. Imaging findings of mucinous type of cholangiocellular carcinoma. J Comput Assist Tomogr 1996;20(3):386–9.

64. King MJ, et al. Outcomes assessment in intrahepatic cholangiocarcinoma using qualitative and quantitative imaging features. Cancer Imaging 2020;20(1):43.

65. Scarsbrook AF, et al. Anatomic and functional imaging of metastatic carcinoid tumors. Radiographics 2007;27(2):455–77.

66. Touloumis Z, et al. Primary hepatic carcinoid; a diagnostic dilemma: a case report. Cases J 2008; 1(1):314.

67. Quartey B. Primary hepatic neuroendocrine tumor: what do we know now? World J Oncol 2011;2(5): 209–16.

68. Lin CW, et al. Primary hepatic carcinoid tumor: a case report and review of the literature. Cases J 2009;2(1):90.

69. Nikfarjam M, Muralidharan V, Christophi C. Primary hepatic carcinoid tumours. HPB (Oxford) 2004; 6(1):13–7.

70. Gravante G, et al. Primary carcinoids of the liver: a review of symptoms, diagnosis and treatments. Dig Surg 2008;25(5):364–8.

71. Kim JE, et al. Three-phase helical computed tomographic findings of hepatic neuroendocrine tumors: pathologic correlation with revised WHO classification. J Comput Assist Tomogr 2011; 35(6):697–702.

72. Yang K, et al. Primary hepatic neuroendocrine tumors: multi-modal imaging features with pathological correlations. Cancer Imaging 2017;17(1):20.

73. Orlefors H, et al. Whole-body (11)C-5-hydroxytryptophan positron emission tomography as a universal imaging technique for neuroendocrine tumors: comparison with somatostatin receptor scintigraphy and computed tomography. J Clin Endocrinol Metab 2005;90(6):3392–400.

74. Koyama T, et al. Primary hepatic angiosarcoma: findings at CT and MR imaging. Radiology 2002; 222(3):667–73.

75. Yang KF, et al. Primary hepatic angiosarcoma: difficulty in clinical, radiological, and pathological diagnosis. Med J Malaysia 2012;67(1):127–8.

76. Thampy R, et al. Imaging features of rare mesenychmal liver tumours: beyond haemangiomas. Br J Radiol 2017;90(1079):20170373.

77. Chung YE, et al. Varying appearances of cholangiocarcinoma: radiologic-pathologic correlation. Radiographics 2009;29(3):683–700.

78. Epelboym Y, et al. Imaging findings in epithelioid hemangioendothelioma. Clin Imaging 2019;58: 59–65.

79. Alomari AI. The lollipop sign: a new cross-sectional sign of hepatic epithelioid hemangioendothelioma. Eur J Radiol 2006;59(3):460–4.

80. Wu CH, et al. Uncommon liver tumors: case report and literature review. Medicine (Baltimore) 2016; 95(39):e4952.

81. Ito Y, et al. A case report of primary fibrosarcoma of the liver. Gastroenterol Jpn 1990;25(6):753–7.

82. Huang ML, et al. Hepatic fibrosarcoma in a middle-aged man. Int J Clin Exp Pathol 2019;12(9): 3555–9.

83. Ali S, et al. Primary fibrosarcoma of the liver: we don't know much: a case report. Case Rep Gastroenterol 2008;2(3):384–9.

84. Chi M, Dudek AZ, Wind KP. Primary hepatic leiomyosarcoma in adults: analysis of prognostic factors. Onkologie 2012;35(4):210–4.

85. Emile JF, et al. Primary non-Hodgkin's lymphomas of the liver with nodular and diffuse infiltration patterns have different prognoses. Ann Oncol 2001; 12(7):1005–10.

86. Ferrozzi F, et al. Primary liver leiomyosarcoma: CT appearance. Abdom Imaging 1996;21(2):157–60.

87. Yu RS, et al. Primary hepatic sarcomas: CT findings. Eur Radiol 2008;18(10):2196–205.

88. Restrepo CS, et al. Imaging manifestations of Kaposi sarcoma. Radiographics 2006;26(4): 1169–85.

89. Luburich P, et al. Hepatic Kaposi sarcoma in AIDS: US and CT findings. Radiology 1990;175(1):172–4.

90. Kim KA, et al. Unusual mesenchymal liver tumors in adults: radiologic-pathologic correlation. AJR Am J Roentgenol 2006;187(5):W481–9.

91. Caccamo D, Pervez NK, Marchevsky A. Primary lymphoma of the liver in the acquired immunodeficiency syndrome. Arch Pathol Lab Med 1986; 110(6):553–5.

92. Padhan RK, Das P, Shalimar. Primary hepatic lymphoma. Trop Gastroenterol 2015;36(1):14–20.

93. Apter S, et al. Calcification in lymphoma occurring before therapy: CT features and clinical correlation. AJR Am J Roentgenol 2002;178(4):935–8.

94. Ippolito D, et al. Diagnostic approach in hepatic lymphoma: radiological imaging findings and literature review. J Cancer Res Clin Oncol 2020; 146(6):1545–58.

95. Colagrande S, et al. MRI features of primary hepatic lymphoma. Abdom Radiol (NY) 2018;43(9):2277–87.

96. Kharuzhyk S, et al. Comparison of whole-body MRI with diffusion-weighted imaging and PET/CT in lymphoma staging. Eur Radiol 2020;30(7):3915–23.

97. Abbas F, et al. Post-transplantation lymphoproliferative disorders: current concepts and future therapeutic approaches. World J Transpl 2020;10(2): 29–46.

98. Pickhardt PJ, Siegel MJ. Posttransplantation lymphoproliferative disorder of the abdomen: CT evaluation in 51 patients. Radiology 1999;213(1):73–8.

99. Borhani AA, et al. Imaging of posttransplantation lymphoproliferative disorder after solid organ

transplantation. Radiographics 2009;29(4): 981–1000. discussion 1000-2.

100. Tomasian A, et al. Hematologic malignancies of the liver: spectrum of disease. Radiographics 2015; 35(1):71–86.

101. Singh A, et al. Role of diffusion weighted imaging in diagnosis of post transplant lymphoproliferative disorders: Case reports and review of literature. Indian J Nephrol 2016;26(3):212–5.

102. Horn SR, et al. Epidemiology of liver metastases. Cancer Epidemiol 2020;67:101760.

103. Del Poggio P, Buonocore M. Cystic tumors of the liver: a practical approach. World J Gastroenterol 2008;14(23):3616–20.

104. Borhani AA, Wiant A, Heller MT. Cystic hepatic lesions: a review and an algorithmic approach. AJR Am J Roentgenol 2014;203(6):1192–204.

105. Casillas VJ, et al. Imaging of nontraumatic hemorrhagic hepatic lesions. Radiographics 2000;20(2):367–78.

106. Siskind BN, et al. CT features of hemorrhagic malignant liver tumors. J Comput Assist Tomogr 1987;11(5):766–70.

Large Regenerative Nodules and Focal Nodular Hyperplasia-Like Lesions
Definition, Pathogenesis, and Imaging Findings

Paul E. Nolan, MD, Roberta Catania, MD, Camila Lopes Vendrami, MD,
Amir A. Borhani, MD*, Frank H. Miller, MD

KEYWORDS

- FNH • FNH-like lesions • Large regenerative nodules • Magnetic resonance imaging • Liver
- Hepatic vascular abnormalities

KEY POINTS

- Focal nodular hyperplasia-like (FNH-like) lesions and large regenerative nodules (LRNs) are benign hyperplastic lesions of hepatocellular origin, which are often encountered in patients with underlying hepatic vascular abnormalities.
- FNH-like lesions classically have similar imaging findings to FNH. Occasionally, they may show atypical features, different from classic FNHs, on imaging because of their variant histology or altered enhancement of background liver in the setting of abnormal global perfusion.
- FNH-like lesions can mimic hepatocellular carcinoma (HCC). Differentiation of these two entities can be challenging, especially in patients at risk for HCC.

INTRODUCTION

Hypervascular liver lesions, when not obviously a hemangioma, often cause concern and diagnostic dilemma. One classic and generally benign type of hypervascular liver lesion to consider is focal nodular hyperplasia-like (FNH-like) nodule. Unlike FNH, which by definition occurs within a normal background liver, FNH-like lesions are seen in the presence of underlying hepatic disease. Although FNH-like lesions are classically described as having an identical radiologic appearance to FNH (with arterial hyperenhancement and central scar), they may have variable imaging appearances. Particularly, the contrast-enhanced appearance of these lesions could be affected by the changes in the global hepatic perfusion (such as in the setting of venous congestion). Recognition of FNH-like lesions is of clinical importance as many patients with diffuse liver disease are also at increased risk for HCC, and misdiagnosis of an FNH-like lesion as HCC can result in unnecessary interventions and therapies. In this article, we describe the pathophysiology and imaging findings of FNH-like lesions, review the common conditions wherein FNH-like lesions can be seen, and discuss the pitfalls and challenges in differentiating these lesions from HCC.

Histology and Nomenclature

Regenerative lesions refer to hyperplastic lesions of hepatocellular origin that form in response to

Department of Radiology, Northwestern University Feinberg School of Medicine, 676 North Saint Claire Street, Arkes Family Pavillion, Suite 800, Chicago, IL 60611, USA
* Corresponding author. Abdominal Imaging, Northwestern University Feinberg School of Medicine, Medical Director, NMH Computed Tomography, Northwestern Medicine, 676 North Saint Clair Street, Arkes Family Pavilion, Suite 800, Chicago, IL 60611.
E-mail address: amir.borhani@northwestern.edu

Radiol Clin N Am 60 (2022) 795–808
https://doi.org/10.1016/j.rcl.2022.05.004
0033-8389/22/© 2022 Elsevier Inc. All rights reserved.

cellular injury or altered perfusion.[1] They include FNH, large regenerative nodules (LRNs), diffuse nodular hyperplasia, lobar or segmental hyperplasia, and cirrhotic nodules.

Classic FNH is a well-defined lesion composed of benign hyperplastic hepatocytes and portal tracts surrounding a central vascular scar.[2,3] By definition, FNH is found within a normal or nearly normal liver. LRNs, also known as multiacinar regenerative nodules, are typically seen in the setting of cirrhosis or advanced hepatic vascular disorders. They both are composed of benign hepatocytes and portal tracts with occasional scarring. Lesions with identical histologic and radiologic appearances to FNH have been described in diffusely abnormal livers and have been referred to as "FNH-like lesions." Others have categorized these as forms of LRNs given their presence within an abnormal liver.[4] Based on current literature, there is no consensus on how these lesions should be categorized. Despite radiologic and histologic similarities between FNH and FNH-like lesions, there is evidence that they differ in genetic expression suggesting a difference in their pathogenesis.[5] In addition, there is some evidence to support that FNH-like lesions are distinct entities from LRNs.[6] For simplicity, in this article, we refer to these entities as FNH-like nodules.

Pathogenesis

Typical FNH is thought to be a hyperplastic response to abnormal perfusion.[2,3] It is theorized that anomalous intrahepatic vessels result in areas of relatively increased regional arterial blood flow that prompts the hyperplastic response. They are often incidentally discovered in young adults with no history of liver disease or other significant pathology.[7] FNH-like lesions, on the other hand, result from a variety of liver pathologies that alter global perfusion and ultimately increase arterial flow to the liver. There are several proposed mechanisms that can result in increased arterial flow. Impaired venous outflow, such as a result of Budd–Chiari syndrome (BCS) and congestive hepatopathy, increases resistance to both arterial and portal inflow. Owing to the higher pressure of the hepatic artery compared with the portal veins, there is resultant disproportionately increased arterial supply to that part of the liver. This amplified arterial supply increases the propensity for a hyperplastic hepatocellular response, resulting in FNH-like nodules. Similarly, increased portal vein resistance due to cirrhosis or venous thrombosis results in compensatory increased arterial supply and increased likelihood of FNH-like lesion

formation. Primary increased arterial flow is another mechanism of FNH-like lesion development, as seen with hereditary hemorrhagic telangiectasia in which there is diminished arterial resistance secondary to hepatic telangiectases and arteriovenous malformations.

Imaging Findings

FNH-like nodules are classically described to have an imaging appearance similar to that of typical FNH occurring in normal background liver. However, they can have atypical imaging features, either because of their variant histology or altered enhancement kinetics in the setting of abnormal global perfusion. Distinction of atypical lesions from malignancies can be difficult, often requiring further workup including additional imaging studies (for instance, MR imaging with hepatobiliary agents) or biopsy.

FNH-like lesions are classically referred to as "stealth lesions," similar to conventional FNH, with a signal intensity close to that of the background liver on unenhanced T1-weighted (T1w) and T2-weighted (T2w) images.[8,9] Despite this classic description, they often have slightly different signal intensity compared with the background liver parenchyma,[10] in part due to abnormal signal intensity of the diseased background liver. One can consider FNH-like lesions as being small islands of relatively "normal" liver that stand out against a background of the diffusely abnormal liver in unenhanced and even in non-arterial phase contrast-enhanced images. Increased water content in the setting of venous congestion results in increased signal intensity of background liver parenchyma on T2w and decreased signal intensity on T1w images. As a result, FNH-like nodules can appear as mildly hyperintense on T1w (Fig. 1) and mildly hypointense on T2w images, compared with the background liver. Other diffuse processes such as steatosis and iron deposition can affect the relative signal intensity of the nodules. Hyperintensity on T1w images has also been explained by the possible presence of elements such as copper.[11] Hyperintensity on T2w images has been attributed to exaggerated venous congestion and infarction, especially in patients with congestive hepatopathy or BCS.[12] FNH-like nodules may show high signal intensity on diffusion-weighted imaging (DWI), presumably because of their different architecture and higher cellularity compared with the background liver (Fig. 2). After injection of gadolinium-based contrast media, there is brisk and usually homogeneous enhancement during the arterial phase. They remain hyperenhancing or become

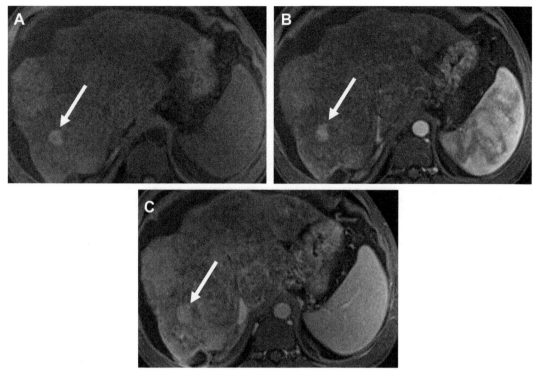

Fig. 1. A 40-year-old man with history of chronic Budd–Chiari syndrome. (*A*). Axial unenhanced T1 FS MR images show hyperintense lesion in segment 8 (*arrow*). Axial T1 FS MR images obtained during hepatic arterial phase (*B*) and venous phase (*C*) show persistent hyperenhancement on both phases. The lesions remained stable for 5 years consistent with benignity.

isointense to the background liver during portal venous and equilibrium phases[8,13,14] (see **Fig. 1**). Their relative signal intensity can be affected by the signal intensity of the diseased background liver. Many of the conditions associated with FNH-like lesions result in a dampened time-enhancement curve with longer time to peak.

The delayed enhancement of the surrounding liver parenchyma during the equilibrium and delayed phases may result in relative hypointensity of the FNH-like lesions mimicking the washout appearance seen in HCC (**Fig. 3**). FNH-like lesions are classically iso- or hyperintense to the background parenchyma during the delayed hepatobiliary

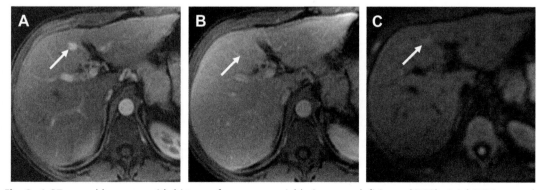

Fig. 2. A 37-year-old woman with history of common variable immune deficiency (CVID). Axial MR image obtained during hepatic arterial phase (*A*) shows an avidly enhancing lesion in segment 2 (*arrow*) which becomes isointense to the background liver during the venous phase (*B*). The lesion showed mild hyperintensity on diffusion-weighted image (b value = 500 s/mm^2) (*C*). Biopsy was consistent with nodular regenerative hyperplasia.

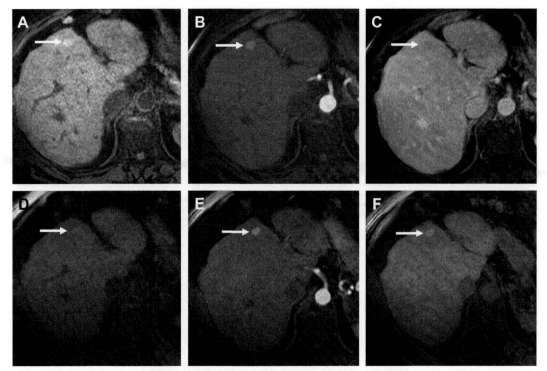

Fig. 3. A 67-year-old woman with history of right heart dysfunction. Axial unenhanced T1w MR (*A*) shows a T1 hyperintense lesion (*arrow*) in segment IV. The lesion showed avid enhancement on arterial phase (*B*) and "wash out" appearance on venous phase (*C*). One-year follow-up MR imaging using hepatobiliary agent (*D–F*) shows stability in size and retention of contrast during the hepatobiliary phase (*F*). Note the decreased signal intensity of liver and delayed excretion of contrast into the biliary tree on hepatobiliary phase (*F*) suggestive of hepatocellular dysfunction in setting of congestive hepatopathy.

phase (when hepatobiliary contrast agents used) owing to overexpression of organic anion-transporting polypeptide (OATP), the main transporter of gadoxetic acid in hepatocytes[15] (**Fig. 4**). A hypointense rim (attributed to peri-lesional sinusoidal dilatation or atrophic tissue) during this phase has also been described.[13] The FNH-like nodules may have a central scar which helps in the diagnosis. The scar tissue typically hyperintense on T2w images and is hypoenhancing during

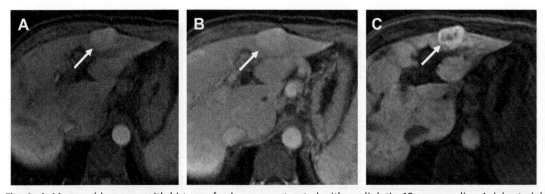

Fig. 4. A 44-year-old woman with history of colon cancer treated with oxaliplatin 13 years earlier. Axial arterial phase T1w MR imaging (*A*) shows an enhancing lesion (*arrow*) in hepatic segment 3 which remained hyperintense on portal venous phase (*B*) and had retention of contrast during the hepatobiliary phase (*C*). Also note the central scar which is slightly hypointense in A and B, becoming more evident on hepatobiliary phase. Percutaneous biopsy was consistent with FNH-like lesion. Lesion differs from metastasis from colon cancer which tends to be hypovascular and hypointense on hepatobiliary phase and not having a central scar.

the arterial, venous, and equilibrium phases while showing delayed enhancement (when extracellular agents used) owing to its larger extracellular compartment. The central scar remains hypointense during hepatobiliary phase (when hepatobiliary contrast agents used) and may appear larger compared with images obtained with extracellular contrast agents, similar to the appearance seen in conventional FNHs (**Fig. 5**).

FNH-like lesions can have variable appearances on ultrasound (US), mostly isoechoic or mildly hypoechoic compared with the liver parenchyma. Contrast-enhanced US is more helpful for characterization by identifying more specific features such as centrifugal arterial enhancement with persistent enhancement during portal venous and late phases.[16] When present, a non-enhancing central scar may be seen.

On CT, FNH-like lesions are typically isodense or slightly hypodense to liver parenchyma on unenhanced phase. After injection of iodinated contrast agents, brisk homogeneous enhancement is usually seen during the arterial phase with persistent homogeneous enhancement during portal venous phase[9,17] (**Fig. 6**). Their appearance on delayed phase is variable ranging from hyperenhancement to hypoenhancement with "washout" appearance (mimicking HCC).[18] As stated earlier, the washout appearance may be due to delayed enhancement of the background liver in the setting of venous congestion. A hypodense central scar may occasionally be seen.

Natural History

Once considered a rare phenomenon, FNH-like lesions are now commonly encountered. Several factors are attributed to this higher incidence. Advances in the medical and surgical management of right heart dysfunction and congenital heart disease (such as the Fontan procedure) have resulted in an increased number of adult patients living with long-standing congestive hepatopathy and with resultant FNH-like lesion formation. Moreover, an increased longevity of oncologic patients treated with oxaliplatin can account for the rising number of FNH-like lesions in these patients. These lesions are believed to have no risk of malignant transformation. Majority of the lesions remain stable over time[19] although growth, regression, and hemorrhagic necrosis have also been reported.[14,20] Despite this preliminary evidence, their natural history and growth rate are not well understood yet, and more longitudinal studies are needed to better clarify the evolution and size changes of these nodules.

DISEASES ASSOCIATED WITH FNH-LIKE LESIONS

Although FNH-like nodules can occur in many scenarios, several disease entities are more classically described to be associated with these nodules and will be discussed in the following.

Budd–Chiari Syndrome

BCS is a heterogeneous group of diseases resulting from hepatic venous outflow obstruction in the absence of right heart failure or constrictive pericarditis.[21] It is more common in women (in countries outside of Asia) and is usually diagnosed in the third or fourth decade of life, although it can occur at any age.[22] The obstruction may occur at any level along the venous outflow from the smaller hepatic veins to the junction of the inferior vena cava to the right atrium. Primary BCS, the most common type, occurs when a predominantly endoluminal venous process (such as thrombus or

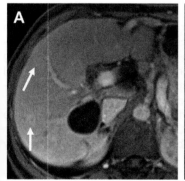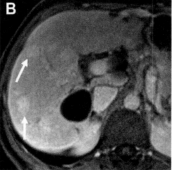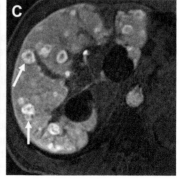

Fig. 5. A 51-year-old woman with history of autoimmune hepatitis. Axial portal venous phase MR imaging (*A*) shows indistinct hepatic lesions (*arrows*). The lesions became more conspicuous during the transitional phase (*B*). All lesions demonstrated intense retention of contrast and central scar during the hepatobiliary phase and central scar (*C*), compatible with FNH-like nodules.

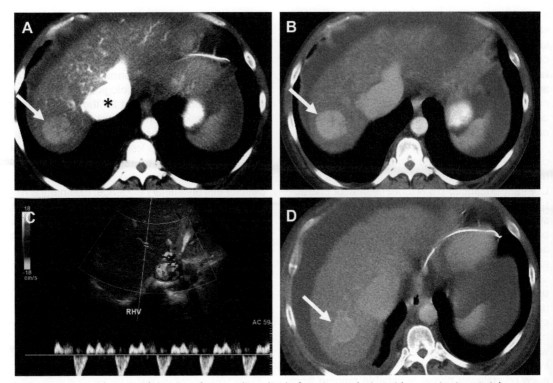

Fig. 6. A 45-year-old man with history of severe diastolic dysfunction and tricuspid regurgitation. Axial contrast-enhanced CT (*A*) shows an avidly arterially enhancing lesion in segment 7 (*arrow*) which remained hyperdense during the venous phase (*B*). Note the reflux of contrast into IVC (*asterisk*) during the arterial phase. Doppler US (*C*) shows abnormal hepatic venous waveform classic for severe tricuspid regurgitation. Contrast-enhanced CT obtained 3 years later (*D*) shows mild decrease in size of the lesion over time.

phlebitis) leads to hepatic venous outflow obstruction. This type is often associated with hypercoagulable states. Secondary BCS applies to hepatic venous outflow obstruction caused by vascular invasion or extrinsic compression. BCS can be also classified as acute (fulminant or not fulminant), subacute, or chronic, based on the chronicity and severity of disease. The majority of the cases are subacute or chronic, associated with dysmorphism of the liver and variable degree of hepatic fibrosis.

Regenerative nodules are commonly seen in the setting of chronic BCS and usually represent FNH-like lesions[23] (**Fig. 7**). Regenerative nodules larger than 5 mm have a reported prevalence of up to 60% to 80% in some pathology series.[12,16,24] No association with any specific etiology of BCS or vascular interventional measures (such as transjugular intrahepatic portosystemic shunt [TIPS]) has been shown.[23] Although their exact pathogenesis remains uncertain, it is thought that they develop as a response to focal loss of portal perfusion and hyper-arterialization in regions of the liver with maintained hepatic venous outflow.[13,17] Patients with BCS are also at risk of developing

HCC, accounting for 0.7% of all cases.[8–10] Patients with long-term inferior vena cava obstruction have a higher risk of developing HCC than those with only hepatic vein involvement.

FNH-like lesions in the setting of BCS are usually hyperintense on fat-suppressed T1w images (see **Fig. 1**) and show more variable signal intensity on T2w MR imaging.[13,23] A slightly hyperenhancing rim mimicking a capsule has also been described.[13] Given their inherent T1 hyperintensity, subtraction images may be helpful to confirm their hypervascularity.[13,23] Some lesions may depict a "pseudo-washout" appearance, mimicking HCC.[13] The larger lesions often have a central scar. No predisposition for a specific hepatic location has been identified.

There is overlap in imaging findings of FNH-like nodules and HCC and differentiation of these two entities could be challenging. HCCs are usually heterogeneous and solitary, whereas benign nodules are usually multiple and small (usually <3 cm).[23] The presence of intralesional fat, hemorrhage, or calcification is atypical for FNH-like nodules and should suggest a different process, including HCC. MR imaging with the use of

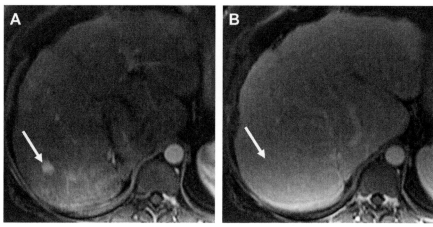

Fig. 7. A 60-year-old man with history of Budd–Chiari syndrome secondary to polycythemia vera. Axial T1 FS arterial phase MR image obtained during hepatic arterial phase (*A*) shows an avidly enhancing lesion in segment 7 (*arrow*). The lesion became isointense to the liver parenchyma on portal venous phase (*B*). The lesion remained stable for 3 years consistent with benignity.

hepatobiliary contrast agents is particularly useful for accurate diagnosis of FNH-like lesions.[23] Retention of contrast during hepatobiliary phase is a common finding with FNH-like nodules while much less common in HCCs. Contrast-enhanced US has also been suggested as a method to distinguish these two entities in the setting of BCS. In a study by Zhang and colleagues most FNH-like lesions showed centrifugal arterial enhancement with persistent enhancement during venous and delayed phases, whereas most HCCs showed heterogeneous enhancement on arterial phase with washout.[16]

Congestive Hepatopathy and Fontan-Associated Liver Disease

Congestive hepatopathy is the umbrella term applied to any hepatic injury as a result of chronic passive hepatic congestion.[25,26] A myriad of diseases (such as myocardial infarction, cardiomyopathy, valvular disease, constrictive pericarditis, and pulmonary hypertension) can result in right-sided heart dysfunction and increased central venous pressure which subsequently transmits to the hepatic venous system.[19] Initial pathologic changes include sinusoidal dilatation with perisinusoidal edema followed by thrombosis, hemorrhage, and loss of hepatocytes surrounding the central veins. Repeated injury results in bridging fibrosis between central veins and regenerating hepatocytes growing along the preserved portal triads, yielding a characteristic fibrosis pattern referred to as reverse lobulation that differs from the more common periportal fibrosis associated with other causes of liver fibrosis.[27] The

diminished portal venous flow, as a result of increased sinusoidal pressure, and the compensatory increased arterial flow result in hepatocellular hyperplasia and development of FNH-like nodules (see **Figs. 3** and **6**).

Fontan-associated liver disease (FALD) is a subset of congestive hepatopathy seen in patients with congenital cardiac anomalies who underwent Fontan procedure. First described in 1971, the Fontan procedure results in direct connection of systemic venous return to the pulmonary circulation in patients with univentricular defects and creates a unique blood flow physiology ("Fontan physiology") with the single ventricle pumping blood into the systemic circulation and the pulmonary blood flow being passively driven from the inferior vena cava.[28,29] The resultant increased systemic venous pressure is the main trigger leading to FALD.[30,31] Initially, the hepatic arterial blood flow increases in response to the higher hepatic venous resistance and, similar to other etiologies of congestive hepatopathy, can lead to the development of FNH-like lesions. With time, these patients may develop a low cardiac output that results in decreased arterial hepatic flow.[32] The complexity of inflow and outflow circulation that post-Fontan patients progressively develop explains the complexity of liver lesions reported in FALD.[32] The end result of this chronic hepatic insult is the progressive development of pericentral and perisinusoidal fibrosis.[33–35]

FNH-like lesions are the most common focal liver lesions in post-Fontan patients with a reported prevalence of 27%[36] (**Fig. 8**). A wide variety of other liver lesions (including hepatic adenomas and HCC) also occurs in FALD as a result of the complexity of

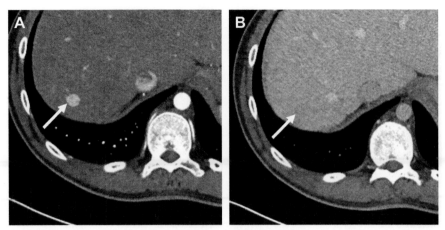

Fig. 8. A 26-year-old boy with history of Fontan procedure as a child for transposition of the great arteries. Axial contrast-enhanced CT (*A*) obtained during hepatic arterial phase shows an avidly enhancing lesion in segment 7 (*arrow*). No convincing associated washout or "capsule" is seen during venous phase (*B*). The lesion remained stable for at least 3 years suggestive of an FNH-like nodule.

the hepatic insult post-Fontan procedure.[31,36] These patients are at increased risk of HCC (**Fig. 9**). In a large multicenter retrospective study involving 2470 patients who had Fontan surgery, the prevalence of biopsy-proven HCC was reported at 1.3%.[35] More recently, Sagawa and colleagues reported a higher prevalence of HCC among patients with FALD, up to 9.8%.[37] Given the multitude of liver lesions encountered in these patients and the increased risk of HCC, confident diagnosis of FNH-like lesions can be challenging because of overlap in imaging features of these lesions, including washout appearance after contrast administration.[5] Stability, uniform homogenous arterial enhancement with central scar appearance and retention of contrast on the hepatobiliary phase

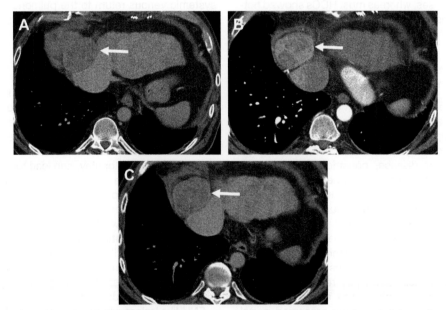

Fig. 9. A 44-year-old man with history of tricuspid atresia status post-Fontan procedure. Axial unenhanced CT (*A*) shows a large hypoattenuating mass in hepatic dome (*arrow*). The lesion shows heterogeneous enhancement during the hepatic arterial phase (*B*) with subsequent washout during the venous phase (*C*). The lesion is heterogeneous and does not have central scar, unlike FNH-like nodules. Percutaneous biopsy was consistent with hepatocellular carcinoma.

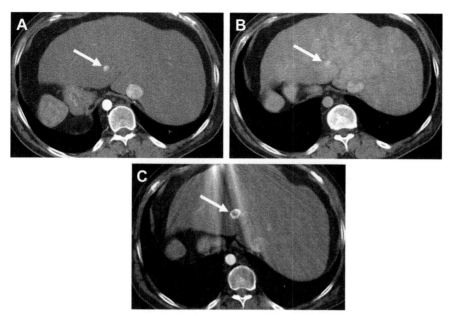

Fig. 10. A 40-year-old man with history of situs inversus and prior Fontan procedure. Axial contrast-enhanced CT images show gradual increase in size of FNH-like nodules over a period of 5 years. Note the homogeneous enhancement and central scar of the dominant lesion (*arrow*) typical of FNH-like nodule.

are features suggestive of FNH-like lesions[32] (**Figs. 10** and **11**). Washout during the portal venous phase (as opposed to washout during delayed phase), mosaic architecture, elevated serum AFP, and higher central vein pressure (CVP) were shown to be associated with a higher risk of HCC.[19] Short-term imaging follow-up (in 3–6 months) and/or

tissue biopsy should be considered for atypical lesions.[32]

Sinusoidal Obstruction Syndrome

Sinusoidal obstruction syndrome (SOS), previously known as hepatic veno-occlusive disease,

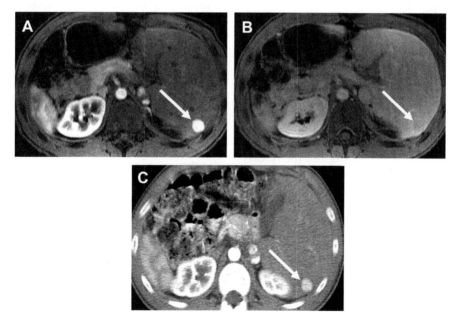

Fig. 11. An 18-year-old boy with history of Fontan procedure and situs inversus. Axial MR imaging shows avidly enhancing lesion (*arrow*) on hepatic arterial phase (*A*) with subsequent washout and enhancing capsule on venous phase (*B*). Contrast-enhanced CT obtained 5 years later (*C*) shows stable size of the lesion suggestive of benignity (despite the worrisome enhancement pattern).

occurs as a result of injury to sinusoidal endothelial cells and is characterized by dilated sinusoids filled with erythrocytes, often associated with centrilobular vein occlusion and perisinusoidal fibrosis.[38] Common causes of SOS include medications, particularly chemotherapy, bone marrow transplantation, and high-dose radiation. Oxaliplatin is one such chemotherapy agent with a known association with SOS.[39] FNH-like lesions have been reported in adults who previously received oxaliplatin for colorectal and pancreatic cancers, with evidence of SOS on pathology.[14] Local perfusion abnormalities related to SOS and centrilobular vein occlusion may account for subsequent FNH-like lesion development in these patients.

FNH-like lesions and nodular regenerative hyperplasia have been reported in 22% of patients treated with oxaliplatin, based on histopathologic examination of hepatectomy specimens.[20] It usually occurs at least 3 to 4 years after the completion of therapy, which is usually later than the interval for the development of hepatic metastases.[14] In addition, they can be distinguished from metastases based on their imaging appearance as these lesions are typically hypervascular often with central scars (FNH-like) and with the retention of hepatobiliary agents during the hepatobiliary phase (see **Fig. 4**), unlike metastases from GI adenocarcinomas that tend to be hypovascular, lack a central scar, and are hypointense on hepatobiliary phase MR imaging.[14] Although oxaliplatin is the most well-documented chemotherapeutic agent associated with FNH-like lesions, these nodules have also been reported in association with other agents including cyclophosphamide-based chemotherapy.[40] FNH-like lesions have also been reported in patients previously treated with chemotherapy for neuroblastoma in childhood. One imaging-based study found FNH-like lesions in 15% of patients who previously received chemotherapy for neuroblastoma.[41]

FNH-like lesions are also reported in the setting of hematopoietic stem cell transplant (SCT). One study reported FNH-like lesion development in 17 of 138 patients who received SCT.[42] All FNH-like lesions were seen in patients who received SCT as children, which may suggest that younger patients are more prone to FNH-like lesion development in the setting of SCT.

Hereditary Hemorrhagic Telangiectasia

Hereditary hemorrhagic telangiectasia (HHT), also known as Osler–Weber–Rendu disease, is an autosomal dominant disorder characterized by arteriovenous malformations and other vascular abnormalities involving multiple organ systems.

Liver involvement is common, with one study demonstrating hepatic vasculature abnormalities in 74% of patients.[43] Liver manifestations include intrahepatic shunts (arterioportal, arteriovenous, and portovenous shunts), telangiectases, regenerative nodular hyperplasia, and FNH-like lesions.[44] In severe cases, intrahepatic shunting can result in diminished distal arterial perfusion and peribiliary necrosis, sometimes necessitating liver transplantation.[45]

Hepatocellular regeneration in HHT can present as nodular regenerative hyperplasia, LRNs, or FNH-like lesions[46] (**Fig. 12**). These patients are not considered at increased risk for primary liver malignancies. As such and given the high prevalence of regenerative lesions in patients with HHT, the diagnosis of FNH-like lesions can be made with higher confidence. It has been suggested that lesions with features indicative of FNH should not undergo biopsy or excision, particularly given presence of vascular abnormalities that may predispose to bleeding.[46]

Cavernous Transformation of the Portal Vein

Cavernous transformation of the portal vein (CTPV) occurs as a response to occlusive portal vein thrombosis in an attempt to restore portal blood flow. Etiologies for portal vein thrombosis include slow flow in the setting of cirrhosis, myeloproliferative syndromes, autoimmune diseases such as antiphospholipid syndrome, and hypercoagulability syndromes. Compensatory increased arterial flow due to reduced portal flow is a possible explanation for the formation of FNH-like lesions in these patients. One study reported a prevalence of 21% of FNH-like lesions in patients with non-cirrhosis-related CTPV.[47] Chronic portal venous thrombosis may result in dysmorphic liver and portal hypertension, even in the absence of fibrosis. FNH-like lesions in this setting can pose a diagnostic challenge because some of these patients are erroneously labeled as having cirrhosis and the lesions may be suspected to be HCC. Familiarity with the association between CTPV and FNH-like lesions and recognizing the typical features of these nodules can help with appropriate management (**Fig. 13**).

Autoimmune Hepatitis

Autoimmune hepatitis (AIH) is one of the rare etiologies of hepatitis characterized by chronic nonspecific inflammation of liver parenchyma, thought to be due to an autoimmune reaction against the liver.[48] Patients are usually female and have circulating autoantibodies (antinuclear and/or anti-smooth muscle antibodies in type I

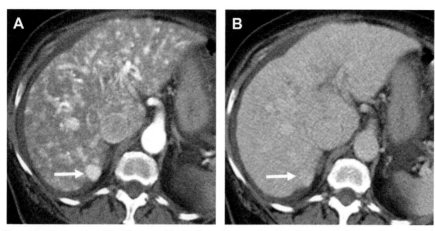

Fig. 12. A 72-year-old woman with history of hereditary hemorrhagic telangiectasia (HHT). Axial hepatic arterial phase CT (*A*) shows an enhancing lesion in hepatic segment VII (*arrow*). The lesion remains mildly hyperdense compared with the background liver on 150-s delayed phase (*B*). Note numerous areas of arterioportal shunting as well as enlargement of hepatic arteries consistent with history of HHT. The segment VII lesion remained stable on follow-up imaging.

antibodies against liver–kidney microsome and/or liver cytosol in type II). FNH-like lesions have been reported in patients with AIH[49] (see **Fig. 5**), although the exact prevalence is unknown. The mechanism for the development of these nodules in AIH is uncertain. A proposed mechanism is alterations in hepatic microcirculation secondary to diffuse parenchymal inflammation.[49] AIH can progress to cirrhosis. The incidence of HCC in patients with AIH (in absence of other etiologies of chronic liver disease), however, is thought to be lower than other etiologies of cirrhosis, estimated to be less than 1%.[50,51] Given the lower chance of malignancy in these patients, differentiation of FNH-like lesions from HCC should be less of a challenge. Awareness of the association of FNH-like nodules with AIH is critical so that there is not misdiagnosis of HCC. The presence of multiple lesions and stability also favor benignity.[49]

Common Variable Immunodeficiency

Common variable immunodeficiency (CVID) is the most common primary immunodeficiency in adults, characterized by decreased serum levels of immunoglobulin and antibody production in response to vaccines and pathogens.[52] Besides an increased susceptibility to infections, CVID presents a broad

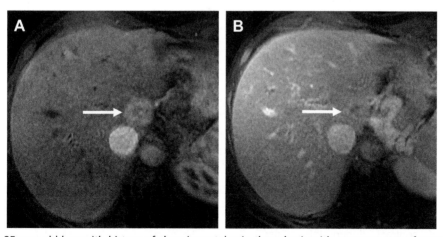

Fig. 13. A 25-year-old boy with history of chronic portal vein thrombosis with cavernous transformation. Axial contrast-enhanced MR imaging obtained during hepatic arterial phase (*A*) shows arterially enhancing lesion (*arrow*) with central scar. The lesion became iso-intense to the background liver on equilibrium phase (*B*). The lesion was stable for 3 years consistent with benign etiology. Of note, this lesion was new compared with prior examinations (not shown).

spectrum of clinical manifestations related to immune dysregulation-related complications. Nodular regenerative hyperplasia is considered the most common form of liver involvement in CVID[53] (see **Fig. 2**). NRH can lead to chronic cholestasis, non-cirrhotic portal hypertension, or cirrhosis.[54] FNH-like lesions seen in these patients likely represent the spectrum of nodular regenerative hyperplasia. These nodules usually have typical radiologic features of FNH-like nodules described earlier. In the absence of risk factor for primary liver malignancies (such as cirrhosis), these lesions can confidently be diagnosed by imaging.

Diagnostic Challenges

Many of the conditions associated with FNH-like lesions are also risk factors for the development of other liver lesions. Furthermore, certain comorbidities (such as history of concomitant chronic liver disease) place the patient at higher risk of HCC development. Confident differentiation of FNH-like lesions from premalignant and malignant lesions (especially HCC) is clinically relevant and critical to guide the management. Clinical and laboratory findings (such as serum AFP level and probability of HCC based on underlying disease) should be considered when making this distinction as in many cases the imaging findings of FNH-like lesions are not specific and overlap those of HCC.[23] Classically described radiologic features of HCC such as arterial phase hyperenhancement and washout appearance are not specific in the setting of global hepatic vascular disorders. Hence, Liver Imaging Reporting and Data System (LI-RADS) classification cannot be applied in this setting.[55] Washout appearance can be seen with FNH-like lesions, with a reported prevalence of up to 10%,[56] although this appearance is likely reflective of abnormal enhancement of the background liver rather than deranged de-enhancement of the lesion (see **Fig. 3**).

Hyperintensity during the delayed hepatobiliary phase (when hepatobiliary MR imaging contrast agents are used) and presence of central scar are the most helpful features to differentiate FNH-like lesions from HCC. Although most HCCs are hypointense during hepatobiliary phase, FNH-like lesions typically show homogeneous iso- to hyperintensity during this phase.[13] This finding, however, is not definitive as hepatic adenomas and well differentiated HCCs may show retention of contrast during this phase.[57,58] HCCs, however, tend to have more heterogenous signal intensity (on unenhanced and contrast-enhanced T1w and T2w sequences) and lack central scar.[59] Intrahepatic cholangiocarcinoma and some metastases can show central retention of hepatobiliary contrast agent that is thought to be due to aberrant expression of OATP1B3 in their fibrotic stroma. This "targetoid" appearance with peripheral hypointense rim and inhomogeneous central uptake of contrast agent during hepatobiliary phase, however, is different from FNH-like nodules that have more homogeneous iso- to hyperintensity with a hypointense central scar.[60]

Patients with atypical imaging features (such as heterogeneity or significant changes of the nodule on serial imaging) and the ones with elevated serum AFP should be discussed by a multidisciplinary team and may require tissue sampling. Patients with lesions typical for FNH-like nodules should also be considered for follow-up by serial imaging and clinical/laboratory assessment.

SUMMARY

FNH-like lesions, and other similar benign nodules, can be seen in association with multiple liver diseases and are increasingly encountered in daily practice. Their imaging findings overlap with other entities, such as HCC. Familiarity with their pathogenesis and their imaging findings will help with a more informed diagnosis.

CLINICS CARE POINTS

- In cancer patients recieving oxaliplatin-based chemotherapy regimen, FNH-like lesion should be considered as differential diagnosis for new hepatic lesions.

- Signal characteristics similar to FNH, presence of central scar, and retention of contrast during hepatobiliary phase are key features helpful for diagnosing FNH-like lesion and differentiation from other hepatic pathologies.

DISCLOSURE

The authors have nothing to disclose.

REFERENCES

1. International Working Party. Terminology of nodular hepatocellular lesions. Hepatology 1995;22(3): 983–93.
2. Wanless IR, Mawdsley C, Adams R. On the pathogenesis of focal nodular hyperplasia of the liver. Hepatology 1985;5(6):1194–200.

3. Wanless IR, Albrecht S, Bilbao J, et al. Multiple focal nodular hyperplasia of the liver associated with vascular malformations of various organs and neoplasia of the brain: a new syndrome. Mod Pathol 1989;2(5):456–62.

4. Hytiroglou P. Well-differentiated hepatocellular nodule: Making a diagnosis on biopsy and resection specimens of patients with advanced stage chronic liver disease. Semin Diagn Pathol 2017;34(2):138–45.

5. Rebouissou S, Couchy G, Libbrecht L, et al. The beta-catenin pathway is activated in focal nodular hyperplasia but not in cirrhotic FNH-like nodules. J Hepatol 2008;49(1):61–71.

6. Nakashima O, Kurogi M, Yamaguchi R, et al. Unique hypervascular nodules in alcoholic liver cirrhosis: identical to focal nodular hyperplasia-like nodules? J Hepatol 2004;41(6):992–8.

7. Cherqui D, Rahmouni A, Charlotte F, et al. Management of focal nodular hyperplasia and hepatocellular adenoma in young women: a series of 41 patients with clinical, radiological, and pathological correlations. Hepatology 1995;22(6):1674–81.

8. Brancatelli G, Federle MP, Grazioli L, et al. Large regenerative nodules in Budd-Chiari syndrome and other vascular disorders of the liver: CT and MR imaging findings with clinicopathologic correlation. AJR Am J Roentgenol 2002;178(4):877–83.

9. Maetani Y, Itoh K, Egawa H, et al. Benign hepatic nodules in Budd-Chiari syndrome: radiologic-pathologic correlation with emphasis on the central scar. AJR Am J Roentgenol 2002;178(4):869–75.

10. Vilgrain V, Lewin M, Vons C, et al. Hepatic nodules in Budd-Chiari syndrome: imaging features. Radiology 1999;210(2):443–50.

11. Wanless IR. Micronodular transformation (nodular regenerative hyperplasia) of the liver: a report of 64 cases among 2,500 autopsies and a new classification of benign hepatocellular nodules. Hepatology 1990;11(5):787–97.

12. Tanaka M, Wanless IR. Pathology of the liver in Budd-Chiari syndrome: portal vein thrombosis and the histogenesis of veno-centric cirrhosis, veno-portal cirrhosis, and large regenerative nodules. Hepatology 1998;27(2):488–96.

13. Mamone G, Carollo V, Di Piazza A, et al. Budd-Chiari Syndrome and hepatic regenerative nodules: Magnetic resonance findings with emphasis of hepatobiliary phase. Eur J Radiol 2019;117:15–25.

14. Furlan A, Brancatelli G, Dioguardi Burgio M, et al. Focal Nodular Hyperplasia After Treatment With Oxaliplatin: A Multiinstitutional Series of Cases Diagnosed at MRI. AJR Am J Roentgenol 2018;210(4):775–9.

15. Grazioli L, Bondioni MP, Haradome H, et al. Hepatocellular adenoma and focal nodular hyperplasia: value of gadoxetic acid-enhanced MR imaging in differential diagnosis. Radiology 2012;262(2):520–9.

16. Zhang R, Qin S, Zhou Y, et al. Comparison of imaging characteristics between hepatic benign regenerative nodules and hepatocellular carcinomas associated with Budd-Chiari syndrome by contrast enhanced ultrasound. Eur J Radiol 2012;81(11):2984–9.

17. Flor N, Zuin M, Brovelli F, et al. Regenerative nodules in patients with chronic Budd-Chiari syndrome: a longitudinal study using multiphase contrast-enhanced multidetector CT. Eur J Radiol 2010; 73(3):588–93.

18. Van Wettere M, Purcell Y, Bruno O, et al. Low specificity of washout to diagnose hepatocellular carcinoma in nodules showing arterial hyperenhancement in patients with Budd-Chiari syndrome. J Hepatol 2019; 70(6):1123–32.

19. Wells ML, Hough DM, Fidler JL, et al. Benign nodules in post-Fontan livers can show imaging features considered diagnostic for hepatocellular carcinoma. Abdom Radiol (Ny) 2017;42(11):2623–31.

20. Wicherts DA, de Haas RJ, Sebagh M, et al. Regenerative nodular hyperplasia of the liver related to chemotherapy: impact on outcome of liver surgery for colorectal metastases. Ann Surg Oncol 2011; 18(3):659–69.

21. DeLeve LD, Valla DC, Garcia-Tsao G. American Association for the Study Liver D. Vascular disorders of the liver. Hepatology 2009;49(5):1729–64.

22. Ludwig J, Hashimoto E, McGill DB, et al. Classification of hepatic venous outflow obstruction: ambiguous terminology of the Budd-Chiari syndrome. Mayo Clin Proc 1990;65(1):51–5.

23. Vilgrain V, Paradis V, Van Wettere M, et al. Benign and malignant hepatocellular lesions in patients with vascular liver diseases. Abdom Radiol (Ny) 2018;43(8):1968–77.

24. Wanless IR. Benign liver tumors. Clin Liver Dis 2002; 6(2):513–526, ix.

25. Louie CY, Pham MX, Daugherty TJ, et al. The liver in heart failure: a biopsy and explant series of the histopathologic and laboratory findings with a particular focus on pre-cardiac transplant evaluation. Mod Pathol 2015;28(7):932–43.

26. Giallourakis CC, Rosenberg PM, Friedman LS. The liver in heart failure. Clin Liver Dis 2002;6(4): 947–967, viii-ix.

27. Sherlock S. The liver in heart failure; relation of anatomical, functional, and circulatory changes. Br Heart J 1951;13(3):273–93.

28. Fontan F, Baudet E. Surgical repair of tricuspid atresia. Thorax 1971;26(3):240–8.

29. Rodriguez FH, Book WM. Management of the adult Fontan patient. Heart 2020;106(2):105–10.

30. Daniels CJ, Bradley EA, Landzberg MJ, et al. Fontan-Associated Liver Disease: Proceedings from the American College of Cardiology Stakeholders Meeting, October 1 to 2, 2015, Washington DC. J Am Coll Cardiol 2017;70(25):3173–94.

31. Ghaferi AA, Hutchins GM. Progression of liver pathology in patients undergoing the Fontan

procedure: Chronic passive congestion, cardiac cirrhosis, hepatic adenoma, and hepatocellular carcinoma. J Thorac Cardiovasc Surg 2005;129(6): 1348–52.

32. Dillman JR, Trout AT, Alsaied T, et al. Imaging of Fontan-associated liver disease. Pediatr Radiol 2020;50(11):1528–41.

33. Goldberg DJ, Surrey LF, Glatz AC, et al. Hepatic Fibrosis Is Universal Following Fontan Operation, and Severity is Associated With Time From Surgery: A Liver Biopsy and Hemodynamic Study. J Am Heart Assoc 2017;6(5):e004809.

34. Wu FM, Kogon B, Earing MG, et al. Liver health in adults with Fontan circulation: A multicenter cross-sectional study. J Thorac Cardiovasc Surg 2017; 153(3):656–64.

35. Egbe AC, Poterucha JT, Warnes CA, et al. Hepatocellular Carcinoma After Fontan Operation: Multicenter Case Series. Circulation 2018;138(7):746–8.

36. Engelhardt EM, Trout AT, Sheridan RM, et al. Focal liver lesions following Fontan palliation of single ventricle physiology: A radiology-pathology case series. Congenit Heart Dis 2019;14(3):380–8.

37. Sagawa T, Kogiso T, Sugiyama H, et al. Characteristics of hepatocellular carcinoma arising from Fontan-associated liver disease. Hepatol Res 2020;50(7): 853–62.

38. Rubbia-Brandt L. Sinusoidal obstruction syndrome. Clin Liver Dis 2010;14(4):651–68.

39. Rubbia-Brandt L, Audard V, Sartoretti P, et al. Severe hepatic sinusoidal obstruction associated with oxaliplatin-based chemotherapy in patients with metastatic colorectal cancer. Ann Oncol 2004;15(3):460–6.

40. Xue DQ, Yang L. Development of Focal Nodular Hyperplasia after Cyclophosphamide-Based Chemotherapy in a Patient with Breast Cancer. Case Rep Hepatol 2018;2018:5409316.

41. Benz-Bohm G, Hero B, Gossmann A, et al. Focal nodular hyperplasia of the liver in longterm survivors of neuroblastoma: how much diagnostic imaging is necessary? Eur J Radiol 2010;74(3):e1–5.

42. Sudour H, Mainard L, Baumann C, et al. Focal nodular hyperplasia of the liver following hematopoietic SCT. Bone Marrow Transplant 2009;43(2):127–32.

43. Ianora AA, Memeo M, Sabba C, et al. Hereditary hemorrhagic telangiectasia: multi-detector row helical CT assessment of hepatic involvement. Radiology 2004;230(1):250–9.

44. Brenard R, Chapaux X, Deltenre P, et al. Large spectrum of liver vascular lesions including high prevalence of focal nodular hyperplasia in patients with hereditary haemorrhagic telangiectasia: the Belgian Registry based on 30 patients. Eur J Gastroenterol Hepatol 2010;22(10):1253–9.

45. Felli E, Addeo P, Faitot F, et al. Liver transplantation for hereditary hemorrhagic telangiectasia: a systematic review. HPB (Oxford) 2017;19(7):567–72.

46. Buscarini E, Gandolfi S, Alicante S, et al. Liver involvement in hereditary hemorrhagic telangiectasia. Abdom Radiol (Ny) 2018;43(8):1920–30.

47. Marin D, Galluzzo A, Plessier A, et al. Focal nodular hyperplasia-like lesions in patients with cavernous transformation of the portal vein: prevalence, MR findings and natural history. Eur Radiol 2011; 21(10):2074–82.

48. European Association for the Study of the L. EASL Clinical Practice Guidelines: Autoimmune hepatitis. J Hepatol 2015;63(4):971–1004.

49. Qayyum A, Graser A, Westphalen A, et al. CT of benign hypervascular liver nodules in autoimmune hepatitis. AJR Am J Roentgenol 2004;183(6):1573–6.

50. Park SZ, Nagorney DM, Czaja AJ. Hepatocellular carcinoma in autoimmune hepatitis. Dig Dis Sci 2000;45(10):1944–8.

51. Teufel A, Weinmann A, Centner C, et al. Hepatocellular carcinoma in patients with autoimmune hepatitis. World J Gastroenterol 2009;15(5):578–82.

52. Pecoraro A, Crescenzi L, Varricchi G, et al. Heterogeneity of Liver Disease in Common Variable Immunodeficiency Disorders. Front Immunol 2020;11:338.

53. Bonilla FA, Barlan I, Chapel H, et al. International Consensus Document (ICON): Common Variable Immunodeficiency Disorders. J Allergy Clin Immunol Pract 2016;4(1):38–59.

54. Song J, Lleo A, Yang GX, et al. Common Variable Immunodeficiency and Liver Involvement. Clin Rev Allergy Immunol 2018;55(3):340–51.

55. American College of Radiology Committee on LI-RADS®. CT/MRI Liver Imaging Reporting and Data System v2018. 2018. Available at: https://www.acr.org/Clinical-Resources/Reporting-and-Data-Systems/LI-RADS/CT-MRI-LI-RADS-v2018. Accessed September 2 2021.

56. Choi JY, Lee HC, Yim JH, et al. Focal nodular hyperplasia or focal nodular hyperplasia-like lesions of the liver: a special emphasis on diagnosis. J Gastroenterol Hepatol 2011;26(6):1004–9.

57. Narita M, Hatano E, Arizono S, et al. Expression of OATP1B3 determines uptake of Gd-EOB-DTPA in hepatocellular carcinoma. J Gastroenterol 2009;44(7):793–8.

58. Ba-Ssalamah A, Antunes C, Feier D, et al. Morphologic and Molecular Features of Hepatocellular Adenoma with Gadoxetic Acid-enhanced MR Imaging. Radiology 2015;277(1):104–13.

59. Kim JW, Lee CH, Kim SB, et al. Washout appearance in Gd-EOB-DTPA-enhanced MR imaging: A differentiating feature between hepatocellular carcinoma with paradoxical uptake on the hepatobiliary phase and focal nodular hyperplasia-like nodules J Magn Reson Imaging 2017;45(6):1599–608.

60. Vernuccio F, Gagliano DS, Cannella R, et al. Spectrum of liver lesions hyperintense on hepatobiliary phase: an approach by clinical setting. Insights Imaging 2021;12(1):8.

Gallbladder Imaging Interpretation Pearls and Pitfalls

Ultrasound, Computed Tomography, and Magnetic Resonance Imaging

Sergio P. Klimkowski, MD[a], Alice Fung, MD[b], Christine O. Menias, MD[c], Khaled M. Elsayes, MD[a],*

KEYWORDS

• Cholelithiasis • Cholecystitis • Gallstones • Gallbladder carcinoma • Adenomyomatosis

KEY POINTS

• Gallbladder disease is very common and presents in a wide variety of ways.
• Pitfalls in the evaluation of gallbladder disease broadly fall into 3 categories: technical, anatomic, and diagnostic.
• Technical pitfalls are related to issues with scanning technique, artifacts and patient positioning.
• Anatomic pitfalls usually result from misidentification of structures or physiologic variants.
• Diagnostic pitfalls often arise due to diagnostic dilemmas stemming from significant overlap in imaging features of both benign and malignant etiologies.

INTRODUCTION

Gallbladder disease is very common and presents in a variety of ways due to a wide range of pathologies. Most common forms of disease can be broadly classified into several categories: calculous disease, infection, inflammation, neoplasia, iatrogenic complications, and trauma. Calculous disease encompasses gallstones and their complications. Gallbladder infection results in suppurative cholecystitis, emphysematous cholecystitis, and gangrenous cholecystitis, while additional forms of cholecystitis and porcelain gallbladder are related to inflammatory causes. Gallbladder neoplasia includes a myriad of benign and malignant lesions. Finally, iatrogenic and traumatic processes can result in complications such as abscess formation, fistulas, hematomas, bile leaks, perforation, and torsion. This article will not focus on iatrogenic and traumatic etiologies of gallbladder disease.

Gallstone formation plays an important role in gallbladder disease pathophysiology and affects 10% to 15% of the adult population.[1–4] Although up to 80% of patients with gallstones will never be symptomatic or require treatment, complications related to gallstones result in a significant health care burden of approximately $6.2 billion annually, an increase of more than 20% over the past 3 decades.[2,5,6] Despite the indolent course of typical gallstone disease, patients at high risk for biliary complications may require intervention. These groups include patients with large gallstones greater than 3 cm or gallbladders packed with gallstones, patients with sickle cell disease, solid organ transplant recipients, and/or high-risk patients undergoing abdominal surgery for other

a Department of Abdominal Imaging, The University of Texas MD Anderson Cancer Center, Houston, TX 77030, USA; b Department of Diagnostic Radiology, Oregon Health & Science University, Portland, OR 97239, USA; c Department of Radiology, Mayo Clinic, Scottsdale, AZ 85259, USA
* Corresponding author.
E-mail address: kmelsayes@mdanderson.org

Radiol Clin N Am 60 (2022) 809–824
https://doi.org/10.1016/j.rcl.2022.05.002

reasons (eg, morbidly obese patients undergoing bariatric surgery).[1,7–10]

Typically, patients with right upper quadrant pain, jaundice, or obstructive symptoms are evaluated using a multimodality approach to include ultrasound and cross-sectional modalities, namely MRCP. Ultrasound is commonly the first-line modality of choice for the imaging evaluation of right upper quadrant pain. This is primarily due to its high sensitivity and specificity for both stone disease and gallbladder inflammation.[11] However, CT has become the most common initial imaging modality in evaluating patients presenting with an acute abdomen (particularly in the United States) due to added benefit of simultaneously evaluating nongallbladder pathologies.[12] Cross-sectional imaging provides a more global view of the right upper quadrant with the benefit of evaluating the entire abdomen. This can be helpful when evaluating for entities related to gallbladder disease, but with findings outside the gallbladder fossa, such as dropped stones, collections, and even gallstone ileus. MRI has also become an important imaging adjunct and problem-solving tool in the evaluation of the right upper quadrant and entire biliary system,[11] while hepatobiliary scintigraphy scans are routinely used to evaluate gallbladder function and cystic duct patency.

Pitfalls in the evaluation of gallbladder disease broadly fall into 3 categories: technical, anatomic, and diagnostic.[13]

TECHNICAL FACTORS PITFALLS

The technical pitfalls include errors of (1) misidentification due to error in scanning technique, such as mistaking bowel or a right upper quadrant collection for the gallbladder; (2) technique, such as improper transducer selection, poor gain settings, poor sonographic windows, and patient immobility; (3) artifacts, including pseudo-sludge and incorrect identification of gallstones related to side lobe artifact.[13] Proper patient preparation can facilitate gallbladder evaluation and avoid misidentification of the gallbladder. Fasting allows for adequate gallbladder distention to optimize the evaluation of the lumen and gallbladder wall. This can help decrease the risk of gallbladder misidentification for an adjacent organ such as bowel, stomach, or duodenum.[14] However, fasting is not practical in acute ER settings and duration of fasting before scheduled examinations varies widely among different institutions. In cases when gallbladder is difficult to identify or poorly distended, evaluation of major regional landmarks and multimodality approach using cross-sectional imaging can be helpful. For example, cross-sectional

imaging would be very useful in E.J. Fitzgerald case report of torsed ovarian dermoid with a long pedicle and migration to the right upper quadrant mimicking acute cholecystitis (internal debris misidentified as gallstones).[13]

Characteristic appearance of bowel on ultrasound is useful when distinguishing bowel from gallbladder. Normal "gut signature" sign represents a typical multi-lamellated sonographic appearance of viscera resulting from high organized and stratified wall histology.[15] The lamellated appearance consists of 5 alternating concentric hyperechoic and hypoechoic bands. The innermost echogenic layer corresponds to the mucosa, followed by hypoechoic muscularis mucosa, hyperechoic submucosa, hypoechoic muscularis propria, and finally hyperechogenic serosal surface.[15] (**Fig. 1**)

Appearance of posterior acoustic shadowing can be helpful in distinguishing gallbladder from adjacent gas-containing bowel and reduce errors of misidentification. Although, the presence of intraluminal or intramural gallbladder gas can be seen in patients with a history of CBD stenting or sphincterotomy or cases of emphysematous cholecystitis. The presence of gas should always be distinguished from gallstones. Posterior acoustic shadowing seen with gallstones should be "clean" and sharply defined. In contrast, acoustic shadowing related to bowel gas will seem indistinctly marginated and "dirty" due to reverberation echoes associated with sound beam and gas bubbles interaction (**Fig. 2**). The reverberation echoes within acoustic shadows deep to gas collections result almost exclusively from total sound reflection at tissue-gas interfaces, whereas shadowing deep to calculi is predominately due to sound absorption.[16] Appearance of shadowing helps distinguish bowel or other gas-containing structures from gallbladder under normal physiologic conditions.

Gallbladder fossa collections or adjacent intrahepatic abscesses can be mistaken for a gallbladder filled with stones or sludge (**Fig. 3**). Careful examination of the liver, gallbladder, and gallbladder contents is essential. The presence of intraluminal dirty shadowing may signify gas. Clinical history, white count and liver function tests (LFTs) should always be considered when evaluating the gallbladder fossa, particularly in cases when the gallbladder is not reliably identified. Ultimately, cross-sectional imaging maybe needed to confirm the diagnosis and to evaluate the abdomen more broadly (see **Fig. 3**).

Examination of right upper quadrant requires curvilinear or convex body transducers which are characterized by wide footprint, convex beam

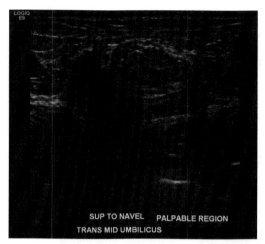

Fig. 1. Multi-lamellated appearance of bowel represents a gut signature sign. This loop of bowel is located within a palpable supraumbilical hernia.

shape, and low frequency of 2.5 to 7.5 MHz. These low-frequency transducers allow for greater penetration and increased depth at the cost of decreased resolution.[17] Adequate penetration is very important in abdominal applications, particularly in larger or obese patients. Poor sonographic windows maybe improved with subcostal or intercoastal approaches and/or changes in patient positioning. Sharply angling the transducer can also help in increasing the field of view.

Patient repositioning allows for the determination of lesion mobility which may be a key clue when distinguishing small calculi from polyps, particularly in cases when vascular stalk is not clearly seen. Furthermore, repositioning often affords better sonographic windows and improved image quality by bringing the gallbladder closer to the transducer. Gallbladder fossa should be thoroughly scanned in cases whereby the gallbladder is not clearly identified. Correlation with cross-sectional imaging and patient history may be helpful to determine if the gallbladder is surgically absent, very contracted, or even ectopic (Fig. 4).

Problems related to artifact are common with ultrasound. Artifactual side lobes from adjacent structures can be mistaken for gallbladder sludge or calculi (Figs. 5 and 6).[18] Ultrasound beam exits the transducer with most of the energy concentrated in the center and additional off-axis low-energy sidelobe beams along periphery. Furthermore, the main ultrasound beam narrows as it approaches the focal zone and then diverges.[19] Side lobe artifacts are caused by transducer detection of echoes generated by strong reflectors (eg, echogenic tissue interfaces) located

outside of the main ultrasound beam, usually located deep to the focal zone whereby the ultrasound beam widens past the width of the transducer.[19] The ultrasound software assumes incoming reflected echoes originate from within the narrow imaging plane corresponding to the width of the transducer. This assumption results in the display of reflected echoes of strong reflectors beyond the width of the transducer resulting in a sidelobe artifact (see Fig. 5). Adjusting the focal zone depth to place the object of interest within the center of the focal zone should help reduce or eliminate this artifact (Fig. 6).

Anatomic and Physiologic Variant Pitfalls

Knowledge of normal anatomic structures and variants is key to preventing misidentifying the gallbladder. The radiologist must be aware of the expected appearances of several entities, such as prominent gallbladder folds mimicking a dilated bile duct, sludge-filled gallbladder mimicking liver parenchyma, gallbladder agenesis and/or ectopia, and missed fundal and Hartmann's stones. For example, an elongated gallbladder that is folded on itself may produce echoes that can be mistaken for gallstones.[20] Alternatively, redundant fold or a folded gallbladder neck may mimic a dilated common bile duct.[21]

Gallbladder agenesis is rare, occurring only in 1/2500 to 1/5000 patients, and is a diagnosis of exclusion after careful assessment of common gallbladder ectopia sites.[22] The most common sites of gallbladder ectopia include beneath the left hepatic lobe, intrahepatic location, transversely positioned, and retroplaced positions into the retrohepatic or retroperitoneal spaces.[23] Fundal and Hartmann stones can be easily missed if the gallbladder fundus and neck are not carefully evaluated. Hartmann's pouch refers to the dilated appearance of the gallbladder neck whereby stones can collect and cause enlargement, inflammation, and adherence of the gallbladder to surrounding structures.[24] In the gallbladder fundus, gallstones can be missed due to the narrowed appearance of the fundus either related to a prominent fold that results in a Phrygian cap appearance or due to adenomyomatosis. In these scenarios, the "waist" can be mistaken for the fundal tip, and the actual bile and gallstone-filled fundus distal to the "waisted" region can be misinterpreted for adjacent colon (Fig. 7).

DIAGNOSTIC PITFALLS

A key step in the evaluation of the gallbladder is the accurate assessment of its wall. For a fasting patient in whom the gallbladder is adequately

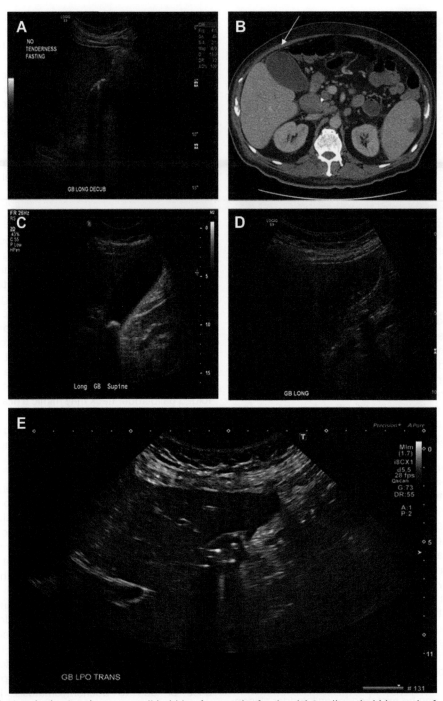

Fig. 2. (*A*) Dirty shadowing due to a small bubble of gas at the fundus. (*B*) Small gas bubbles at the fundus from the same patient (*white arrow*). Patient has an indwelling CBD stent. (*C*) Gallstone laying at the gallbladder neck. (*D*) Layering low-level echoes consistent with sludge. Differences in shadowing are related to the way sound beam interacts with a given structure (beam absorption, reflection, or combination of both to various degrees). (*E*) Dirty shadowing of gas within duodenum.

distended, the wall is typically no thicker than 3 mm. Diffuse abnormal gallbladder wall thickening, however, is nonspecific and can occur in a wide variety of conditions, including heart failure, hypoproteinemia, or even in decompressed states.[25] Thus, gallbladder wall thickening should be interpreted in conjunction with other findings when evaluating the right upper quadrant. I

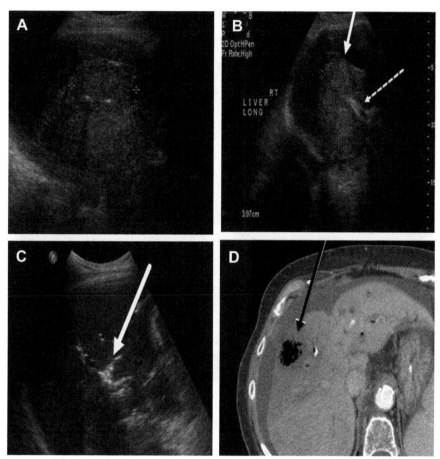

Fig. 3. (*A* and *B*) Hyperechoic collection at gallbladder fossa can be easily mistaken for gallbladder full of stones. This collection (*solid white arrow* in pane B) represents an intraparenchymal abscess related to cholangitis in patient with occluded biliary stent (*dotted white arrow*). (*C*) Branching "dirty shadowing" represents pneumobilia (*solid white arrow*). (*D*) CT image of hepatic abscess containing predominately air (*solid black arrow*).

additional findings of pericholecystic fluid, positive sonographic Murphy's sign, and stones or sludge are present, then the etiology is more likely to be acute cholecystitis. If the diffuse wall thickening is found in isolation, then the finding is likely reactive to an underlying systemic process, or inflammatory conditions. Oftentimes, the patient's history and laboratory values are helpful, as well.

In cases of chronically sick, debilitated, or ICU patients with suspected acalculous cholecystitis, the presence of gallbladder wall thickening and pericholecystic fluid can be helpful in suggesting the diagnosis (**Fig. 8**). However, these nonspecific findings are not always reliable in diagnosing acute cholecystitis, particularly in patients with edematous states/anasarca and ascites. Evaluation for acute cholecystitis can be further complicated by the presence of viscous bile or sludge that maybe slow to move or nonmoving on repositioning. Worse yet, the appearance of sludge may even

mimic a polyp or gallbladder tumor (**Fig. 9**).[26] Careful evaluation with Doppler is recommended to assess for any intralesional vascular flow. Ultimately, a hepatobiliary scintigraphy scan may be needed to confirm cystic duct occlusion (or patency), if clinical picture remains unclear (see **Fig. 8**).

The term gallstone ileus is a misnomer as this entity represents a true mechanical bowel obstruction due to the impaction of one or more gallstones in the gastrointestinal tract.[27,28] Mechanical obstruction occurs due to erosion of a gallstone(s) through a fistula to the adjacent duodenum, gastric pylorus, or hepatic flexure with subsequent migration of the eroded stone into the more distal gastrointestinal tract (**Figs. 10 and 11**). The potential point of obstruction depends on stone size. Most gallstones less than 2.5 cm can pass through the gastrointestinal tract to be expelled in the stool.[28,29] The most common

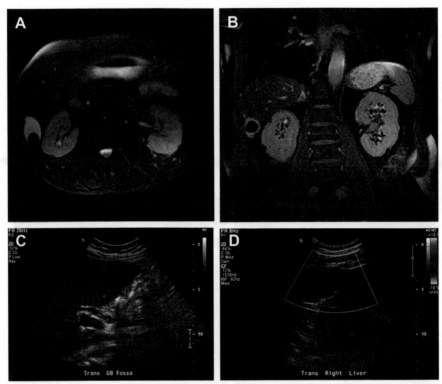

Fig. 4. Gallbladder ectopia. (*A, B*): Gallbladder containing a single gallstone is located along the inferior–posterior margin of the liver, adjacent to the right kidney. (*C, D*): US images showing empty gallbladder fossa (*C*) and cystic structure representing the ectopic gallbladder near the right kidney (*D*).

site of obstruction is the ileocecal valve, assuming the biliary fistula is at the level of duodenum or proximal small bowel.[27] Underlying conditions, such as inflammatory bowel disease resulting in strictures, neoplasms, and adhesive disease, increase the risk of stone impaction and mechanical obstruction.[28–30] Sonographic evaluation of the gallbladder can be challenging in gallstone ileus

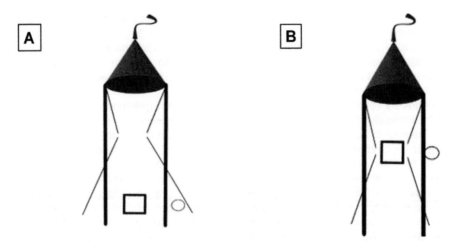

Fig. 5. (*A*) Imaged object (*square*) is beyond the focal zone represented by angulated lines. Strong reflector outside the main beam is represented by the oval. (*B*) Adjust focal zone to the level of imaged structure to decrease side lobe artifact.

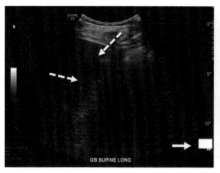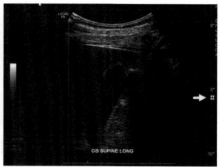

Fig. 6. (*Left*) Sidelobe artifact within the gallbladder mimicking possible sludge (*dashed white arrows*). Note that the focal zone is set deep to the gallbladder level (*white arrow* indicates focal zone). (*Right*) Focal zone adjusted to the level of gallbladder results in the elimination of the sidelobe artifact.

due to a potentially contracted gallbladder that has decompressed through the fistula with the gastrointestinal tract. The gallbladder may no longer contain any stones, and the actual fistulous tract may be difficult to see. Furthermore, bowel obstruction can be missed if cross-sectional imaging is not performed. Impacted gallstones causing the mechanical obstruction may be difficult to identify by CT, particularly if they are not radiopaque (see **Fig. 11**). The GI tract should be carefully examined for potential transition points, including obstructing intraluminal contents. Patients with gallstone ileus typically present with symptoms of bowel obstruction and history of right upper quadrant pain that has recently improved. Improvement in right upper quadrant pain coincides with the passage of stone into the GI tract. Clinical picture may also be complicated by intermittent obstructive symptoms which are related to intermittent gallstone movement until impaction occurs. Differential considerations aside from gallstone ileus include small bowel

obstruction related to other etiology such as adhesive disease or carcinomatosis.

Bouveret syndrome is an uncommon proximal variant of gallstone ileus consisting of gastric outlet obstruction due to an impacted gallstone in the distal stomach or proximal duodenum.

Mirizzi syndrome is a condition caused by extrinsic compression of the common bile duct by an impacted gallbladder neck, Hartmann's pouch, or infundibular stone resulting in obstructive jaundice and the possible later development of a cholecystobiliary or cholecystoenteric fistula (**Fig. 12**). Classification schemes proposed by Csendes and Beltran are based on the presence, size, and location of cholecystobiliary or bilioenteric fistulas.[31–33] Long cystic duct parallel to the CBD or low cystic duct insertion have been described as predisposing factors.[34,35] Diagnostic challenges are related to the relatively low sensitivity on ultrasound ranging from 8% to 27%.[36–38] MRCP and ERCP are particularly useful in characterizing potential fistulas, identifying filling

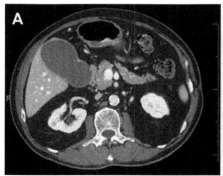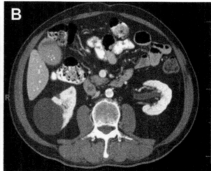

ig. 7. (*A*) Axial CECT shows a gallbladder with a prominent waist at the fundus. (*B*) Stones and sludge in gallbladder fundus which are more inferior can easily be missed on ultrasound or be mistaken for colonic contents due to proximity to adjacent hepatic flexure).

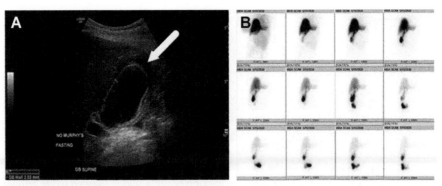

Fig. 8. (A) Mildly dilated gallbladder without gallbladder wall thickening. Trace pericholecystic fluid is present (*solid white arrow*) (B) Nonvisualization of gallbladder on HIDA. Findings are consistent with acalculous cholecystitis.

defects and extent of ductal dilatation of the biliary tree. CT and MRI/MRCP are very helpful in delineating anatomy, defining the extent of inflammatory changes, and evaluating the bowel. Both modalities are also helpful in excluding a possible neoplastic etiology.

Adenomyomatosis is a benign gallbladder condition characterized by epithelial, mucosal, and muscular hyperplastic changes in the gallbladder wall. Three main forms may be present: diffuse (<5%), fundal (30%), or segmental (>60%).[39] In this entity, the thickened gallbladder wall exhibits dilated Rokitansky–Aschoff sinuses which represent prominent invaginations into the muscularis layer of smooth muscle. These cystic pockets can contain calculi or cholesterol crystals.[40] Adenomyomatosis represents one of the 2 hyperplastic cholecystosis entities with the other type being cholesterolosis or "strawberry gallbladder," as the mucosal surface of the gallbladder resembles a strawberry due to the cholesterol esters that collect in the lamina propria.[41] Ultrasound

findings include gallbladder wall thickening, intramural cystic spaces, and mural echogenic foci with short "comet tail" reverberation artifact (Fig. 13).[39] The presence of "comet tail" confirms the diagnosis of adenomyomatosis and no further imaging is typically necessary.[42] Sometimes, distinguishing fundal or even segmental adenomyomatosis from gallbladder cancer can be challenging and sometimes presents a diagnostic dilemma. This usually occurs when gallbladder thickening is not adequately characterized either due to a partially decompressed state, obscuration by bowel gas, or extensive sludge/gallstones. Doppler interrogation should show no increased vascular flow of the thickened gallbladder wall. If present or unclear, then further imaging with MRI or CT should be performed to evaluate for a potential gallbladder mass with MR helpful in the distinction which can be challenging with CT.[43] Rokitansky–Aschoff sinuses appear as T2 hyperintense spaces on MR that align in curvilinear fashion and represent the "pearl necklace" sign

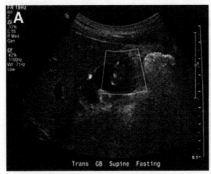
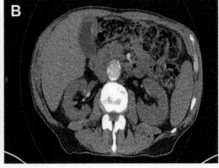

Fig. 9. (A) Rounded echogenic material at the gallbladder fundus represents tumefactive sludge. This can be confused for a potential gallbladder mass. Doppler demonstrates no increased vascular flow. (B) Axial CT image demonstrating tumefactive sludge versus stones adherent to the fundal wall.

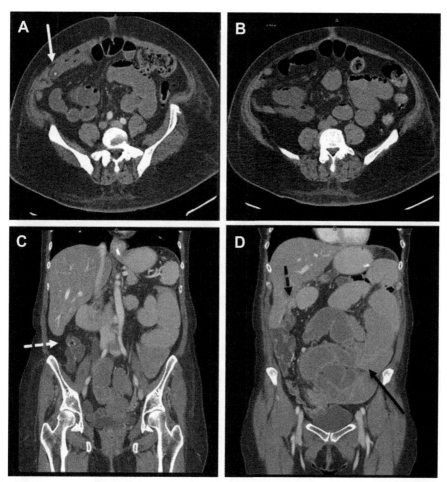

Fig. 10. (*A, B*) Radiopaque gallstone impacted in the distal small bowel (*solid white arrow*) with dilated upstream small bowel consistent with gallstone ileus. (*C, D*) Different patients with gallstones in the ascending colon (*dotted white arrow*) due to cholecystocolonic fistula (*dotted black arrow*). Small bowel obstruction in this patient was due to multifocal transition points related to peritoneal carcinomatosis from recurrent serous ovarian cancer (*solid black arrow*).

on MRI which can help in the distinction from cancer (**Fig. 14**).[40]

Gallbladder cancer can present as focal wall thickening, a mass, or a polyp, and distinguishing benign gallbladder disease from gallbladder cancer is sometimes challenging. This presents a significant diagnostic dilemma with an impact on patient management, specifically because resectable gallbladder cancer requires resection of hepatic segments 4 and 5 at the time of cholecystectomy to offer the best surgical outcome.[44] Common risk factors for gallbladder cancer include gallstone disease, polyps greater than 1.5 cm, chronic gallbladder inflammatory changes, chronic cholecystitis, obesity, and porcelain gallbladder.[44] Clinical presentations are nonspecific and overlap with benign gallbladder

disease. Patients with gallbladder cancer commonly present with biliary colic and indigestion. Weight loss and obstructive jaundice herald advanced disease that is likely metastatic and unresectable.[44] Gallbladder carcinoma often coexists with benign gallbladder disease and over half of new gallbladder cancer cases are diagnosed at or after cholecystectomy performed for benign disease.[45,46] A high level of suspicion for gallbladder carcinoma should be maintained. Elderly patients with a dilated common bile duct elevated alkaline phosphatase, and gallbladder wall thickening with suspected cholecystitis but no pericholecystic fluid are more commonly found with gallbladder cancer than those patients without such findings.[47] Another common pitfall in diagnosing gallbladder cancer is patients with

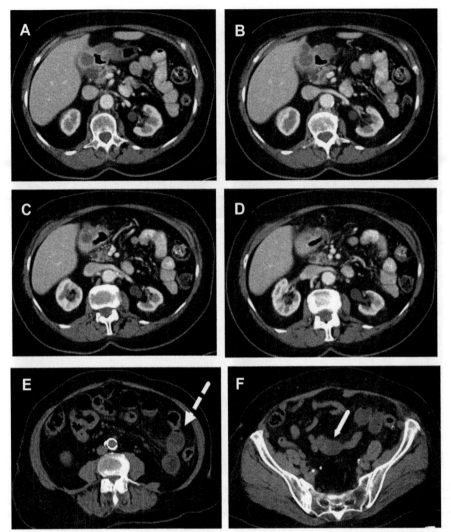

Fig. 11. (*A, B, C,* and *D*) Thickened gallbladder with pericholecystic inflammatory changes is inseparable from duodenal bulb secondary to both chronic duodenitis and chronic cholecystitis. (*E, F*) The same patient imaged a month later demonstrates difficulty to identify radiolucent gallstone (*solid white arrow*) impacted in the distal small bowel with mild upstream bowel dilatation (*dotted white arrow*).

chronic cholecystitis or perforated cholecystitis with pericholecystic abscesses due to an obstructing mass at the gallbladder neck. Inflammatory changes, hyperemia, and possible intramural hematomas may obscure the detection of potential obstructing masses. Cross-sectional imaging may help in further characterizing the gallbladder fossa, but detection of these masses may be very difficult on preoperative imaging. Gallbladder carcinoma can be very difficult to delineate in the setting of acute or chronic cholecystitis unrelated to the presence of carcinoma. Inflammatory changes and hyperemia can obscure potential masses, particularly if small. Kim and colleagues[48] analyzed enhancement

characteristics of the gallbladder wall on CT and found that inner wall layer thickness of greater or equal to 2.6 mm, outer wall layer thickness less than or equal to 3.4 mm, marked enhancement of the inner wall layer and irregular contour of the thickened wall represent features that can be used to predict malignancy (**Fig. 15**). Some present with pericholecystic abscesses on imaging (US and CT), and can be diagnostically challenging, as they look perforated on imaging but often, these patients are often elderly and clinically "not sick" with no WBC elevation and symptoms may improve after perforation.[49]

Another important imaging pitfall is confusing potential xanthogranulomatous cholecystitis with

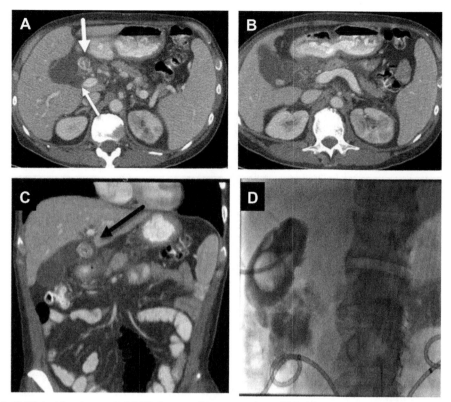

Fig. 12. (*A, B*) Mirizzi Syndrome Axial CT shows gallstones at the gallbladder neck causing extrinsic compression of the common bile duct resulting in intrahepatic biliary ductal dilatation. (*C*) Coronal CT imaging showing extrinsic compression of CBD with upstream biliary ductal dilatation. (*D*) Cholecystostomy images showing no opacification of cystic or common bile duct. Contrast within right upper quadrant bowel is due to oral contrast from prior CT (partially seen on both axial and coronal images).

gallbladder cancer. Distinguishing these 2 entities can be challenging as both entities can show diffusion restriction on MRI. In case of xanthogranulomatous cholecystitis, the pattern of restriction tends to be circumferential corresponding to the inflamed gallbladder wall and ADC values are typically higher than gallbladder cancer.[50,51] Irregular margins, invasive appearance such as invasion of the adjacent structures, and enlarged rounded regional lymph nodes tend to favor malignancy.[25]

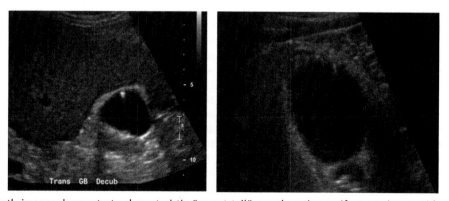

ig. 13. Both images demonstrate characteristic "comet tail" reverberation artifact consistent with segmental denomyomatosis.

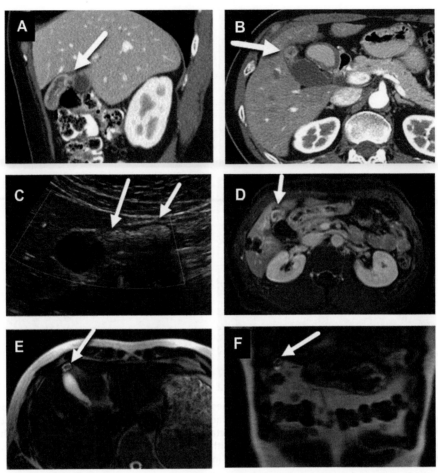

Fig. 14. (*A, B, C, D*) Sagittal (*A*) and axial (*B*) CECT images of fundal form of adenomyomatosis, showing focal soft-tissue attenuation of the fundus with tiny cystic spaces outlining the wall on the axial image (*B*) (*solid white arrow*). (*C, D*) US and MRI T1 postcontrast images of the same patient with the fundal form of adenomyomatosis. No increased vascular flow or mass is seen at the fundus. Note that there is mild posterior acoustic shadowing (without comet tail artifact) on the US image that should not be confused with gallstones (*E, F*) Axial and coronal T2s of fundal adenomyomatosis in a different patient. This characteristic appearance with T2 bright mural foci is called the "pearl necklace" sign.

Other important mimics of gallbladder cancer include lymphoma, hepatocellular carcinoma, intrahepatic cholangiocarcinoma, metastasis, and carcinoid tumor.

Porcelain gallbladder is poorly characterized on ultrasound due to circumferential calcifications. Sonographically, it can be difficult to distinguish from a partially contracted gallbladder filled with stones. Evaluation of the gallbladder wall on Doppler is also limited due to aliasing caused by wall calcifications. In these cases, CT or MR would be helpful to visualize the gallbladder contents and evaluate the right upper quadrant (**Fig. 16**) with MR potentially helpful as calcifications are not seen which may help show an underlying mass more effectively.

Gallbladder polyps are very common incidental findings in the evaluation of the gallbladder. Generally, the gallbladder polyps are small and mimic small gallstones adherent to the gallbladder wall. Doppler interrogation should reveal the presence of vascular flow in the polyp stalk. However, this is not always the case, especially when the potential polyp is very small or if the Doppler velocity scale is set too high. Evaluation of these lesions should include assessment for mobility with patient repositioning. If available, the review of old multiphasic cross-sectional imaging may help in identifying a small enhancing polyp. Ultimately, distinguishing small polyps from gallstones may be difficult. Risk factors for malignancy in gallbladder polyps are cholelithiasis, history of

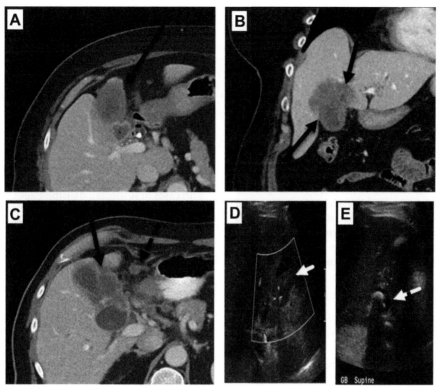

Fig. 15. (*A* and *B*) Axial (*A*) and coronal (*B*) CECT shows gallbladder mass invading the adjacent liver consistent with gallbladder carcinoma. Note irregular wall thickening, particularly on image B. (*C*) Another patient with nodular thickening of gallbladder wall (*long black arrow*). Peritoneal implant at the gallbladder fossa (*dotted black arrow*). Findings represent advanced gallbladder cancer. This patient also had liver and ascending colon serosal metastasis. (*D*) The same patient with irregular wall thickening shows no discernible color Doppler despite a very aggressive appearance on CT with the invasion of adjacent liver. (*E*) This patient also has gallstones layering at the gallbladder neck on ultrasound.

primary sclerosing cholangitis, age greater than 50 year old, Indian ethnicity, polyp size greater than 1 cm, sessile polyp morphology and/or wall thickening greater than 4 mm.[44,52–54] Surgical management guidelines account for these risk factors. For example, polyps equal to or greater than 15 mm are usually resected due to elevated risk of malignancy (45%–65%).[52]

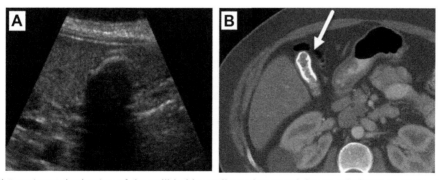

Fig. 16. (*A*) Prominent shadowing of the gallbladder wall on ultrasound due to calcifications. Sonographically it is unclear whether this represents gallstones ("WES" sign) or mural calcifications seen in porcelain gallbladder. (*B*) CT of the same patient performed for further evaluation demonstrates circumferential calcification of the gallbladder wall consistent with "porcelain gallbladder."

SUMMARY

Gallbladder disease is a common clinical problem in both emergent and nonemergent settings and includes both malignant and benign etiologies. Imaging evaluation of the right upper quadrant plays a key role in establishing the correct diagnosis. Clinical history, physical examination, and laboratory values are important in the accurate imaging assessment of the right upper quadrant. Significant overlap in imaging features of both benign and malignant etiologies can pose diagnostic dilemmas. Additionally, inherent limitations of ultrasound and cross-sectional techniques may lead to diagnostic pitfalls preventing accurate diagnosis. Knowledge of these pitfalls and their solutions help in the accurate assessment of the gallbladder.

CLINICS CARE POINTS

- Clinical history, physical examination, and laboratory values are important in the accurate imaging assessment of the right upper quadrant due to significant overlap in imaging features of both benign and malignant etiologies.

- Ultrasound is commonly the first-line modality of choice for the imaging evaluation of right upper quadrant pain.

- Cross-sectional imaging provides a more global view of the right upper quadrant with the benefit of evaluating the entire abdomen.

- Examination of right upper quadrant requires curvilinear or convex body transducers which are characterized by wide footprint, convex beam shape, and low frequency of 2.5 to 7.5 MHz.

- Appearance of posterior acoustic shadowing can be helpful in distinguishing gallbladder from adjacent gas-containing bowel and reduce errors of misidentification. "Dirty" posterior acoustic shadowing is usually seen with intraluminal gas suggesting bowel contents versus "clean" shadowing is seen with gallstones.

- Comet tail artifact is seen with adenomyomatosis.

- Doppler and decubitus positioning are very helpful in distinguishing small polyps from gallstones.

- Circumferential wall calcifications may be challenging to distinguish from "WES" sign on ultrasound and CT may help establish the diagnosis.

- Set the focal zone to the level of the gallbladder to avoid or decrease side lobe artifact.

- Gallbladder wall thickening is nonspecific and should be considered with other clinical information including presence of positive Murphy's sign, focality, hemodynamic status, presence or absence of heart failure and hypoproteinemia.

- Small bowel should be carefully examined on cross sectional imaging for obstructing stones in cases of suspected gallstone ileus or in cases of suspected biliary-enteric fistulas (though may be difficult to identify if stones are relatively radiolucent).

- Distinguishing gallbladder neoplasia from chronic inflammatory changes can be difficult. Signs such as high ADC values, irregular margins and invasive appearance tend to favor malignancy.

- Inflammatory changes can mask underlying malignancy.

DISCLOSURE

The authors have nothing to disclose.

REFERENCES

1. Schirmer BD, Winters KL, Edlich RF. Cholelithiasis and cholecystitis. J Long Term Eff Med Implants 2005;15(3):329–38.
2. Shaffer EA. Epidemiology and risk factors for gallstone disease: has the paradigm changed in the 21st century? Curr Gastroenterol Rep 2005;7(2):132–40.
3. Tazuma S. Gallstone disease: Epidemiology, pathogenesis, and classification of biliary stones (common bile duct and intrahepatic). Best Pract Res Clin Gastroenterol 2006;20(6):1075–83.
4. Kratzer W, Mason RA, Kachele V. Prevalence of gallstones in sonographic surveys worldwide. J Clin Ultrasound 1999;27(1):1–7.
5. Sakorafas GH, Milingos D, Peros G. Asymptomatic cholelithiasis: is cholecystectomy really needed? A critical reappraisal 15 years after the introduction of laparoscopic cholecystectomy. Dig Dis Sci 2007;52(5):1313–25.
6. Everhart JE, Ruhl CE. Burden of digestive diseases in the United States part I: overall and upper gastrointestinal diseases. Gastroenterology 2009;136(2):376–86.
7. Kapoor VK. Cholecystectomy in patients with asymptomatic gallstones to prevent gall bladder cancer–the case against. Indian J Gastroenterol 2006;25(3):152–4.

8. Bonatsos G, Birbas K, Toutouzas K, et al. Laparoscopic cholecystectomy in adults with sickle cell disease. Surg Endosc 2001;15(8):816–9.

9. Ebert EC, Nagar M, Hagspiel KD. Gastrointestinal and hepatic complications of sickle cell disease. Clin Gastroenterol Hepatol 2010;8(6):483–9. quiz e470.

10. Kao LS, Kuhr CS, Flum DR. Should cholecystectomy be performed for asymptomatic cholelithiasis in transplant patients? J Am Coll Surg 2003;197(2):302–12.

11. Catalano OA, Sahani DV, Kalva SP, et al. MR imaging of the gallbladder: a pictorial essay. Radiographics 2008;28(1):135–55.

12. Grand D, Horton KM, Fishman EK. CT of the gallbladder: spectrum of disease. AJR Am J Roentgenol 2004;183(1):163–70.

13. Fitzgerald EJ, Toi A. Pitfalls in the ultrasonographic diagnosis of gallbladder diseases. Postgrad Med J 1987;63(741):525–32.

14. Cooperberg PL, Pon MS, Wong P, et al. Real-time high resolution ultrasound in the detection of biliary calculi. Radiology 1979;131(3):789–90.

15. Maturen KE, Wasnik AP, Kamaya A, et al. Ultrasound imaging of bowel pathology: technique and keys to diagnosis in the acute abdomen. Am J Roentgenol 2011;197(6):W1067–75.

16. Sommer FG, Taylor KJW. Differentiation of acoustic shadowing due to calculi and gas collections. Radiology 1980;135(2):399–403.

17. Ploquin M, Basarab A, Kouame D. Resolution enhancement in medical ultrasound imaging. J Med Imaging (Bellingham) 2015;2(1):017001.

18. Mattson MW, Sterchi JM, Myers RT. Accuracy of ultrasonography and oral cholecystography in the diagnosis of cholelithiasis. Am Surg 1981;47(2):80–1.

19. Feldman MK, Katyal S, Blackwood MS. US Artifacts. Radiographics 2009;29(4):1179–90.

20. Arnon S, Rosenquist CJ. Gray scale cholecystosonography: an evaluation of accuracy. AJR Am J Roentgenol 1976;127(5):817–8.

21. Laing FC, Jeffrey RB. The pseudo-dilated common bile duct: ultrasonographic appearance created by the gallbladder neck. Radiology 1980;135(2):405–7.

22. Mouzas G, Wilson AK. Congenital absence of the gall-bladder with stone in the common bile-duct. Lancet 1953;1(6761):628–9.

23. Rafailidis V, Varelas S, Kotsidis N, et al. Two congenital anomalies in one: an ectopic gallbladder with phrygian cap deformity. Case Rep Radiol 2014;2014:246476.

24. Khan KS, Sajid MA, McMahon RK, et al. Hartmann's pouch stones and laparoscopic cholecystectomy: the challenges and the solutions. JSLS 2020;24(3).

25. Runner GJ, Corwin MT, Siewert B, et al. Gallbladder wall thickening. AJR Am J Roentgenol 2014;202(1):W1–12.

26. Anastasi B, Sutherland GR. Biliary sludge-ultrasonic appearance simulating neoplasm. Br J Radiol 1981;54(644):679–81.

27. Nuno-Guzman CM, Marin-Contreras ME, Figueroa-Sanchez M, et al. Gallstone ileus, clinical presentation, diagnostic and treatment approach. World J Gastrointest Surg 2016;8(1):65–76.

28. Abou-Saif A, Al-Kawas FH. Complications of gallstone disease: Mirizzi syndrome, cholecystocholedochal fistula, and gallstone ileus. Am J Gastroenterol 2002;97(2):249–54.

29. Fox PF. Planning the operation for cholecystoenteric fistula with gallstone ileus. Surg Clin North Am 1970;50(1):93–102.

30. Rogers FA, Carter R. Gallstone intestinal obstruction. Calif Med 1958;88(2):140–3.

31. Beltran MA. Mirizzi syndrome: history, current knowledge and proposal of a simplified classification. World J Gastroenterol 2012;18(34):4639–50.

32. Beltran MA, Csendes A, Cruces KS. The relationship of Mirizzi syndrome and cholecystoenteric fistula: validation of a modified classification. World J Surg 2008;32(10):2237–43.

33. Csendes A, Diaz JC, Burdiles P, et al. Mirizzi syndrome and cholecystobiliary fistula: a unifying classification. Br J Surg 1989;76(11):1139–43.

34. Montefusco P, Spier N, Geiss AC. Another facet of Mirizzi's syndrome. Arch Surg 1983;118(10):1221–3.

35. Toscano RL, Taylor PH Jr, Peters J, et al. Mirizzi syndrome. Am Surg 1994;60(11):889–91.

36. Safioleas M, Stamatakos M, Safioleas P, et al. Mirizzi syndrome: an unexpected problem of cholelithiasis. Our experience with 27 cases. Int Semin Surg Oncol 2008;5:12.

37. Yonetci N, Kutluana U, Yilmaz M, et al. The incidence of Mirizzi syndrome in patients undergoing endoscopic retrograde cholangiopancreatography. Hepatobiliary Pancreat Dis Int 2008;7(5):520–4.

38. Al-Akeely MHA, Alam MK, Bismar HA, et al. Mirizzi syndrome: ten years experience from a teaching hospital in Riyadh. World J Surg 2005;29(12):1687–92.

39. Golse N, Lewin M, Rode A, et al. Gallbladder adenomyomatosis: diagnosis and management. J Visc Surg 2017;154(5):345–53.

40. Joshi JK, Kirk L. Adenomyomatosis. In: StatPearls. Treasure Island (FL): StatPearls Publishing; 2022

41. Sandri L, Colecchia A, Larocca A, et al. Gallbladder cholesterol polyps and cholesterolosis. Minerva Gastroenterol Dietol 2003;49(3):217–24.

42. Oh SH, Han HY, Kim HJ. Comet tail artifact on ultrasonography: is it a reliable finding of benign gallbladder diseases? Ultrasonography 2019;38(3):221–30.

43. Ching BH, Yeh BM, Westphalen AC, et al. CT differentiation of adenomyomatosis and gallbladder cancer. AJR Am J Roentgenol 2007;189(1):62–6.

44. Hickman L, Contreras C. Gallbladder cancer: diagnosis, surgical management, and adjuvant therapies. Surg Clin North Am 2019;99(2):337–55.

45. Hueman MT, Vollmer CM Jr, Pawlik TM. Evolving treatment strategies for gallbladder cancer. Ann Surg Oncol 2009;16(8):2101–15.

46. Duffy A, Capanu M, Abou-Alfa GK, et al. Gallbladder cancer (GBC): 10-year experience at memorial sloan-kettering cancer centre (MSKCC). J Surg Oncol 2008;98(7):485–9.

47. Goussous N, Maqsood H, Patel K, et al. Clues to predict incidental gallbladder cancer. Hepatobiliary Pancreat Dis Int 2018;17(2):149–54.

48. Kim SJ, Lee JM, Lee JY, et al. Analysis of enhancement pattern of flat gallbladder wall thickening on MDCT to differentiate gallbladder cancer from cholecystitis. Am J Roentgenol 2008;191(3):765–71.

49. Vendrami CL, Magnetta MJ, Mittal PK, et al. Gallbladder carcinoma and its differential diagnosis at mri: what radiologists should know. Radiographics 2021;41(1):78–95.

50. Gupta P, Marodia Y, Bansal A, et al. Imaging-based algorithmic approach to gallbladder wall thickening. World J Gastroenterol 2020;26(40):6163–81.

51. Kang TW, Kim SH, Park HJ, et al. Differentiating xanthogranulomatous cholecystitis from wall-thickening type of gallbladder cancer: added value of diffusion-weighted MRI. Clin Radiol 2013;68(10):992–1001.

52. Wiles R, Thoeni RF, Barbu ST, et al. Management and follow-up of gallbladder polyps : Joint guidelines between the European Society of Gastrointestinal and Abdominal Radiology (ESGAR), European Association for Endoscopic Surgery and other Interventional Techniques (EAES), International Society of Digestive Surgery - European Federation (EFISDS) and European Society of Gastrointestinal Endoscopy (ESGE). Eur Radiol 2017;27(9):3856–66.

53. Buckles DC, Lindor KD, Larusso NF, et al. In primary sclerosing cholangitis, gallbladder polyps are frequently malignant. Am J Gastroenterol 2002;97(5):1138–42.

54. Park JK, Yoon YB, Kim YT, et al. Management strategies for gallbladder polyps: is it possible to predict malignant gallbladder polyps? Gut Liver 2008;2(2):88–94.

Update on Biliary Cancer Imaging

Dong Wook Kim, MD, PhD[a], So Yeon Kim, MD, PhD[a,*], Changhoon Yoo, MD, PhD[b], Dae Wook Hwang, MD, PhD[c]

KEYWORDS

- Bile duct • Biliary cancer • Cholangiocarcinoma • CT • MR imaging • MRCP

KEY POINTS

- Imaging analysis using computed tomography (CT) and/or MR imaging with magnetic resonance cholangiopancreatography (MRCP) plays an essential role in diagnosis and treatment planning in cholangiocarcinoma.
- Irregular wall thickening in the bile duct or an intraductal mass associated with upstream biliary dilatation is imaging features that indicate extrahepatic cholangiocarcinoma.
- Thin-section (slice thickness ≤3 mm) multiphase CT imaging (noncontrast, arterial, and portal venous phases) with multiplanar reformation is the optimal CT protocol for extrahepatic cholangiocarcinoma.
- MR imaging with MRCP presents additional information for evaluating cholangiocarcinoma. Recent advances in MR imaging techniques provide rapid imaging with high resolution, which can enhance the visualization of cancer extent and complex anatomy.
- For preoperative assessment of extrahepatic cholangiocarcinoma, longitudinal tumor extent, vascular involvement, lymph node and distant metastasis, and future remnant liver volume should be carefully evaluated on imaging.

INTRODUCTION

Biliary cancer, also known as cholangiocarcinoma (CC), is a primary malignant epithelial neoplasm arising in any location of the biliary tree from the intrahepatic bile ductule to the common bile duct, and adenocarcinoma comprises 95% of CC. Although approximately 80% of CC occurs sporadically without a definite risk factor, the known risk factors for CC include choledochal cyst and chronic biliary inflammation such as primary sclerosing cholangitis or recurrent pyogenic cholangitis, with the latter being commonly caused by liver fluke infection or hepatolithiasis.[1] A wide geographic variation in the prevalence of CC is noted, with the highest incidence occurring in Asian countries such as Thailand, China, and Korea.[1] The worldwide incidence of CC has recently been increasing. CC is usually asymptomatic in the early stage, but patients with advanced extrahepatic CC commonly present with jaundice. Elevation of carbohydrate antigen 19-9 is a useful laboratory finding, reportedly having high diagnostic performance (80%–90%) for CC in patients with primary sclerosing cholangitis.[2,3]

Complete resection is the only curative treatment of CC. Given that the surgical techniques for CC are highly demanding and involve a wide

[a] Department of Radiology and Research Institute of Radiology, University of Ulsan College of Medicine, Asan Medical Center, 88 Olympic-ro 43-gil, Songpa-gu, Seoul 05505, Republic of Korea; [b] Department of Oncology, University of Ulsan College of Medicine, Asan Medical Center, 88 Olympic-ro 43-gil, Songpa-gu, Seoul 05505, Republic of Korea; [c] Division of Hepatobiliary and Pancreatic Surgery, Department of Surgery, University of Ulsan College of Medicine, Asan Medical Center, 88 Olympic-ro 43-gil, Songpa-gu, Seoul 05505, Republic of Korea

* Corresponding author. Department of Radiology and Research Institute of Radiology, University of Ulsan College of Medicine, Asan Medical Center, 88 Olympic-ro 43-gil, Songpa-gu, Seoul 05505, Republic of Korea.
E-mail address: sykim.radiology@gmail.com

Radiol Clin N Am 60 (2022) 825–842
https://doi.org/10.1016/j.rcl.2022.05.001
0033-8389/22/© 2022 Elsevier Inc. All rights reserved.

surgical field that includes important organs such as the liver or pancreas, biliary structures with small caliber, and adjacent critical vascular structures, and the comprehensive imaging evaluation is imperative for treatment planning. Computed tomography (CT) with multiphase imaging plays a fundamental role in the workup for CC, and magnetic resonance (MR) imaging with magnetic resonance cholangiopancreatography (MRCP) allows more detailed information. An understanding of the recent advances in MR imaging techniques will empower radiologists to obtain an upgraded tool in the hard-fought battle to beat CC, which has a notoriously poor prognosis.

In this review, we provide a brief clinical overview of CC, including classification, current treatment options, and prognosis, which all need to be taken into account in its imaging analysis. This article then comprehensively reviews the imaging techniques for evaluating CC, including their performance and recent updates, the imaging characteristics of CC, and the key points for preoperative imaging. This article mainly focuses on extrahepatic CC including perihilar CC (pCC) and distal CC (dCC).

CLASSIFICATION OF CHOLANGIOCARCINOMA

Anatomic classification and morphologic classification form the two major classifications of CC. In the anatomic classification, CC is most commonly subdivided into the following three subtypes[4] (**Fig. 1**): (a) intrahepatic CC (iCC), located from the bile ductule to the secondary bile duct confluence; (b) pCC, located from the secondary bile duct confluence to the common hepatic duct; and (c) dCC, located in the common bile duct. The most common type is pCC (50%–60%), followed by dCC (20%–30%), and iCC (10%–20%).[4,5] The different anatomic subtypes of CC require different surgical resection methods (see **Fig. 1**).

The Liver Cancer Group of Japan classification is the most common morphologic classification,[6] and its classes consist of (a) mass-forming CC; (b) periductal infiltrating CC; (c) intraductal growing CC; and (d) combined-type CC (eg, mass-forming CC + periductal infiltrating CC) (**Fig. 2**). Mass-forming CC is the most common type of iCC, whereas periductal infiltrating CC is the most common type of pCC and dCC. Less common is intraductal growing CC, which sometimes presents synchronously in any of the anatomic locations. Mass-forming and intraductal growing CC both show mucosal spread, whereas periductal infiltrating CC shows submucosal spread.[7] CC also has different prognoses according to its morphologic classification. Intraductal CC generally has a more favorable prognosis than CC of other morphologic types,[8] whereas combined mass-forming and periductal infiltrating CC have a poorer prognosis than mass-forming CC.[9,10]

TREATMENT AND PROGNOSIS

Surgical resection with a negative resection margin is by far the only curative option for CC.

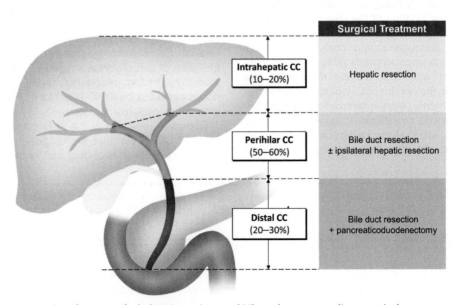

Fig. 1. Anatomic classification of cholangiocarcinoma (CC) and corresponding surgical treatment options. Numbers in parenthesis indicate the incidence of each type of CC.

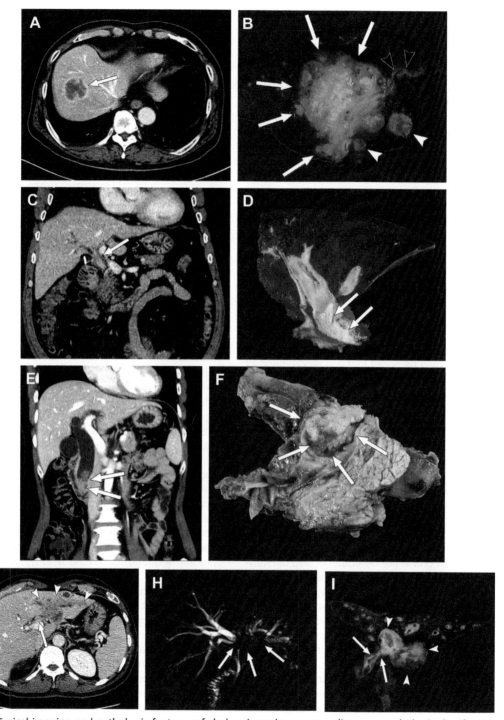

Fig. 2. Typical imaging and pathologic features of cholangiocarcinoma according to morphologic classification. (A, B) Mass-forming type. (A) A peripheral-enhancing mass in the right lobe of the liver (*arrow*) is noted on a portal venous phase axial CT image. (B) Gross photography of the hepatectomy specimen reveals a lobulating, contoured mass (*arrows*) with adjacent small daughter nodules (*white arrowheads*). Bile duct dilatation (*black arrowheads*) is noted in the distal portion of the mass. (C, D) Periductal infiltrating type. (C) Coronal image of a portal venous CT scan shows an infiltrative mass involving the perihilar bile duct (*arrow*), which causes intrahepatic bile duct dilatation. (D) A surgical specimen obtained after partial hepatectomy and bile duct resection depicting the mass along the bile duct (*arrows*). (E, F) Intraductal growing type. (E) A polypoid mass (*arrows*) in the distal bile duct with upstream bile duct dilatation is seen on the coronal image of the portal venous phase CT. (F)

Unfortunately, less than 25% of patients are suitable candidates for curative-intent surgery at presentation.[11] Adjuvant chemotherapy such as capecitabine is recommended for patients with a high-risk of recurrence after resection.[12] Liver transplantation is traditionally contraindicated because of the high recurrence rate.[13-15] In patients with unresectable or metastatic CC, systemic chemotherapy is the standard of care: gemcitabine plus cisplatin is the standard first-line chemotherapy[16,17] and FOLFOX (folinic acid, 5-fluorouracil, and oxaliplatin) is the recommended second-line therapy.

The overall prognosis for CC is very poor, with 5 year survival of less than 20%.[18-21] Even after curative resection, postoperative recurrence is reported to be as high as 70%.[22,23]

IMAGING TECHNIQUES FOR PERIHILAR AND DISTAL CHOLANGIOCARCINOMA

For extrahepatic CC, the major imaging roles are assessment of tumor resectability and preoperative planning, given that surgery is the only curative option. It should be noted that it is recommended to obtain imaging before biliary drainage because the drainage catheter or stent may obscure or overestimate the lesion (Fig. 3).[24,25]

Computed Tomography

Multiphasic contrast-enhanced CT is the imaging modality of choice for preoperative assessment of extrahepatic CC because of its excellent temporal and spatial resolution.[26,27] A recent consensus statement by the Korean Society of Abdominal Radiology[26] recommends obtaining three phasic images with slice thickness ≤3 mm, including a non-contrast phase (for detection of and differentiation from intraductal stones), arterial phase (for increasing the conspicuity of tumor against the background and for evaluation of arterial invasion), and portal venous phase (for evaluation of disease extent and detection of distant metastasis) (Fig. 4). In addition, multiplanar reconstruction is recommended to better identify the tumor extent and the relationships between tumors and neighboring structures (see Fig. 4).[28,29] It is recommended to include the pelvic cavity in the scan range of the

initial staging, preferably in the portal venous phase imaging, to detect peritoneal seeding.[26] An example of CT protocol is summarized in Table 1, and the diagnostic performance of CT in the evaluation of extrahepatic bile duct cancer is summarized in Table 2.[30,31] As pCC and dCC present as microscopic submucosal extension, CT has a tendency to underestimate the longitudinal tumor extent in these types.[7,32]

MR Imaging with Magnetic Resonance Cholangiopancreatography

MR imaging with MRCP is increasingly being used because of its better demonstration of tumor extent and bile duct anatomy in comparison with CT. MR imaging also facilitates the differentiation of dCC from benign biliary diseases as well as dCC from pancreas cancer.[26,33] Differentiating dCC and pancreas cancer is important, as treatment strategies including preoperative chemotherapy differ (Fig. 5). MR imaging with MRCP is reported to have good diagnostic performance for assessing biliary cancer extent (see Table 2).[31,34-36]

Examples of MR imaging with MRCP protocols are provided in Table 3. MR imaging sequences include T2-weighted imaging and multiphasic (eg, precontrast, arterial, portal venous, and delayed phases) three-dimensional (3D) fat-saturated contrast-enhanced T1-weighted imaging. Diffusion-weighted imaging is also recommended, as it enhances detection of tumor, evaluation of tumor extent, and detection of intrahepatic metastasis.[37-40] The choice of contrast agent for extrahepatic CC is a topic requiring discussion. A conventional extracellular contrast agent is preferred over a hepatocyte-specific contrast agent (ie, gadoxetic acid [Eovist or Primovist, Bayer Schering Pharma, Berlin, Germany]), particularly in patients with biliary obstruction. Although gadoxetic acid can be useful for detecting hepatic metastasis,[40,41] extrahepatic biliary cancer often causes bile duct obstruction that prohibits the hepatocyte uptake and biliary excretion of gadoxetic acid, thus mitigating its potential advantages.[42] In addition, gadoxetic acid-enhanced MR imaging may underestimate the extent of tumor because of the

---

A pancreaticoduodenectomy specimen reveals a nodular mass in the distal bile duct (*arrows*). (G–I) Combined type (mass-forming type + periductal infiltrating type). (G) An axial portal venous phase image shows an ill-defined mass (*white arrowheads*) obliterating the left portal vein, extending to the common hepatic ducts as a periductal infiltrating type (*arrow*). In the peripheral portion of the left lobe, two hepatic abscesses are also visible (*black arrowheads*). (H) On MRCP, the extent of the mass and periductal extension is clearly visualized (*arrows*). (I) Gross photography obtained after partial hepatectomy and bile duct resection reveals the intrahepatic mass (*arrowheads*) extending along the adjacent bile duct (*arrows*).

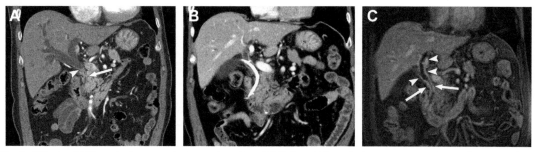

Fig. 3. Effects of biliary drainage catheter on imaging. (A) Before biliary drainage, a coronal portal venous phase CT image clearly depicts the extent of the distal cholangiocarcinoma with growth indicative of the periductal infiltrating type (proximal extent, *arrowhead*; distal extent, *arrow*). The perihilar and intrahepatic bile ducts look normal without definite enhancement or wall thickening. (B) After biliary drainage, the tumor is obscured by the presence of biliary stent, which presents as hyperdense linear material on the coronal CT image. (C) Coronal portal venous phase MR imaging after biliary drainage reveals diffuse enhancement of the proximal duct (*arrowheads*) beyond the cancer-involved segment (*arrows*), possibly due to postinterventional inflammatory changes.

relatively weak enhancement of tumor but strong enhancement of background liver.[26,43] The arterial motion artifacts that are sometimes present in gadoxetic acid-enhanced MR imaging can further deteriorate image quality.[44,45]

MRCP is basically T2-weighted imaging with a long echo time, on which the high signal of bile within the biliary system is accentuated, although the background tissue is suppressed. MRCP comprises the following three main sequences:

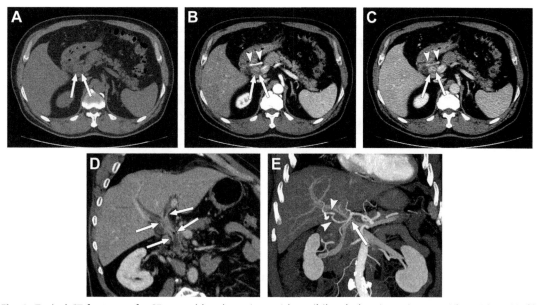

Fig. 4. Typical CT features of a 65-year-old male patient with perihilar cholangiocarcinoma with periductal infiltrating growth pattern. (A–C) An axial un-enhanced CT image (A) and dynamic contrast-enhanced axial CT images on arterial (B) and portal venous phase (C) depict progressive enhancing wall thickening in the perihilar bile duct (*arrows*) with subtle peribiliary infiltration. The right hepatic artery (*arrowheads* in B and C) aberrantly arising from the gastroduodenal artery runs anterior to the tumor (*arrows*). (D) Multiplanar reconstruction of the CT image on portal venous phase clearly visualizes the longitudinal tumor extent (*arrows*). (E) Maximal intensity projection of arterial phase image demonstrates the anatomic variation of the right hepatic artery (*arrowheads*) aberrantly arising from the gastroduodenal artery (*arrow*). This type of anatomic variation should be noted before surgery because the aberrant artery traverses just above the pancreas, which can be possibly damaged when the distal tumor margin is resected.

Table 1
Example CT protocol for evaluation of bile duct cancer

Characteristics	Value
Number of channels	128
Tube voltage	100 kVp
Tube current	200 reference mAs (Care dose 4D, Siemens Medical Solutions)
Pitch	0.6
Reconstruction Kernel	B30
Reconstruction algorithm	SAFIRE 2 (Siemens Medical Solutions)
Reconstruction slice thickness	5 mm (non-enhanced phase) 3 mm (arterial and portal venous phases) 1.25 mm thin section data (arterial and portal venous phases) for MRP reconstruction
Contrast administration	
Dose	100–130 mL
Rate	3 mL/s
Phases of imaging (axis of imaging)	
Un-enhanced (axial)	Before contrast administration
Arterial (axial and coronal planes and MPR)	10 s after reaching peak enhancement of abdominal aorta at 100 Hounsfield units
Portal venous (axial and coronal planes and MPR)	70 s after contrast administration

Abbreviations: MPR, multiplanar reconstruction; SAFIRE, sonogram-affirmed iterative reconstruction.

(a) two-dimensional (2D) thick-slab MRCP; (b) 2D thin-slice MRCP; and (c) 3D MRCP (**Fig. 6**). The advantages and disadvantages of each MRCP sequence are summarized in **Table 4**.

Updated MR Imaging Techniques

Recent advances in abdominal MR imaging enable reduced scan times and enhanced image resolution. An understanding of these updated techniques is essential to obtain high-quality MR images for better delineation of the fine details required for biliary cancer analysis.

First, the undersampling of k-space using parallel imaging techniques or compressed sensing markedly improves the quality of MR imaging for biliary cancer (**Fig. 7**). Parallel imaging (eg, generalized autocalibrating partially parallel acquisition [Siemens Healthineers, Erlangen, Germany],[46] sensitivity encoding [Philips Healthcare, Best, The Netherlands],[47] autocalibrating reconstruction for cartesian imaging [GE healthcare, Waukesha, WI, USA],[48] and array coil spatial sensitivity encoding [ASSET; GE Healthcare, Waukesha, WI, USA][49]) enables the acquisition of images from partial k-space data by using variations in the sensitivity profiles of multiple phased-array

Table 2
Diagnostic performance of CT in the diagnosis of extrahepatic cholangiocarcinoma

Characteristic	CT		MR imaging	
	Sensitivity	Specificity	Sensitivity	Specificity
Resectability	95% (91%–97%)[31]	69% (63%–75%)[31]	94% (90%–97%)[31]	71% (60%–81%)[31]
Portal vein invasion	89% (80%–94%)[30]	92% (85%–96%)[30]	40%–80%[a35,36]	91%–99%[a35,36]
Hepatic artery invasion	84% (63%–94%)[30]	93% (69%–99%)[30]	28%–73%[a34,36]	93%–99%[a34,36]
Lymph node metastasis	61% (28%–86%)[30]	88% (74%–95%)[30]	Not available	Not available

Unless otherwise specified, data are meta-analytic pooled estimates with 95% confidence interval in parentheses.
[a] Ranges of values from the published reports.[34–36]

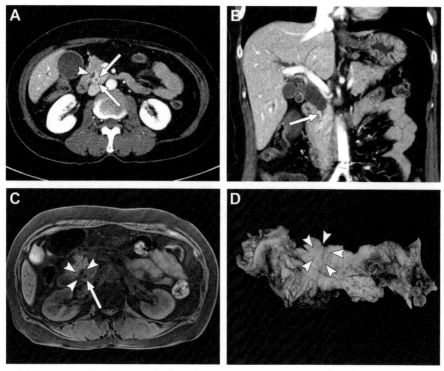

Fig. 5. CT and MR images of a 61-year-old female patient with pancreatic ductal adenocarcinoma mimicking distal cholangiocarcinoma. (A, B) Axial (A) and coronal (B) portal venous phase CT images show abrupt narrowing of the intrapancreatic common bile duct with short-segmental bile duct wall thickening (arrows). Of note, no definite mass is observed in the pancreas parenchyma on CT. A small cystic lesion (arrowhead in A) is also noted. (C, D) Axial unenhanced T1-weighted image (C) clearly depicts a pancreatic mass showing an ill-defined low-signal intensity area (arrowheads) around the involved intrapancreatic common bile duct (arrow), which are confirmed as pancreatic ductal adenocarcinoma on a surgical specimen (arrowheads, D).

MR imaging coils.[50] Compressed sensing, which has recently been applied to abdominal MR imaging, is based on the concept that incoherent or pseudorandomized samples are sufficient to acquire qualified images.[50,51] Considering that MRCP data consist of high-contrast fluid-containing structures and suppressed background signal, which is sparse in the image domain, compressed sensing is an effective tool for 3D MRCP. Many studies reported that a combination of compressed sensing and parallel imaging markedly reduces scan time,[52–54] and it can even enable single breath-hold 3D MRCP.[52,55] Adding breath-hold 3D MRCP with parallel imaging and compressed sensing to conventional navigation-triggered MRCP is likely to guarantee 3D MRCP with stable image quality, regardless of the patient's respiratory pattern.[56] These techniques can also be implemented to acquire high-resolution 3D contrast-enhanced T1-weighted imaging with thin sections, which enables better evaluation of the extent and vascular involvement of CC and multiplanar reformation (Fig. 8).[50]

Second, the gradient and spin-echo technique, which fills the center of k-space with signal from the spin-echo and peripheral k-space with signal from the gradient-echo using echo-planar imaging readouts, vastly improves the speed of data sampling.[57] This technique can also be used to obtain high-quality breath-hold 3D MRCP.[57–59]

Third, the acquisition of a small field of view covering only the biliary system (eg, ZOOMit [Siemens Healthineers, Erlangen, Germany], dS-Zoom [Philips Healthcare, Best, The Netherlands], and FOCUS [GE Healthcare, Waukesha, WI, USA]) with the use of focused radiofrequency excitation and overvolume suppression techniques with multichannel transmit technology facilitates high-resolution MRCP or diffusion weighted imaging (DWI) in a reduced time frame (see Fig. 7).[60]

Fourth, simultaneous multi-slice excitation (SMS), which refers to the excitation of multiple 2D slices at the same time using a multiband radiofrequency pulse,[61] can reduce the scan time. In the field of hepatobiliary imaging, this

Table 3
Example MR imaging with MRCP protocols for evaluation of bile duct cancer

Protocol	Repetition Time (ms)	Echo Time (ms)	Angle (°)	Matrix	Field of View (mm)	Section Thickness (mm)	Acceleration Factor
Axial dual-echo GRE	133	1.33 (opposed phase) 2.63 (in phase)	70	320 × 250	380 × 380	5	2
Axial T2-weighted HASTE	1100	150	90	320 × 260	380 × 380	5	2
Axial T2-weighted TSE	3000	87	90	352 × 352	380 × 380	5	3
MR cholangiopancreatography (MRCP)							
2D radial coronal thick-slab RARE	5000	928	90	384 × 384	270 × 270	40	2
2D coronal thin-slice HASTE	1100	147	90	256 × 256	300 × 300	3	3
3D coronal MRCP (navigator-triggered)	4207.5	701	90	512 × 336	400 × 262	0.9	3
3D coronal MRCP (breath-hold)[a]	1700	484	90	320 × 320	329 × 218	0.85	2
Axial diffusion-weighted imaging (b = 0, 50, 500, 900 s/mm^2)	6900	47	90	140 × 112	380 × 380	5	2
Axial contrast-enhanced 3D T1-weighted GRE[a] (precontrast, arterial, portal venous, and delayed phases)	3.8	1.36	11	384 × 300	384 × 350	1.5	1

Abbreviations: GRE, gradient recalled echo; HASTE, half-Fourier acquisition single-shot turbo-spin echo; TSE, turbo-spin echo.

[a] Compressed sensing is used, and coronal reconstruction images are also provided on each phase of contrast-enhanced 3D T1-weighted GRE.

technique is now beginning to be implemented to acquire DWI with reduced susceptibility and motion artifacts by reducing scan time.[62,63]

Last, deep-learning techniques are starting to be applied to various MR imaging techniques to achieve better imaging quality. Deep-learning techniques have been applied to both T2-weighted and DWI,[64–67] which traditionally demanded long acquisition times.

IMAGING CHARACTERISTICS OF PERIHILAR AND DISTAL CHOLANGIOCARCINOMA

Infiltrating type CC, which is the most common type of extrahepatic CC, usually manifests as irregular thickening of the bile duct wall, showing progressive enhancement with luminal narrowing (see **Figs. 2–4**, **Fig. 9**). Benign diseases such as primary sclerosing cholangitis, recurrent pyogenic cholangitis, and IgG4-related sclerosing disease

sometimes also present with biliary wall thickening similar to infiltrative type CC.[68] However, long segmental involvement, a thick wall, indistinct margin, luminal irregularity and asymmetry, great enhancement, prominent upstream dilation, and high diffusion restriction are all reported to favor malignant strictures caused by CC over benign biliary disease.[37,38,69–71] Intraductal growing CC typically manifests as a papillary or irregular polypoid mass without bile duct thickening or stricture (see **Figs. 2, 6,** and **8**).[72] Upstream and downstream duct dilatation or cyst formation may be particularly found in mucin-producing intraductal growing CC.[73] Because multiplicity of intraductal growing CC (and its precursor, intraductal papillary neoplasm of the bile duct) is not uncommon, careful exploration is required to detect other diminutive intraductal lesions when radiologists evaluate intraductal growing CC (see **Figs. 6** and **8**).

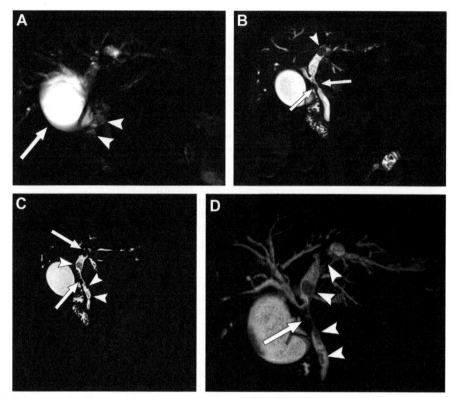

Fig. 6. MRCP images of a 68-year-old male patient with intraductal growing type cholangiocarcinoma (CC) in the background of intraductal papillary neoplasm of the bile duct. (*A*) 2D thick-slab MRCP techniques present a good overview of the dilated biliary system. However, the gallbladder (*arrow*) and fluid in the duodenum (*arrowheads*) partially obscure the bile ducts. (*B*) On 2D thin-slab MRCP obtained with moderate T2-weighted imaging (TE = 96 msec), the adjacent soft tissue structures such as the liver and pancreas are better visualized than heavily T2-weighted MRCP techniques. Irregular luminal narrowing of the perihilar duct (*arrows*) is clearly seen as well as another polypoid lesion in the left hepatic duct (*arrowhead*). (*C*) Thin-section navigator-triggered 3D MRCP with a slice thickness of 1 mm reveals more details of biliary abnormalities. In addition to the abnormalities (*arrows*) detected on 2D thin-slab MRCP, additional intraductal filling defects (*arrowheads*) are found. (*D*) A volume-rendering reconstructed image from the thin-section 3D MRCP data shows irregular luminal narrowing (*arrow*) involving the perihilar bile duct, confirmed as an intraductal growing type CC. Multifocal variable-sized filling defects in the intrahepatic and extrahepatic bile ducts (*arrowheads*) are also well-defined, which were confirmed as intraductal papillary neoplasm of the bile duct.

INTERPRETATION OF PREOPERATIVE IMAGING FOR PERIHILAR AND DISTAL CHOLANGIOCARCINOMA

Longitudinal tumor extent, vascular involvement, lymph node and distant metastasis, and future remnant liver volume are the key factors to be taken into account in the preoperative imaging assessment (**Table 5**). In addition, the vascular and biliary anatomy which may affect surgical techniques should also be scrutinized (see **Figs. 4** and **8, Table 6**).

Longitudinal Tumor Extent: Proximal and Distal Resection Margins

Regarding the proximal resection margin, the involvement of the primary and secondary confluence of the bile duct primarily influences the extent of surgery. The Bismuth–Corlette classification is the most widely used system,[74] and its categories and their recommended surgical options are described in **Table 7**. However, the Bismuth–Corlette classification does not consider bile duct variation and only includes the proximal extents of the tumor,[75,76] nor imply different prognoses.[77,78] In addition, advances in surgical techniques enable curative resection for conventionally unresectable pCC (eg, type IV or type III with contralateral vascular involvement) by resecting the intrahepatic portion beyond the secondary confluence, in combination with multiple bilio-enteric anastomosis and extended hepatectomy (eg, right or left trisectionectomy).[79–81] In these cases, tumor involvement extent at the level

Table 4
Common MRCP sequences and their advantages and disadvantages

Sequence	Slice Thickness	Breath Management	Advantages	Disadvantages
2D thick slab MRCP	40–60 mm (rotating 15°–20° per image)	Multiple breath hold	• Overview of biliary anatomy	• Low resolution: obscuring complex anatomy and small abnormality
2D thin slice MRCP	2–5 mm	Multiple (eg, 2–4) breath hold	• Good resolution • Simultaneous visualization of biliary tree and adjacent organs with relatively short echo time (TE) <150 msec	• Relatively lower resolution than 3D MRCP
3D MRCP	≤1 mm	Navigation-triggered (breath hold, if using recent rapid imaging techniques)	• Best resolution allowing for detection of diminutive abnormality • Isometric voxel enabling multiplanar and volumetric reformatting	• Long scan time (4–5 min) • Susceptible to motion artifact

Abbreviation: MRCP, magnetic resonance cholangiopancreatography.

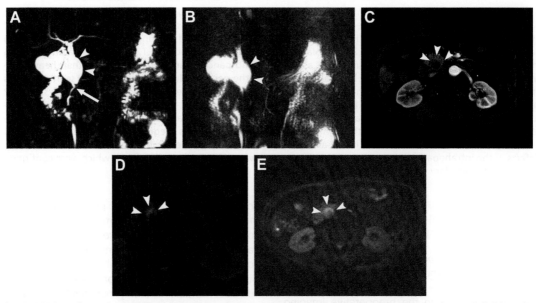

Fig. 7. MR imaging using updated imaging techniques. (*A, B*) Undersampling of *k*-space using parallel imaging and compressed sensing. In a 55-year-old female patient with an irregular respiratory cycle, a maximal intensity projection image from single breath-hold 3D MRCP using parallel imaging and compressed sensing techniques (compressed sensing factors = 25) (*A*) shows superior image quality to that from conventional navigation-trigged 3D MRCP (*B*). The patient has a choledochal cyst (*arrowheads*). An anomalous union of the bile duct and pancreatic duct is well demonstrated on breath-hold 3D MRCP (*arrow* in *A*), whereas navigation-trigged 3D MRCP (*B*) fails to define it due to blurring. (*C–E*) Small field of view (FOV) imaging. (*C*) An axial T1 contrast-enhanced image in an 80-year-old male patient with distal cholangiocarcinoma shows an eccentrically thickened bile duct wall (*arrowheads*). (*D, E*) Small FOV diffusion-weighted imaging (*D*) better depicts the involvement of the tumor showing diffusion restriction (*arrowheads*) compared with conventional diffusion-weighted imaging (*E*).

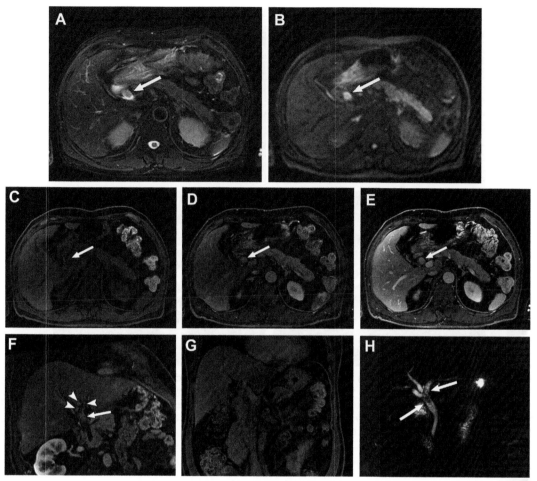

Fig. 8. Typical MR imaging features of intraductal growing perihilar cholangiocarcinoma in a 64-year-old male patient in the background of intraductal papillary neoplasm of the bile duct. (*A–C*) An intraductal polypoid mass (*arrows*) is noted in the perihilar duct showing subtle hyperintensity on T2-weighted (*A*) and diffusion-weighted images (*B*), and hypointensity on T1-weighted images (*C*). (*D, E*) Axial T1-weighted images reveal prominent enhancement of the intraductal mass (*arrows*) on arterial (*D*) and portal venous (*E*) phase images. (*F*) An oblique coronal reconstruction image from thin section (slice thickness = 1.5 mm) contrast-enhanced T1-weighted images depicts other small intraductal lesions in the left hepatic ducts (*arrowheads*) in addition to the perihilar intraductal mass (*arrow*). The small intraductal masses are considered as intraductal papillary neoplasms of the bile duct. Compressed sensing techniques enable thin section axial data on MR imaging in a single breath hold, which aids detection of fine abnormalities and reconstruction in multiplanar planes. (*G*) Conventional coronal T1-weighted coronal imaging fails to detect fine abnormalities due to its relatively thicker slice thickness (3 mm). (*H*) A maximal intensity projection image from 3D MRCP reveals the overall extent of intraductal lesions (*arrows*). Biliary anatomic variation as trifurcation is also noted.

of umbilical portion of left portal vein and at the level of right posterior sectional pedicle should be described in detail.

Evaluation of the distal tumor extent is as important as evaluation of the proximal tumor extent because involvement of intrapancreatic bile duct may require resection of the pancreas for curative-intent surgery, that is, hepatopancreato-duodenectomy, which results in higher mortality and morbidity.[82,83]

Vascular Involvement

Hepatic artery and portal vein involvement are crucial factors in the assessment of resectability. In this regard, the major classification systems for CC,[75,84,85] other than the Bismuth–Corlette classification, take vascular involvement into account. However, the definition of vascular involvement of CC is not well established. The Korean Society of Abdominal Radiology[26] recently suggested classifying vascular contact in a similar

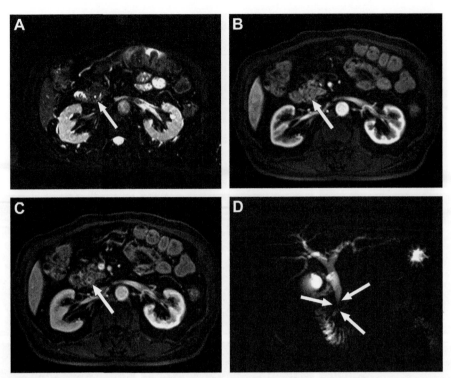

Fig. 9. Typical MR imaging features in a 76-year-old male patient with periductal infiltrating distal cholangiocarcinoma. (*A*) On T2-weighted imaging, the involved segment shows subtle hyperintensity (*arrow*). (*B, C*) Contrast-enhanced T1-weighted images on arterial (*B*) and portal venous (*C*) phases show progressively enhancing wall thickening in the involved segment (*arrows*). (*D*) 2D thick-slab MRCP shows abrupt narrowing of the intrapancreatic common bile duct caused by the tumor (*arrows*).

Table 5
Key components for preoperative imaging interpretation of perihilar and distal cholangiocarcinoma

Component	Key Interpretation Points
Longitudinal tumor extent	
Proximal margin	• Tumor involvement of 1st and 2nd confluence of right/left bile duct • Tumor involvement extent at the level of umbilical portion of left portal vein and at the level of right posterior sectional pedicle
Distal margin	Tumor involvement of intrapancreatic bile duct
Vascular involvement (hepatic artery and portal vein)	Any vascular involvement affecting operability and surgical planning
Regional lymph node metastasis	Detection of suspected lymph nodes beyond routine surgical fields
Distant metastasis	Scrutiny of prevalent locations of distant metastasis (eg, liver, lung, peritoneum, and distant lymph nodes)
Future liver remnant	Measurement of total and future remnant liver volume

Table 6
Vascular and biliary variations potentially affecting surgical techniques

Anatomy	Variation
Hepatic artery	Origin of middle hepatic artery (either from left or right hepatic artery) Separate origin of right anterior and posterior hepatic arteries Replaced or accessory right hepatic artery Replaced or accessary left hepatic artery
Portal vein	Trifurcation of RAPV, RPPV, and LPV RPPV from main portal vein RAPV from LPV Portal vein anomaly associated with right-sided ligamentum teres
Hepatic vein	Right hepatic vein into middle hepatic vein Right inferior hepatic vein
Bile duct	Triple confluence of RAHD, RPHD, and LHD RPHD into LHD RPHD into common bile duct/common hepatic duct RPHD into cystic duct Accessory RAHD or RPHD

Abbreviations: LHD, left hepatic duct; LPV, left portal vein; RAHD, right anterior hepatic duct; RAPV, right anterior portal vein; RPHD, right posterior hepatic duct; RPPV, right posterior portal vein.

manner to the definition of vascular involvement in patients with pancreatic cancer[86]: (a) no contact; (b) abutment, tumor involvement $\leq 180°$ of vascular circumference; and (c) invasion, tumor involvement $\leq 180°$ of vascular circumference or with occlusion, contour deformity, or tumor thrombosis. However, this categorization of vascular involvement needs to be further validated. Traditionally, contralateral vascular involvement was regarded as a contraindication to curative-intent surgery. However, curative-intent surgery with vascular resection is now more regularly performed and shows good long-term survival.[87,88] Thus, the location and length

Table 7
Bismuth–Corlette classification

Type	Tumor Involvement	Suggested Treatment
Type I	Common hepatic duct below primary confluence of bile duct	Bile duct resection
Type II	Primary confluence of bile duct without involvement of either secondary confluence	Bile duct resection + caudate lobectomy
Type IIIa	Right secondary confluence of bile duct without involvement of left secondary confluence	Bile duct resection + right hepatectomy + caudate lobectomy
Type IIIb	Left secondary confluence of bile duct without involvement of right secondary confluence	Bile duct resection + left hepatectomy + caudate lobectomy
Type IV	Bilateral secondary confluences of bile duct	Conventionally unresectable, but extended hepatectomy can be attempted

of contralateral vascular involvement should be reported in detail, as there may be a chance for curative resection.

Lymph Node Metastasis

Current imaging modalities do not show sufficient performance in the diagnosis of lymph node metastasis, with inconsistent diagnostic criteria for lymph node involvement.[89,90] A false-positive diagnosis commonly occurs with obstructive cholangitis. Regional lymph node metastasis confined to the hepatic pedicle and hepatoduodenal ligament does not significantly affect the surgical decision.[91] By contrast, the presence of lymph node metastasis beyond regional lymph nodes is deemed a contraindication to surgery given the dismal postoperative survival (5 year survival, 0%–12%) in such patients.[92] Positron emission tomography with ^{18}F-fluorodeoxyglucose may help to diagnose distant lymph node metastasis.[92]

Distant Metastasis

Along with distant lymph node metastasis, other distant metastases are an absolute contraindication to curative-intent surgery. Common locations of distant metastasis include liver (11.9%–23.2%), lung (2.7%–5.8%), and peritoneum (no reported prevalence).[93] In the presence of biliary obstruction caused by extrahepatic CC, the diagnosis of metastases in the liver is sometimes challenging because small abscesses can mimic metastases. Previous studies suggested imaging features favoring abscess over metastasis, such as patchy enhancement, arterial rim and persistent enhancement, perilesional hyperemia, and size discrepancy between different MR imaging sequences.[94,95] Short-term imaging follow-up after biliary decompression is very important in difficult cases to differentiate abscess and metastasis.

Future Remnant Liver

The future remnant liver also needs to be taken into account in patients with pCC who require major hepatectomy.[75,84] In general, a remnant liver volume greater than 25–30% of the total liver volume in patients with normal liver function, or greater than 40% of total liver volume in patients with impaired liver function, is required to avoid postsurgical liver failure and to yield favorable outcomes.[96,97] The total and estimated remnant liver volume can be analyzed via virtual liver segmentation on CT and MR imaging.[98] Portal vein embolization can be considered as an option to enlarge the remnant liver volume by 35% to 40% and enable hepatectomy in an additional 20% of cases.[96] In the case of biliary obstruction, the reliability of liver function evaluation using gadoxetic acid-enhanced MR imaging [99,100] and elastography[101,102] is questionable, as the degree of liver enhancement and the stiffness values can be affected by biliary obstruction.

SUMMARY

For the best outcomes in patients with biliary cancer, optimal imaging quality is a prerequisite. Radiologists need to be fully aware of the currently available imaging techniques for diagnosis and treatment planning for CC, in addition to having a thorough knowledge of therapeutic methods. Resectability assessment and surgical planning are important parts of the imaging workup of extrahepatic CC. Longitudinal tumor extent, vascular involvement, lymph node metastasis, distant metastasis, and future remnant liver volume are the key factors requiring scrutiny in the preoperative imaging of extrahepatic CC.

CLINICS CARE POINTS

- Multiphase CT is the imaging modality of choice for preoperative assessment of extrahepatic cholangiocarcinoma.

- MR imaging with magnetic resonance cholangiopancreatography has strength in evaluation of tumor extent and bile duct anatomy.

- Updated MR imaging techniques, including parallel imaging, compressed sensing, gradient and spin-echo technique, small field of view technique, simultaneous multi-slice excitation, and deep-learning techniques, enable better MR images with reduced scan time.

DISCLOSURE

Conflict of Interest: None of the authors have any conflicts of interest to declare.

REFERENCES

1. Clements O, Eliahoo J, Kim JU, et al. Risk factors for intrahepatic and extrahepatic cholangiocarcinoma: A systematic review and meta-analysis. J Hepatol 2020;72:95–103.
2. Nichols JC, Gores GJ, LaRusso NF, et al. Diagnostic role of serum CA 19-9 for

cholangiocarcinoma in patients with primary sclerosing cholangitis. Mayo Clin Proc 1993;68:874–9.

3. Ramage JK, Donaghy A, Farrant JM, et al. Serum tumor markers for the diagnosis of cholangiocarcinoma in primary sclerosing cholangitis. Gastroenterology 1995;108:865–9.

4. Nakeeb A, Pitt HA, Sohn TA, et al. Cholangiocarcinoma. A spectrum of intrahepatic, perihilar, and distal tumors. Ann Surg 1996;224:463–73.

5. DeOliveira ML, Cunningham SC, Cameron JL, et al. Cholangiocarcinoma: thirty-one-year experience with 564 patients at a single institution. Ann Surg 2007;245:755–62.

6. Yamasaki S. Intrahepatic cholangiocarcinoma: macroscopic type and stage classification. J Hepatobiliary Pancreat Surg 2003;10:288–91.

7. Sakamoto E, Nimura Y, Hayakawa N, et al. The pattern of infiltration at the proximal border of hilar bile duct carcinoma: a histologic analysis of 62 resected cases. Ann Surg 1998;227:405–11.

8. Yeh CN, Jan YY, Yeh TS, et al. Hepatic resection of the intraductal papillary type of peripheral cholangiocarcinoma. Ann Surg Oncol 2004;11:606–11.

9. Guglielmi A, Ruzzenente A, Campagnaro T, et al. Intrahepatic cholangiocarcinoma: prognostic factors after surgical resection. World J Surg 2009; 33:1247–54.

10. Shimada K, Sano T, Sakamoto Y, et al. Surgical outcomes of the mass-forming plus periductal infiltrating types of intrahepatic cholangiocarcinoma: a comparative study with the typical mass-forming type of intrahepatic cholangiocarcinoma. World J Surg 2007;31:2016–22.

11. van Vugt JLA, Gaspersz MP, Coelen RJS, et al. The prognostic value of portal vein and hepatic artery involvement in patients with perihilar cholangiocarcinoma. HPB (Oxford) 2018;20:83–92.

12. Primrose JN, Fox RP, Palmer DH, et al. Capecitabine compared with observation in resected biliary tract cancer (BILCAP): a randomised, controlled, multicentre, phase 3 study. Lancet Oncol 2019; 20:663–73.

13. Meyer CG, Penn I, James L. Liver transplantation for cholangiocarcinoma: results in 207 patients. Transplantation 2000;69:1633–7.

14. Robles R, Figueras J, Turrión VS, et al. Spanish experience in liver transplantation for hilar and peripheral cholangiocarcinoma. Ann Surg 2004;239: 265–71.

15. Seehofer D, Thelen A, Neumann UP, et al. Extended bile duct resection and [corrected] liver and transplantation in patients with hilar cholangiocarcinoma: long-term results. Liver Transpl 2009; 15:1499–507.

16. Valle J, Wasan H, Palmer DH, et al. Cisplatin plus gemcitabine versus gemcitabine for biliary tract cancer. N Engl J Med 2010;362:1273–81.

17. Okusaka T, Nakachi K, Fukutomi A, et al. Gemcitabine alone or in combination with cisplatin in patients with biliary tract cancer: a comparative multicentre study in Japan. Br J Cancer 2010; 103:469–74.

18. Kamsa-Ard S, Luvira V, Suwanrungruang K, et al. Cholangiocarcinoma Trends, Incidence, and Relative Survival in Khon Kaen, Thailand From 1989 Through 2013: A Population-Based Cancer Registry Study. J Epidemiol 2019;29:197–204.

19. Strijker M, Belkouz A, van der Geest LG, et al. Treatment and survival of resected and unresected distal cholangiocarcinoma: a nationwide study. Acta Oncol 2019;58:1048–55.

20. Groot Koerkamp B, Wiggers JK, Allen PJ, et al. Recurrence Rate and Pattern of Perihilar Cholangiocarcinoma after Curative Intent Resection. J Am Coll Surg 2015;221:1041–9.

21. Lindnér P, Rizell M, Hafström L. The impact of changed strategies for patients with cholangiocarcinoma in this millennium. HPB Surg 2015;2015: 736049.

22. Wang Y, Li J, Xia Y, et al. Prognostic nomogram for intrahepatic cholangiocarcinoma after partial hepatectomy. J Clin Oncol 2013;31:1188–95.

23. Zhang XF, Beal EW, Bagante F, et al. Early versus late recurrence of intrahepatic cholangiocarcinoma after resection with curative intent. Br J Surg 2018; 105:848–56.

24. Masselli G, Gualdi G. Hilar cholangiocarcinoma: MRI/MRCP in staging and treatment planning. Abdom Imaging 2008;33:444–51.

25. Jhaveri KS, Hosseini-Nik H. MRI of cholangiocarcinoma. J Magn Reson Imaging 2015;42:1165–79.

26. Lee DH, Kim B, Lee ES, et al. Radiologic Evaluation and Structured Reporting Form for Extrahepatic Bile Duct Cancer: 2019 Consensus Recommendations from the Korean Society of Abdominal Radiology. Korean J Radiol 2021;22:41–62.

27. National Comprehensive Cancer network. Biliary Tract Cancers, Version 3. 2021, NCCN Clinical Practice Guidelines in Oncology. Available at: https://www.nccn.org/professionals/physician_gls/pdf/pancreatic.pdf. Accessed July 15, 2021.

28. Yamada Y, Mori H, Hijiya N, et al. Extrahepatic bile duct cancer: invasion of the posterior hepatic plexuses–evaluation using multidetector CT. Radiology 2012;263:419–28.

29. Kim HJ, Park DI, Park JH, et al. Multidetector computed tomography cholangiography with multiplanar reformation for the assessment of patients with biliary obstruction. J Gastroenterol Hepatol 2007;22:400–5.

30. Ruys AT, van Beem BE, Engelbrecht MR, et al. Radiological staging in patients with hilar cholangiocarcinoma: a systematic review and meta-analysis. Br J Radiol 2012;85:1255–62.

31. Zhang H, Zhu J, Ke F, et al. Radiological Imaging for Assessing the Respectability of Hilar Cholangiocarcinoma: A Systematic Review and Meta-Analysis. Biomed Res Int 2015;2015:497942.

32. Lee HY, Kim SH, Lee JM, et al. Preoperative assessment of resectability of hepatic hilar cholangiocarcinoma: combined CT and cholangiography with revised criteria. Radiology 2006;239:113–21.

33. Kim JH, Kim MJ, Chung JJ, et al. Differential diagnosis of periampullary carcinomas at MR imaging. Radiographics 2002;22:1335–52.

34. Lee MG, Park KB, Shin YM, et al. Preoperative evaluation of hilar cholangiocarcinoma with contrast-enhanced three-dimensional fast imaging with steady-state precession magnetic resonance angiography: comparison with intraarterial digital subtraction angiography. World J Surg 2003;27: 278–83.

35. Masselli G, Manfredi R, Vecchioli A, et al. MR imaging and MR cholangiopancreatography in the preoperative evaluation of hilar cholangiocarcinoma: correlation with surgical and pathologic findings. Eur Radiol 2008;18:2213–21.

36. Ryoo I, Lee JM, Chung YE, et al. Gadobutrol-enhanced, three-dimensional, dynamic MR imaging with MR cholangiography for the preoperative evaluation of bile duct cancer. Invest Radiol 2010;45:217–24.

37. Park HJ, Kim SH, Jang KM, et al. The role of diffusion-weighted MR imaging for differentiating benign from malignant bile duct strictures. Eur Radiol 2014;24:947–58.

38. Lee NK, Kim S, Seo HI, et al. Diffusion-weighted MR imaging for the differentiation of malignant from benign strictures in the periampullary region. Eur Radiol 2013;23:1288–96.

39. Kim YK, Lee MW, Lee WJ, et al. Diagnostic accuracy and sensitivity of diffusion-weighted and of gadoxetic acid-enhanced 3-T MR imaging alone or in combination in the detection of small liver metastasis ($\leq$ 1.5 cm in diameter). Invest Radiol 2012;47:159–66.

40. Park MJ, Kim YK, Lim S, et al. Hilar cholangiocarcinoma: value of adding DW imaging to gadoxetic acid-enhanced MR imaging with MR cholangiopancreatography for preoperative evaluation. Radiology 2014;270:768–76.

41. Sun HY, Lee JM, Park HS, et al. Gadoxetic acid-enhanced MRI with MR cholangiography for the preoperative evaluation of bile duct cancer. J Magn Reson Imaging 2013;38:138–47.

42. Higaki A, Tamada T, Sone T, et al. Potential clinical factors affecting hepatobiliary enhancement at Gd-EOB-DTPA-enhanced MR imaging. Magn Reson Imaging 2012;30:689–93.

43. Choi JY, Lee JM, Sirlin CB. CT and MR imaging diagnosis and staging of hepatocellular carcinoma: part II. Extracellular agents, hepatobiliary agents, and ancillary imaging features. Radiology 2014;273:30–50.

44. Kim DW, Choi SH, Park T, et al. Transient Severe Motion Artifact on Arterial Phase in Gadoxetic Acid-Enhanced Liver Magnetic Resonance Imaging: A Systematic Review and Meta-analysis. Invest Radiol 2022;57:62–70.

45. Davenport MS, Viglianti BL, Al-Hawary MM, et al. Comparison of acute transient dyspnea after intravenous administration of gadoxetate disodium and gadobenate dimeglumine: effect on arterial phase image quality. Radiology 2013;266:452–61.

46. Griswold MA, Jakob PM, Heidemann RM, et al. Generalized autocalibrating partially parallel acquisitions (GRAPPA). Magn Reson Med 2002;47: 1202–10.

47. Pruessmann KP, Weiger M, Scheidegger MB, et al. SENSE: sensitivity encoding for fast MRI. Magn Reson Med 1999;42:952–62.

48. Brau AC, Beatty PJ, Skare S, et al. Comparison of reconstruction accuracy and efficiency among autocalibrating data-driven parallel imaging methods. Magn Reson Med 2008;59:382–95.

49. King KF. ASSET–parallel imaging on the GE scanner. Second International Workshop on Parallel MRI, Zurich, Switzerland;2004. p. 15–7.

50. Yoon JH, Nickel MD, Peeters JM, et al. Rapid Imaging: Recent Advances in Abdominal MRI for Reducing Acquisition Time and Its Clinical Applications. Korean J Radiol 2019;20:1597–615.

51. Welle CL, Miller FH, Yeh BM. Advances in MR Imaging of the Biliary Tract. Magn Reson Imaging Clin N Am 2020;28:341–52.

52. Yoon JH, Lee SM, Kang HJ, et al. Clinical Feasibility of 3-Dimensional Magnetic Resonance Cholangiopancreatography Using Compressed Sensing: Comparison of Image Quality and Diagnostic Performance. Invest Radiol 2017;52:612–9.

53. Seo N, Park MS, Han K, et al. Feasibility of 3D navigator-triggered magnetic resonance cholangiopancreatography with combined parallel imaging and compressed sensing reconstruction at 3T. J Magn Reson Imaging 2017;46:1289–97.

54. Nagata S, Goshima S, Noda Y, et al. Magnetic resonance cholangiopancreatography using optimized integrated combination with parallel imaging and compressed sensing technique. Abdom Radiol (Ny) 2019;44:1766–72.

55. Chandarana H, Doshi AM, Shanbhogue A, et al. Three-dimensional MR Cholangiopancreatography in a Breath Hold with Sparsity-based Reconstruction of Highly Undersampled Data. Radiology 2016;280:585–94.

56. Tokoro H, Yamada A, Suzuki T, et al. Usefulness of breath-hold compressed sensing accelerated three-dimensional magnetic resonance cholangiopancreatography (MRCP) added to respiratory-

gating conventional MRCP. Eur J Radiol 2020;122: 108765.

57. Nam JG, Lee JM, Kang HJ, et al. GRASE Revisited: breath-hold three-dimensional (3D) magnetic resonance cholangiopancreatography using a Gradient and Spin Echo (GRASE) technique at 3T. Eur Radiol 2018;28:3721–8.

58. Yoshida M, Nakaura T, Inoue T, et al. Magnetic resonance cholangiopancreatography with GRASE sequence at 3.0T: does it improve image quality and acquisition time as compared with 3D TSE? Eur Radiol 2018;28:2436–43.

59. He M, Xu J, Sun Z, et al. Comparison and evaluation of the efficacy of compressed SENSE (CS) and gradient- and spin-echo (GRASE) in breath-hold (BH) magnetic resonance cholangiopancreatography (MRCP). J Magn Reson Imaging 2020; 51:824–32.

60. Tanabe M, Onoda H, Higashi M, et al. Three-Dimensional (3D) Breath-Hold Zoomed MR Cholangiopancreatography (MRCP): Evaluation of Additive Value to Conventional 3D Navigator Triggering MRCP in Patients With Branch Duct Intraductal Papillary Mucinous Neoplasms. J Magn Reson Imaging 2022;55:1234–40.

61. Barth M, Breuer F, Koopmans PJ, et al. Simultaneous multislice (SMS) imaging techniques. Magn Reson Med 2016;75:63–81.

62. Taron J, Martirosian P, Erb M, et al. Simultaneous multislice diffusion-weighted MRI of the liver: Analysis of different breathing schemes in comparison to standard sequences. J Magn Reson Imaging 2016;44:865–79.

63. Tavakoli A, Attenberger UI, Budjan J, et al. Improved Liver Diffusion-Weighted Imaging at 3 T Using Respiratory Triggering in Combination With Simultaneous Multislice Acceleration. Invest Radiol 2019;54:744–51.

64. Herrmann J, Gassenmaier S, Nickel D, et al. Diagnostic Confidence and Feasibility of a Deep Learning Accelerated HASTE Sequence of the Abdomen in a Single Breath-Hold. Invest Radiol 2021;56:313–9.

65. Herrmann J, Nickel D, Mugler JP 3rd, et al. Development and Evaluation of Deep Learning-Accelerated Single-Breath-Hold Abdominal HASTE at 3 T Using Variable Refocusing Flip Angles. Invest Radiol 2021;56:645–52.

66. Shanbhogue K, Tong A, Smereka P, et al. Accelerated single-shot T2-weighted fat-suppressed (FS) MRI of the liver with deep learning-based image reconstruction: qualitative and quantitative comparison of image quality with conventional T2-weighted FS sequence. Eur Radiol 2021;31:8447–57.

67. Hu Z, Wang Y, Zhang Z, et al. Distortion correction of single-shot EPI enabled by deep-learning. Neuroimage 2020;221:117170.

68. Seo N, Kim SY, Lee SS, et al. Sclerosing Cholangitis: Clinicopathologic Features, Imaging Spectrum, and Systemic Approach to Differential Diagnosis. Korean J Radiol 2016;17:25–38.

69. Kim JY, Lee JM, Han JK, et al. Contrast-enhanced MRI combined with MR cholangiopancreatography for the evaluation of patients with biliary strictures: differentiation of malignant from benign bile duct strictures. J Magn Reson Imaging 2007;26:304–12.

70. Choi SH, Han JK, Lee JM, et al. Differentiating malignant from benign common bile duct stricture with multiphasic helical CT. Radiology 2005;236: 178–83.

71. Park MS, Kim TK, Kim KW, et al. Differentiation of extrahepatic bile duct cholangiocarcinoma from benign stricture: findings at MRCP versus ERCP. Radiology 2004;233:234–40.

72. Kim JE, Lee JM, Kim SH, et al. Differentiation of intraductal growing-type cholangiocarcinomas from nodular-type cholangiocarcinomas at biliary MR imaging with MR cholangiography. Radiology 2010;257:364–72.

73. Park HJ, Kim SY, Kim HJ, et al. Intraductal Papillary Neoplasm of the Bile Duct: Clinical, Imaging, and Pathologic Features. AJR Am J Roentgenol 2018; 211:67–75.

74. Bismuth H, Corlette MB. Intrahepatic cholangioenteric anastomosis in carcinoma of the hilus of the liver. Surg Gynecol Obstet 1975;140:170–8.

75. Deoliveira ML, Schulick RD, Nimura Y, et al. New staging system and a registry for perihilar cholangiocarcinoma. Hepatology 2011;53:1363–71.

76. Ji GW, Zhu FP, Wang K, et al. Clinical Implications of Biliary Confluence Pattern for Bismuth-Corlette Type IV Hilar Cholangiocarcinoma Applied to Hemihepatectomy. J Gastrointest Surg 2017;21:666–75.

77. Paul A, Kaiser GM, Molmenti EP, et al. Klatskin tumors and the accuracy of the Bismuth-Corlette classification. Am Surg 2011;77:1695–9.

78. Suarez-Munoz MA, Fernandez-Aguilar JL, Sanchez-Perez B, et al. Risk factors and classifications of hilar cholangiocarcinoma. World J Gastrointest Oncol 2013;5:132–8.

79. Han IW, Jang JY, Kang MJ, et al. Role of resection for Bismuth type IV hilar cholangiocarcinoma and analysis of determining factors for curative resection. Ann Surg Treat Res 2014;87:87–93.

80. Matsumoto N, Ebata T, Yokoyama Y, et al. Role of anatomical right hepatic trisectionectomy for perihilar cholangiocarcinoma. Br J Surg 2014;101: 261–8.

81. Natsume S, Ebata T, Yokoyama Y, et al. Clinical significance of left trisectionectomy for perihilar cholangiocarcinoma: an appraisal and comparison with left hepatectomy. Ann Surg 2012;255:754–62.

82. Ebata T, Yokoyama Y, Igami T, et al. Hepatopancreatoduodenectomy for cholangiocarcinoma: a

single-center review of 85 consecutive patients. Ann Surg 2012;256:297–305.

83. Aoki T, Sakamoto Y, Kohno Y, et al. Hepatopancreaticoduodenectomy for Biliary Cancer: Strategies for Near-zero Operative Mortality and Acceptable Long-term Outcome. Ann Surg 2018;267:332–7.

84. Burke EC, Jarnagin WR, Hochwald SN, et al. Hilar Cholangiocarcinoma: patterns of spread, the importance of hepatic resection for curative operation, and a presurgical clinical staging system. Ann Surg 1998;228:385–94.

85. Amin MB, Edge S, Greene F, et al. AJCC cancer staging manual. 8th edition. New York: Springer; 2017.

86. Al-Hawary MM, Francis IR, Chari ST, et al. Pancreatic ductal adenocarcinoma radiology reporting template: consensus statement of the Society of Abdominal Radiology and the American Pancreatic Association. Radiology 2014;270:248–60.

87. Schimizzi GV, Jin LX, Davidson JTt, et al. Outcomes after vascular resection during curative-intent resection for hilar cholangiocarcinoma: a multi-institution study from the US extrahepatic biliary malignancy consortium. HPB (Oxford) 2018;20:332–9.

88. de Jong MC, Marques H, Clary BM, et al. The impact of portal vein resection on outcomes for hilar cholangiocarcinoma: a multi-institutional analysis of 305 cases. Cancer 2012;118:4737–47.

89. Noji T, Kondo S, Hirano S, et al. Computed tomography evaluation of regional lymph node metastases in patients with biliary cancer. Br J Surg 2008;95:92–6.

90. Ruys AT, Kate FJ, Busch OR, et al. Metastatic lymph nodes in hilar cholangiocarcinoma: does size matter? HPB (Oxford) 2011;13:881–6.

91. Ramos E. Principles of surgical resection in hilar cholangiocarcinoma. World J Gastrointest Oncol 2013;5:139–46.

92. Kim JY, Kim MH, Lee TY, et al. Clinical role of 18F-FDG PET-CT in suspected and potentially operable cholangiocarcinoma: a prospective study compared with conventional imaging. Am J Gastroenterol 2008;103:1145–51.

93. Wang X, Yu GY, Chen M, et al. Pattern of distant metastases in primary extrahepatic bile-duct cancer: A SEER-based study. Cancer Med 2018;7:5006–14.

94. Choi SY, Kim YK, Min JH, et al. The value of gadoxetic acid-enhanced MRI for differentiation between hepatic microabscesses and metastases in patients with periampullary cancer. Eur Radiol 2017; 27:4383–93.

95. Oh JG, Choi SY, Lee MH, et al. Differentiation of hepatic abscess from metastasis on contrast-enhanced dynamic computed tomography in patients with a history of extrahepatic malignancy: emphasis on dynamic change of arterial rim enhancement. Abdom Radiol (Ny) 2019;44:529–38.

96. van Mierlo KM, Schaap FG, Dejong CH, et al. Liver resection for cancer: New developments in prediction, prevention and management of postresectional liver failure. J Hepatol 2016;65:1217–31.

97. Wiggers JK, Groot Koerkamp B, Cieslak KP, et al. Postoperative Mortality after Liver Resection for Perihilar Cholangiocarcinoma: Development of a Risk Score and Importance of Biliary Drainage of the Future Liver Remnant. J Am Coll Surg 2016; 223:321–31.e1.

98. Gotra A, Sivakumaran L, Chartrand G, et al. Liver segmentation: indications, techniques and future directions. Insights Imaging 2017;8:377–92.

99. Sato Y, Matsushima S, Inaba Y, et al. Preoperative estimation of future remnant liver function following portal vein embolization using relative enhancement on gadoxetic acid disodium-enhanced magnetic resonance imaging. Korean J Radiol 2015;16:523–30.

100. Yoon JH, Choi JI, Jeong YY, et al. Pre-treatment estimation of future remnant liver function using gadoxetic acid MRI in patients with HCC. J Hepatol 2016;65:1155–62.

101. Cescon M, Colecchia A, Cucchetti A, et al. Value of transient elastography measured with FibroScan in predicting the outcome of hepatic resection for hepatocellular carcinoma. Ann Surg 2012;256: 706–12.

102. Lee DH, Lee JM, Yi NJ, et al. Hepatic stiffness measurement by using MR elastography: prognostic values after hepatic resection for hepatocellular carcinoma. Eur Radiol 2017;27:1713–21.

MR Imaging in Primary Sclerosing Cholangitis and Other Cholangitis

Ciara O'Brien, MB, BCh, BAO, FFRRCSI[a], Mikail Malik[b],
Kartik Jhaveri, MD, FRCPC, DABR[c],*

KEYWORDS

• Primary sclerosing cholangitis (PSC) • MR imaging • Cholangitis

KEY POINTS

• Sclerosing cholangitis describes several chronic, cholestatic diseases that involve the intrahepatic and extrahepatic bile ducts.
• Primary sclerosing cholangitis (PSC) is an idiopathic slowly progressive inflammatory biliary disease that is refractory to medical treatment.
• The gold standard diagnostic test for PSC and other cholangitis is MR imaging.

Abbreviations	
MRCP	Magnetic resonance cholangiopancreatography
ALP	Alkaline phosphatase
CBD	Common Bile Duct
HIV	Human immunodeficiency virus
RUQ	Right upper QuadrantIg

INTRODUCTION

Sclerosing cholangitis (SC) describes several chronic, cholestatic diseases that involve the intrahepatic and extrahepatic bile ducts. SC is characterized by irregular and ill-defined inflammation, fibrosis, and stricturing of the bile ducts and may be primary or secondary in cause. It causes progressive destruction of the biliary tree, progressive parenchymal cirrhosis, hepatic failure, and malignancy such as cholangiocarcinoma.[1] The subtypes of SC can be broken down into primary sclerosing cholangitis (PSC), immune-mediated SC, infectious cholangitis, ischemic cholangitis

with other causes including metastatic disease and chemotherapy change.

PRIMARY SCLEROSING CHOLANGITIS

PSC is an uncommon, chronic cholestatic liver disease characterized by progressive inflammation and fibrosis resulting in obliteration of normal bile duct architecture. It is characterized by biliary strictures, progressive hepatic fibrosis and is associated with increased risk if hepatobiliary malignancy including cholangiocarcinoma, hepatocellular carcinoma (HCC), and gallbladder malignancy.[2]

The authors have no commercial or financial conflicts of interest to disclose.
ᵃ Department of Medical Imaging, JDMI University Health Network, University of Toronto, 610 University Avenue, Toronto, Ontario M5G 2M9, Canada; ᵇ McMaster University, Hamilton, ON L8S 4L8, Canada; ᶜ Department of Medical Imaging, JDMI University Health Network, University of Toronto, 610 University Avenue, 3-957, Toronto, Ontario M5G 2M9, Canada
* Corresponding author.
E-mail address: kartik.jhaveri@uhn.ca

Categories and Pathogenesis of Primary Sclerosing Cholangitis

There are 3 subtypes of PSC: classic, small duct, and an overlapping disease with autoimmune hepatitis. It is reported that 90% of cases are the classic subtype, whereas the overlapping subtype is most prevalent in children.[3] The pathogenesis of PSC is multifactorial and is related to cholangiocyte injury with an exaggerated cholangiocyte immune response that results in the clinical disease. Patients with PSC maybe asymptomatic.

Investigation of Primary Sclerosing Cholangitis

PSC is suspected clinically when liver function tests (LFTs) show a cholestatic picture. The diagnostic triad for PSC described in the American associated for the study of liver diseases guidelines includes a cholestatic pattern on biochemical LFTs when the MRCP confirms the presence of characteristic biliary changes. Patients with a normal cholangiogram and biochemical and histologic features consistent with PSC are classified with small duct disease.[4] PSC requires a radiological diagnosis, and the gold standard is MR imaging with reported sensitivity of 86% and specificity of 94% for accurate diagnosis.[5] Ideally, an MR imaging of liver with contrast and an MRCP should be performed to investigate for PSC. The recommendations for the study include a field strength of 1.5 T or greater and the patient should fast for a minimum of 4 hours before the study. The MRCP is a T2-weighted sequence and should include a 2D and 3D MRCP, single shot MRCP performed in an orthogonal coronal plane with a thin slice acquisition (~1 mm). MR imaging liver with gadolinium contrast should include an axial and coronal T2-weighted sequence, an axial T1-weighted sequence, diffusion-weighted imaging and postcontrast dynamic T1-weighted sequences.[6]

MR Imaging Features of Primary Sclerosing Cholangitis

Biliary strictures are the hallmark of PSC, commonly affecting both the intrahepatic and extrahepatic ducts or intrahepatic ducts alone; however, isolated extrahepatic duct involvement is rare.[4] Patients with the "small duct" variant of PSC can have a normal MR imaging examination. Intrahepatic strictures are typically multisegmental and bilobar although isolated strictures can be seen uncommonly and may cause variable upstream biliary dilatation. Strictures are graded as low or high grade; low grade is less than 75%

luminal narrowing, whereas high grade is greater than 75% luminal narrowing.[7] A dominant stricture develops in ~50% of patients with PSC during the disease course and up to 25% of dominant strictures develop cholangiocarcinoma. Strictures can be short or long (>10 mm) in length. Peripheral intrahepatic duct obliteration referred to as "pruning" of the ducts is also observed. The bile ducts may be thickened and demonstrate enhancement on the dynamic contrast-enhanced sequences, which may be the first sign of cholangiocarcinoma. Enhancement should be evaluated on all dynamic sequences, and a wall thickness of greater than 2 mm is considered abnormal.[7] Intrahepatic biliary duct stones are observed as intraductal filling defects on the MRCP and T2-weighted sequence, whereas on noncontrast T1-weighted sequence, they are typically seen as high signal foci with the biliary ducts. The liver parenchyma may demonstrate segmental atrophy, often the left lateral and posterior right hepatic segments with compensatory hypertrophy of the caudate lobe. There are often peripheral wedge-shaped areas of T2 hyperintensity with or without enhancement secondary to inflammation and/or fibrosis. In progressive cases, features of cirrhosis will be apparent. An example MR imaging reporting template is provided to help standardize PSC MR imaging reports[8] (Box 1). Magnetic resonance risk scoring systems have been developed to predict disease progression. The Mayo risk score is used to assess the short-term mortality risk of patients with PSC and was derived from a cohort of PSC patients with end-stage disease.[9] The Amsterdam-Oxford model (AOM) is prognostic imaging tool for PSC developed to predict long-term risk of PSC-related death and/or liver transplantation. The AOM is calculated based on the patients PSC subtype, age at diagnosis, ALP, aspartate aminotransferase, total bilirubin, and platelet count. The ANALI risk scores are based on MR imaging findings and were developed to predict radiologic progression of PSC, and these scores demonstrate good prognostic value in PSC patients at different stages of the disease and strength the role for MR imaging. The ANALI 1 to 2 scores are based on MR imaging with gadolinium (ANALI 1) and without gadolinium (ANALI 2).[10] The use of gadolinium in PSC patients is useful for a cohort of patients with severe disease where underlying cancer may be suspected.[9] MRCP+ is a technique using semiautomated software that analyzes 3D MRCP images that provide quantitative measurements for direct assessment of ductal anatomy. Liver stiffness measurement has also been described in the literature as a promising prognostic tool for PSC-derived using

---

Box 1
MR imaging template reporting template

A. Biliary system

- Location: Normal or intrahepatic or extrahepatic or both
- Modified Amsterdam score:
  - Intrahepatic:
  - Extrahepatic:
- Intrahepatic distribution: Localized (<25%) or diffuse (>25%)
- Beading: Yes/No
- Stricture severity: Grade (mild <75%, severe>75%), Length (1–2, 3–10, >10 mm)
  - RHD
  - LHD
  - CBD
- Dominant stricture: Yes or No, if Yes
  - Location: Confluence or extrahepatic CBD
  - Stricture diameter: mm
  - Length: mm
  - Upstream dilatation: mm
  - Downstream duct diameter: mm
- Bile duct calculi: Yes/No Location: Intrahepatic vs extrahepatic ducts versus both
- Cholangiocarcinoma: Yes/No, if yes, location and size

B. Liver parenchyma

- Cirrhosis: yes/no
- Parenchymal signal heterogeneity yes/no, location

C. Pancreas

- Signal: Normal or low
- Duct dilatation: Yes (=5 mm or more) or No (<5 mm)
- Features of autoimmune pancreatitis: Yes or No

D. Gallbadder

- Stones/Polyps/Mass: Yes/No

From Venkatesh SK, Welle CL, Miller FH, et al. Reporting standards for primary sclerosing cholangitis using MR imaging and MR cholangiopancreatography: guidelines from MR Working Group of the International Primary Sclerosing Cholangitis Study Group. *Eur Radiol.* 2021.

---

magnetic resonance elastography (MRE). The liver stiffness value calculated at baseline is used to evaluate the rate of disease progression by correlating fibrosis and histologic stage. MRCP + used in conjunction with MRE shows comparable results to ANALI scores as PSC prognostic indicators.[11–13]

Complications and Treatment of Primary Sclerosing Cholangitis

In patients with PSC, a 10.9% incidence of cholangiocarcinoma is reported[5]; Gallbladder and HCC are reported at lower frequencies. Approximately a third of cholangiocarcinoma is detected within 1 year of MR imaging diagnosis of PSC. Cholangiocarcinoma may be intrahepatic, perihilar, or extrahepatic. It is classified as periductal-infiltrating, mass forming, or intraductal. MR imaging reporting of these tumors should therefore carefully describe these tumor characteristics. The prognosis for cholangiocarcinoma is not favorable with a reported 1% to 5-year survival rate, and surgical resection lengthens the prognosis to a 5-year survival rate of 10% to 30%.[14] The presence of metastasis, lymph node involvement, and advanced liver disease is a contraindication for resection. Liver transplantation is indicated in patients who develop complications such as portal hypertension and chronic liver failure. PSC accounts for approximately 5% of liver transplants in the United States per annum. Liver transplantation is successful with a 5-year survival rate of 80% to 85%. The risk of recurrence in the first year posttransplant is low at 2% but increases to 20% to 25% of cases 5 to 10 years following transplantation.[4,15]

- Key points:
  - PSC is characterized by biliary strictures, progressive hepatic fibrosis.
  - PSC is associated with increased risk of hepatobiliary malignancy.
  - MR imaging is the gold standard diagnostic test.

Case presentations <<**Figs. 1–5**>>

IMMUNE MEDIATED
IgG4-related Sclerosing Cholangitis

IgG4-related sclerosing cholangitis (IgG4SC) is an immune-mediated inflammatory disease of the pancreaticobiliary tract. It most commonly affects the pancreas and is termed autoimmune pancreatitis; the biliary tract is the second most common location for disease. LFT will demonstrate an obstructive pattern with elevated ALP and bilirubin. The serum IgG4 levels will be elevated with approximately 10% greater than the normal level.

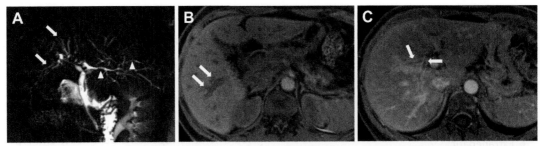

Fig. 1. A 54-year-old woman with longstanding colitis. MR imaging was performed to investigate for PSC. MRCP radial image (*A*) demonstrates diffuse multifocal intrahepatic bile duct strictures causing beading (*white arrows*) and dilatation (*arrowheads*). Noncontrast T1WI (*B*) show high signal intensity foci in the intrahepatic ducts consistent with calculi (*white arrows*). The delayed postcontrast T1WI (*C*) show diffuse thickening and enhancement of the intrahepatic bile ducts (*white arrows*). These MR imaging features are consistent with PSC in the clinical context.

MR Imaging Features

MR imaging is modality of choice for image investigation of IgG4SC. The MR imaging findings include long segment strictures, bile duct wall thickening with a preserved visible lumen of the thickened segments and occasionally prestenotic dilatation of the ducts. There is resulting upstream cholestasis and occasionally intraductal calculi. The thickened duct wall will be isointense to hypointense on T2-weighted imaging with associated diffusion restriction. There is typically homogenous delayed enhancement on the postcontrast sequences of the thickened segments best appreciated on the 3-minute delayed sequence. The disease can affect one duct or be multifocal; isolated extrahepatic duct involvement is reported in 43% of patients.[16] When IgG4SC is localized to one duct, it is often hilar in location and presents as a pseudotumor. Studies have shown the average wall thickness of the affected CBD is 3 mm, compared with patients with PSC with an average reported thickness of 1.89 mm.[17] Gallbladder involvement occurs in approximately 51% of patients.[18] MR imaging features including CBD wall thickening, continuous involvement of the CBD

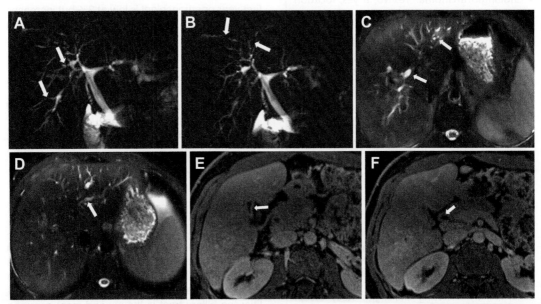

Fig. 2. A 33-year-old man with PSC associated with ulcerative colitis on treatment with ursodiol. MR imaging performed for surveillance demonstrating both intrahepatic and extrahepatic bile duct abnormalities. MRCP radial images (*A*, *B*) show diffuse multifocal intrahepatic bile duct strictures and dilatation (*white arrows*). Axial T2-weighted images (*C*, *D*) demonstrate multifocal peripheral beaded intrahepatic biliary dilatation (*white arrows*). The delayed postcontrast images (*E*, *F*) show diffuse thickening of the common hepatic duct and common bile duct without a focal mass (*white arrows*).

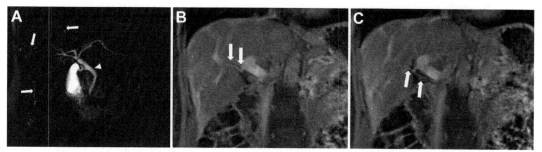

Fig. 3. A 46-year-old woman with PSC associated with inflammatory bowel disease. MRCP radial image (*A*) shows peripheral intrahepatic biliary dilatation with beading (*white arrows*). The extrahepatic bile ducts are smooth without stricturing or dilatation (*arrowhead*). The delayed phase postcontrast T1WI images (*B, C*) show central and extrahepatic bile duct thickening and enhancement (*white arrows*).

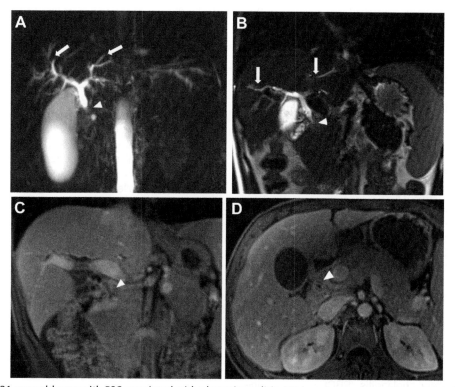

Fig. 4. A 31-year-old man with PSC associated with ulcerative colitis. MR imaging performed to evaluate for worsening liver function tests and right upper quadrant pain. MRCP radial image (*A*) and the coronal T2WI (B) demonstrates a dominant/high grade stricture of the distal CBD (*arrow* heads) with features of PSC throughout the biliary tree (*white arrows*). The coronal and axial T1WIs (*C, D*) demonstrate marked circumferential mural thickening and enhancement at the site of the stricture (*arrow* heads). Ductal cholangiocarcinoma was confirmed with ERCP and pathologic evaluation of the brushings.

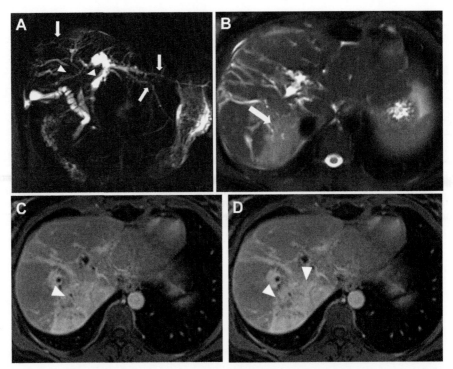

Fig. 5. A 47-year-old patient with PSC and a mass forming cholangiocarcinoma in the posterior right hepatic lobe. MRCP radial image (*A*) shows diffuse intrahepatic biliary dilatation consistent with PSC (*white arrows*) and separation of the ducts centrally (*arrowheads*). On the axial T2WI (*B*) there is regional mass like T2 hyperintense signal (*white arrow*) with heterogeneous enhancement on the delayed axial T1WIs (*red arrows*) (*C, D*).

and an abnormal gallbladder have a statistically significant association with IgG4SC and can be used to differentiate it from PSC on MR imaging.[17]

Treatment and Complications

IgG4SC responds to steroid therapy in up to 97% of cases.[19] Cholangiocarcinoma is rare.

- Key points
  - MR imaging features, including CBD wall thickening, continuous involvement of the CBD, and an abnormal gallbladder have a statistically significant association with IgG4SC. These parameters can be used to differentiate IgG4SC from PSC on MRI.

Case presentation <<**Fig. 6**>>

PRIMARY BILIARY CHOLANGITIS

Primary biliary cholangitis (PBC) is an immune-mediated inflammatory disease of the small intrahepatic bile ducts arising secondary to genetic and environmental factors. The disease is slowly progressive, resulting in chronic cholestasis and cirrhosis.

MR Imaging Features

MR imaging features of PBC include diffuse hepatomegaly, splenomegaly, portal hypertension, T2-weighted periportal hyperintensity, and the periportal halo sign. The periportal halo sign is T1 and T2 low signal intensity surrounding the portal venous branches measuring 1 to 5 mm. PBC does not cause bile duct stricturing, and its detection should raise consideration of an alternative diagnosis or an overlapping condition.

Treatment and Complications

Cholestasis and cirrhosis lead to portal hypertension and increases the incidence of HCC. Therapy is with ursodeoxycholic acid (UDCA), which when started early in the disease course increases the transplant-free survival period. Liver transplant is indicated for decompensated cirrhosis or HCC. Recurrence posttransplant is reported in 25% of patients.[20]

- Key points
  - PBC is an immune-mediated inflammatory disease of the small intrahepatic bile ducts.
  - MR imaging features include diffuse hepatomegaly, splenomegaly, portal hypertension

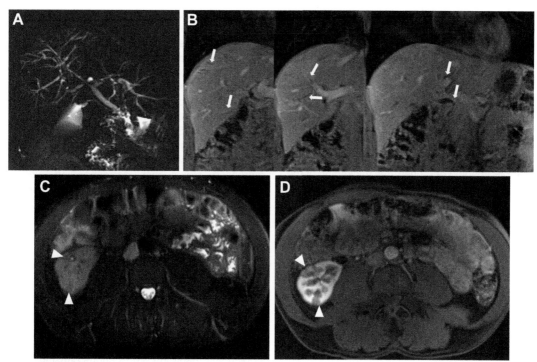

Fig. 6. A 67-year-old man with known IgG4 disease treated with corticosteroids. MRCP radial (*A*) shows multifocal beading and stricturing of bilobar intrahepatic bile ducts with sparing of the extrahepatic duct. Coronal delayed phase T1W postcontrast images (*B*) demonstrates dilated bile ducts with diffuse biliary thickening and enhancement (*white arrows*). The axial T2WI and postcontrast T1W images (*C, D*) show wedge-shaped areas of T2 low signal and hypoenhancement in the right renal cortex consistent with renal IgG4 disease (*arrowheads*).

T2-weighted periportal hyperintensity, and the periportal halo sign.

Case presentation <<**Fig. 7**>>

EOSINOPHILIC CHOLANGITIS

Eosinophilic cholangitis (EC) is a rare benign disease of the biliary tree that is defined as eosinophilic infiltration of the biliary system. The cause is unknown.

MR Imaging Features

MR imaging typically demonstrates thickening of the CBD wall (the gallbladder and cystic duct may also be thickened) with a dominant stricture/narrowing of the CBD to the confluence of the right

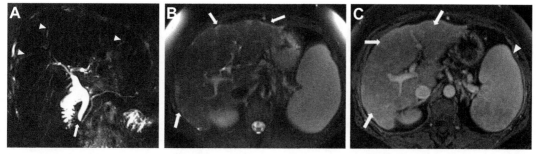

Fig. 7. A 33-year-old man with known primary biliary cholangitis cirrhosis, MR imaging performed to investigate rising bilirubin. MRCP radial image (*A*) shows apparent peripheral biliary dilatation (*arrowheads*). There is dilatation of the CBD with tapering at the ampulla of Vater (*white arrow*). On the T2W1 (*B*) liver shows macronodular contours (*arrow* heads) and heterogeneous T2-weighted signal throughout the parenchyma. The axial T1 postcontrast-weighted image (*C*) demonstrates patchy enhancement (*white arrows*) of the macronodular cirrhotic liver and splenomegaly (*arrowhead*) in keeping with portal hypertension.

and left hepatic ducts. EC mimics ductal chonlangiocarcinoma, and therefore, invasive imaging modalities such as ERCP or cholangioscopy are required to obtain tissue as the definitive diagnosis is made histologically.

Treatment and Complications

EC is often self-limiting and demonstrates a response to corticosteroid therapy.

- Key points
  - MR imaging demonstrates thickening of the CBD wall with a dominant stricture/narrowing of the CBD to the confluence.

Case presentation <<**Fig. 8**>>

INFECTIOUS CHOLANGITIS
Ascending Cholangitis

Ascending cholangitis results from partial or complete biliary obstruction. Infection typically originates from the intestine, ascends the biliary tree, and proliferates within the bile. Infection may also originate from the portal venous system. Obstruction can arise secondary to benign or malignant biliary strictures or choledocholithiasis. The Tokyo Guideline for the diagnosis was derived from international meetings and updated most recently in 2018. It is a published tool used for the diagnosis, classification, and treatment of acute ascending cholangitis. The severity of ascending cholangitis is graded based on a modified expert grading system (2018): grade 1 is mild, grade 2 is moderate disease requiring biliary drainage, and grade 3 is severe with associated organ failure. The degrees of severity are associated with increasing 30 day mortality.[21,22]

MR imaging features

MR imaging is the modality of choice for the assessment of ascending cholangitis. MRCP assesses the biliary tree, identifies biliary obstruction, and evaluates the liver parenchyma. Patients will have intrahepatic biliary dilatation, which may be central, segmental, or diffuse. Ducts seem smoothly thickened with peribiliary enhancement. Typical PSC pattern is not typical of ascending cholangitis; however, recurrent episodes if ascending cholangitis may lead to biliary damage resulting in a PSC like pattern of disease. On T2-weighted images, the liver parenchyma may show wedge-shaped or geographic areas of increased signal with corresponding wedge-shaped enhancement of the dynamic contrast-enhanced sequences.

Treatment and complications

The most effective antimicrobial treatment is with broad-spectrum antibiotics that can pass into the bile duct, 70% of cases respond to medical therapy.[23] Therapeutic biliary drainage and decompression is necessary to avoid septic shock. Complications of ascending cholangitis include acute pancreatitis, hepatic abscesses, and septic shock. Over time recurrent episodes of ascending cholangitis result in complications causing biliary damage resulting in a PSC type picture.

- Key points
  - Ascending cholangitis results from biliary obstruction
  - Recurrent episodes, if ascending cholangitis, may lead to biliary damage resulting in a PSC like pattern of disease.

Case presentation <<**Figs. 9 and 10**>>

RECURRENT PYOGENIC CHOLANGITIS

Recurrent pyogenic cholangitis (RPC) is a biliary disease endemic in Southeast Asia. It is characterized by pigment stones in the intrahepatic and extrahepatic biliary tree with absence of calculi in

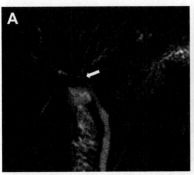
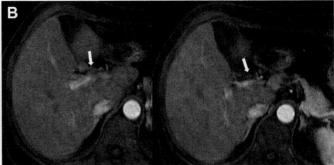

Fig. 8. A 66-year-old woman with biopsy proven necrotizing eosinophilic granulomas in the liver. MR imaging demonstrated a stricture at the confluence of the common duct (*A*) on the MRCP radial with circumferential thickening and enhancement at the confluence of the biliary ducts seen on the axial T1W postcontrast sequences (*B*).

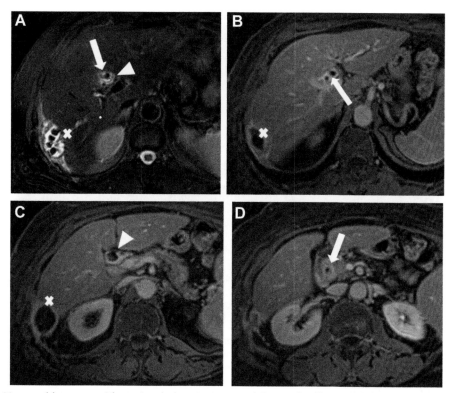

Fig. 9. A 44-year-old woman with a prior cholecystectomy and dropped gallstones with abscess formation posterior to the right hepatic lobe (white x) on the axial T2WI and T1WI (*A–D*). There is diffuse central and extrahepatic bile duct thickening and enhancement (*white arrows*) with choledocholithiasis (*arrow* heads) in keeping with acute cholangitis.

the gallbladder. The cause of the disease is not definitely known; however, it is associated with infections from parasites such as *Ascaris lumbricoides* and *Clonorchis sinensis*. Chronic inflammation of the biliary tree results in inflammation and fibrosis of the bile duct walls, infiltration of the portal tracts and causing strictures, biliary stasis, and periductal abscesses.

MR Imaging Features

MRCP is the most sensitive modality for depicting short segment biliary strictures and calculi described in RPC. The hallmark of RPC is complete obstruction of the intrahepatic ducts secondary to impacted calculi or strictures, this is termed "the missing duct sign." On MRCP stricturing can mimic the appearance of PSC. Typically, the central ducts and extrahepatic ducts are dilated with decreased caliber and tapering of the peripheral ducts. RPC is associated with other hepatic manifestations such as segmental parenchymal atrophy, abscess, bilomas, inflammatory pseudotumor, thrombophlebitis of the portal or hepatic veins and cholangiocarcinoma. Atrophy is most prevalent involving the left lateral and right posterior segments with hypertrophy of the caudate and left medial segment giving

a round liver appearance.[24] If the underlying cause is *C. sinensis* infection, the fluke may be identified within the dilated ducts.

Treatment and Complications

Cholangiocarcinoma occurs in 2% to 6% of cases. Patients who develop cirrhosis have a higher incidence of HCC. Antibiotics are used for an acute flair. The goal of therapy is to alleviate the biliary obstruction and stasis with the removal of the calculi. Interventional biliary drainage and stone evacuation or surgical biliary bypass, segmental liver resection, and transplantation are the therapeutic options available.[25–27]

- Key points
  - The hallmark of RPC is complete obstruction of the intrahepatic ducts secondary to impacted calculi or strictures

Case presentation <<**Figs. 11 and 12**>>

AIDS-RELATED CHOLANGITIS

AIDS-related cholangiopathy or HIV cholangiopathy is seen in patients with a CD4 count of less than 100 cells/mm^3, and the prevalence has decreased with

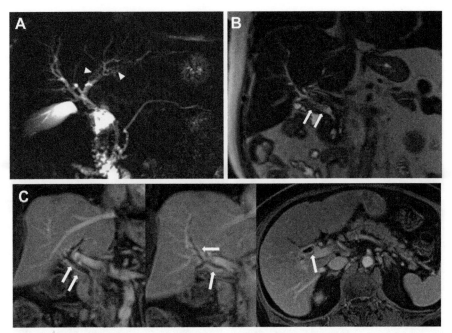

Fig. 10. An 82-year-old woman with fever, right upper quadrant pain and rising liver enzymes, imaging in conjunction with history and laboratory investigations was consistent with ascending cholangitis. MRCP radial image (*A*) shows multifocal intrahepatic biliary stricturing with peripheral biliary dilatation. There are multiple filling defects in the CBD and left intrahepatic ducts (*arrowheads*). The coronal T2WI (*B*) confirms choledocholithiasis with thickening of the bile ducts (*white arrows*). On the T1 postcontrast images (*C*), there is smooth thickening and enhancement of the intrahepatic ducts and CBD.

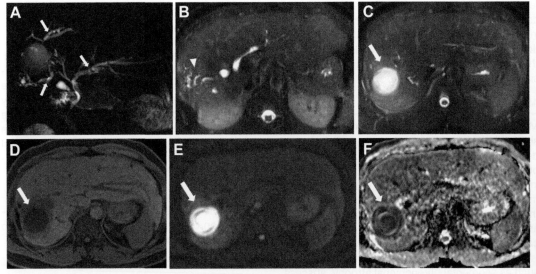

Fig. 11. A 56-year-old man with recurrent RUQ pain, fever, and jaundice. Imaging and laboratory findings were consistent with recurrent pyogenic cholangitis. MRCP radial image (*A*) image shows increased caliber of the intrahepatic ducts predominantly in posterior right lobe and left lateral lobe of liver (*white arrows*). Axial T2WI (*B*) shows irregular peripheral biliary dilatation (*arrow head*). The axial T2WI, T1WI, diffusion, and ADC map (*C–F*) show a T2 hyperintense mass that is T1 hypointense with surrounding edema and diffusion restriction consistent with an intrahepatic abscess (*white arrows*).

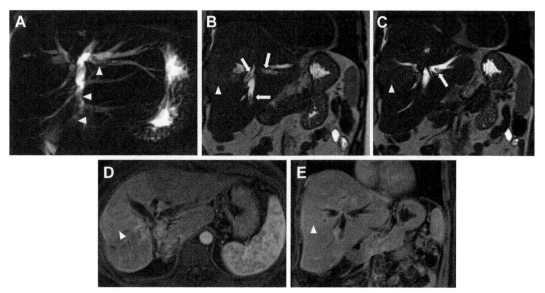

Fig. 12. A 50-year-old woman with worsening right upper quadrant pain and deranged liver function tests and a diagnosis of recurrent pyogenic cholangitis. The MRCP radial image (*A*) shows increased caliber of the intrahepatic ducts throughout the liver with multiple filling defects (*arrow* heads). The coronal T2WI s (*B, C*) demonstrate filling defects in the intrahepatic ducts (*white arrows*), with increased T2W signal of the parenchyma in segments 6 and 8 consistent with active inflammation (*arrow* heads). The axial and coronal T1 postcontrast images (*D, E*) show heterogeneous enhancement of the segment 6 and 8 parenchyma confirming active inflammation (*arrowheads*).

the use of highly active antiretroviral therapy.[28] An ALP level of 5 to 7 times greater than normal is a hallmark sign of AIDS-related cholangiopathy.[3] The most common imaging finding is a long smooth tapered stricture at the distal aspect of the CBD to the level of the ampulla, reported in 75% of cases.[3] Treatment of opportunistic infection is commonly ineffective to reduce the progression of SC or papillary stenosis. In some patient's chronic biliary infection may initiate dysplasia of the biliary epithelium resulting in cholangiocarcinoma.[28]

- Key points
  - Most common imaging finding is a long smooth tapered stricture at the distal aspect of the CBD to the level of the ampulla.

Case presentation <<**Fig. 13**>>

ISCHEMIC CHOLANGITIS

The biliary system is solely dependent on the hepatic arteries for blood supply with more than 50% of the hepatic arterial supply dedicated to the bile ducts.[29] Ischemic cholangitis (IC) arises when the hepatic arteries become compromised. The pattern of IC will vary depending on the volume of hepatic insufficiency and the stage of the

disease. In the acute phase, the patient form biliary casts, later there will be biliary necrosis with break down of the damaged ducts and bile leaks from the damaged duct to form a biloma. Chronically patients develop diffuse stricturing and dilatation of the ducts mimicking PSC.

MR Imaging Features

MR imaging appearances at the early stages demonstrate T1 hyperintensities within dilated bile ducts mimicking stones, and these are the biliary casts. In the intermediate phase, MR imaging will show dilated bile ducts with peripheral enhancement on the dynamic sequences. During the chronic phase of the disease, there is multifocal stricturing and segmental dilatation of the ducts mimicking PSC.[24,30]

Treatment and Complications

Treatment of IC depends on the individual and clinical course. Bacterial sepsis is treated with antimicrobials. In the context of large vessel occlusion, surgical or endovascular restoration of blood flow may be performed. Patients with small ductal disease management are commonly supportive. There is no significant risk of cholangiocarcinoma associated with IC in the literature.

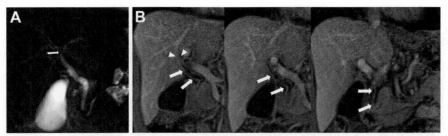

Fig. 13. A 60-year-old man with HIV presenting with elevated LFT and right upper quadrant pain. MRCP radial image shows a focal stricture at the biliary confluence (*white arrow*) with mild upstream biliary dilatation (*A*). There was smooth thickening and enhancement of the common hepatic and common bile ducts to the ampulla of Vater (*white arrows*), a focal narrowing is seen on the postcontrast T1W image (*B*) at the biliary confluence (*arrowheads*). MR imaging findings are most compatible with HIV cholangitis.

- Key points
  - Ischemia-related bile duct injury is called IC and arises when the hepatic arteries become compromised.
  - During the chronic phase of the disease, appearances mimic PSC.

Case presentation <<**Fig. 14**>>

MISCELLANEOUS INFLAMMATORY CHOLANGITIS
Chemotherapy-related Cholangitis

Chemotherapy-related cholangitis most commonly arises secondary to conventional transarterial emulsion-based chemoembolization, drug-eluting bead chemoembolization and hepatic

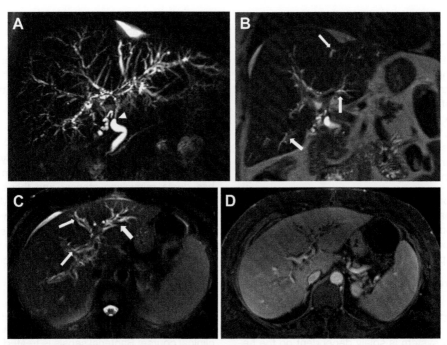

Fig. 14. A 55-year-old man after cadaveric liver transplantation with a bile duct-to-duct anastomosis. There is marked irregularity of the intrahepatic bile ducts with dilatation and strictures extending from the periphery to the common hepatic confluence demonstrated on the MRCP radial image (*A*). The coronal and axial T2WIs (*B,C*) show the normal T2 signal of the liver parenchyma with multifocal biliary structuring and dilatation (white arrows). Axial T1 postcontrast imaging shows no liver parenchymal abnormality (*D*). The biliary anastomosis is depicted with the arrowhead. The clinical, laboratory and imaging findings are compatible with ischemic biliopathy.

arterial infusion chemotherapy with a reported 8% to 55% prevalence.[31] Although rare, there are reports of chemotherapy-related cholangitis arising secondary to systemic chemotherapy from taxanes and bevacizumab. The mechanism of the cholangitis is not clear, although is it postulated that it is due to direct toxicity causing ischemic damage to the peribiliary vascular plexus. To date case reports describe treatment with UDCA, steroids, and biliary drainage.[32,33] MR imaging appearances are similar to IC with strictures predominantly involving the CBD and intrahepatic biliary dilatation.

- Key points
  - MR imaging appearances are similar to IC

METASTATIC DISEASE

Metastatic disease mimicking PSC is rare, although there are case reports of liver, pancreatic, and prostate metastasis simulating SC. In all reported cases, pathologic condition proved underlying adenocarcinoma metastatic disease to the liver. Patients have histologic features suggesting biliary obstruction, which can lead to compression or invasion of the biliary tree by tumor.[34] It is thought that patients with liver metastasis have prolonged biliary obstruction resulting in a pattern of secondary cholangitis.

- Key points
  - Metastatic disease mimicking PSC is rare with reports of liver, pancreatic, and prostate metastasis simulating cholangitis.

SUMMARY

SC describes several chronic, cholestatic diseases that involve the intrahepatic and extrahepatic bile ducts. The subtypes of SC are PSC, immune-mediated SC, infectious cholangitis, and ischemic cholangitis with other causes including metastatic disease and chemotherapy change. MR imaging is the gold standard diagnostic test for the assessment and diagnosis of sclerosing cholangitis. The International PSC study group recently recommended that MR imaging and MRCP should be the first diagnostic imaging modality for people with suspected PSC.

CLINICS CARE POINTS

- PSC is characterized by biliary strictures, progressive hepatic fibrosis.
- MRI is the gold standard test for diagnosis and follow-up of PSC.

- PSC is associated with an increased risk of malignancy, particularly cholangiocarcinoma.
- Secondary sclerosing cholangitis may mimic the appearance of PSC.
- The etioloies of secondary sclerosing cholangitis include; immune-mediated, infectious, ischemic, toxin mediated and malignant associated cholangitis.

REFERENCES

1. Gossard AA, Angulo P, Lindor KD. Secondary sclerosing cholangitis: a comparison to primary sclerosing cholangitis. Am J Gastroenterol 2005; 100(6):1330–3.
2. van Erp LW, Cunningham M, Narasimman M, et al. Risk of gallbladder cancer in patients with primary sclerosing cholangitis and radiographically detected gallbladder polyps. Liver Int 2020;40(2): 382–92.
3. Leake R, Rezvani M, Willmore R, et al. Primary Sclerosing Cholangitis and Its Mimickers: A Review of Disease and MRI Findings. Curr Radiol Rep 2017; 5(6):21.
4. Chapman R, Fevery J, Kalloo A, et al. Diagnosis and management of primary sclerosing cholangitis. Hepatology 2010;51(2):660–78.
5. Karlsen TH, Folseraas T, Thorburn D, et al. Primary sclerosing cholangitis – a comprehensive review. J Hepatol 2017;67(6):1298–323.
6. Schramm C, Eaton J, Ringe KI, et al. Recommendations on the use of magnetic resonance imaging in PSC-A position statement from the International PSC Study Group. Hepatology 2017;66(5):1675–88.
7. Bookwalter CA, Venkatesh SK, Eaton JE, et al. MR elastography in primary sclerosing cholangitis: correlating liver stiffness with bile duct strictures and parenchymal changes. Abdom Radiol 2018; 43(12):3260–70.
8. Venkatesh SK, Welle CL, Miller FH, et al. Reporting standards for primary sclerosing cholangitis using MRI and MR cholangiopancreatography: guidelines from MR Working Group of the International Primary Sclerosing Cholangitis Study Group. Eur Radiol 2022;32(2):923–37.
9. Goet JC, Floreani A, Verhelst X, et al. Validation, clinical utility and limitations of the Amsterdam-Oxford model for primary sclerosing cholangitis. J Hepatol 2019;71(5):992–9.
10. Lemoinne S, Cazzagon N, El Mouhadi S, et al. Simple Magnetic Resonance Scores Associate With Outcomes of Patients With Primary Sclerosing Cholangitis. Clin Gastroenterol Hepatol 2019;17(13): 2785–92.e3.

11. Ismail MF, Hirschfield GM, Hansen B, et al. Evaluation of quantitative MRCP (MRCP+) for risk stratification of primary sclerosing cholangitis: comparison with morphological MRCP, MR elastography, and biochemical risk scores. Eur Radiol 2022;32(1):67–77.

12. Tafur M, Cheung A, Menezes RJ, et al. Risk stratification in primary sclerosing cholangitis: comparison of biliary stricture severity on MRCP versus liver stiffness by MR elastography and vibration-controlled transient elastography. Eur Radiol 2020;30(7):3735–47.

13. Jhaveri KS, Hosseini-Nik H, Sadoughi N, et al. The development and validation of magnetic resonance elastography for fibrosis staging in primary sclerosing cholangitis. Eur Radiol 2019;29(2):1039–47.

14. Ahrendt SA, Nakeeb A, Pitt HA. Cholangiocarcinoma. Clin Liver Dis 2001;5(1):191–218.

15. Astarcioglu I, Egeli T, Unek T, et al. Liver transplant in patients with primary sclerosing cholangitis: long-term experience of a single center. Exp Clin Transplant 2018;16(4):434–8.

16. Zacarias MS, Pria HRFD, Oliveira RASd, et al. Non-neoplastic cholangiopathies: an algorithmic approach. Radiologia Brasileira 2020;53:262–72.

17. Tokala A, Khalili K, Menezes R, et al. Comparative MRI analysis of morphologic patterns of bile duct disease in IgG4-related systemic disease versus primary sclerosing cholangitis. AJR Am J Roentgenol 2014;202(3):536–43.

18. Madhusudhan KS, Das P, Gunjan D, et al. IgG4-Related Sclerosing Cholangitis: A Clinical and Imaging Review. AJR Am J Roentgenol 2019;213(6):1221–31.

19. Hubers LM, de Buy Wenniger LJM, Doorenspleet ME, et al. IgG4-associated cholangitis: a comprehensive review. Clin Rev Allergy Immunol 2015;48(2–3):198–206.

20. Carey EJ, Ali AH, Lindor KD. Primary biliary cirrhosis. Lancet 2015;386(10003):1565–75.

21. Alizadeh AHM. Cholangitis: diagnosis, treatment and prognosis. J Clin Transl Hepatol 2017;5(4):404.

22. Sokal A, Sauvanet A, Fantin B, et al. Acute cholangitis: Diagnosis and management. J Visc Surg 2019;156(6):515–25.

23. Sun Z, Zhu Y, Zhu B, et al. Controversy and progress for treatment of acute cholangitis after Tokyo Guidelines (TG13). Biosci Trends 2016;10(1):22–6.

24. Seo N, Kim SY, Lee SS, et al. Sclerosing Cholangitis: Clinicopathologic Features, Imaging Spectrum, and Systemic Approach to Differential Diagnosis. Korean J Radiol 2016;17(1):25–38.

25. Harris H, Kumwenda Z, Sheen-Chen S-M, et al. Recurrent pyogenic cholangitis. Am J Surg 1998;176(1):34–7.

26. Park M-S, Yu J-S, Kim KW, et al. Recurrent Pyogenic Cholangitis: Comparison between MR Cholangiography and Direct Cholangiography. Radiology 2001;220(3):677–82.

27. Heffernan EJ, Geoghegan T, Munk PL, et al. Recurrent pyogenic cholangitis: from imaging to intervention. AJR Am J Roentgenol 2009;192(1):W28–35.

28. Naseer M, Dailey FE, Juboori AA, et al. Epidemiology, determinants, and management of AIDS cholangiopathy: A review. World J Gastroenterol 2018;24(7):767–74.

29. Deltenre P, Valla D-C. Ischemic cholangiopathy. Paper presented at: Seminars in liver disease2008.

30. Alabdulghani F, Healy GM, Cantwell CP. Radiological findings in ischaemic cholangiopathy. Clin Radiol 2020;75(3):161–8.

31. Sandrasegaran K, Alazmi WM, Tann M, et al. Chemotherapy-induced sclerosing cholangitis. Clin Radiol 2006;61(8):670–8.

32. Kusakabe A, Ohkawa K, Fukutake N, et al. Chemotherapy-Induced Sclerosing Cholangitis Caused by Systemic Chemotherapy. ACG Case Rep J 2019;6(7):e00136.

33. von Figura G, Stephani J, Wagner M, et al. Secondary sclerosing cholangitis after chemotherapy with bevacizumab and paclitaxel. Endoscopy 2009;41(S 02):E153–4.

34. Vilgrain V, Erlinger S, Belghiti J, et al. Cholangiographic appearance simulating sclerosing cholangitis in metastatic adenocarcinoma of the liver. Gastroenterology 1990;99(3):850–3.

Imaging Vascular Disorders of the Liver

Nandan Keshav, MD, MS[a], Michael A. Ohliger, MD, PhD[b,c],*

KEYWORDS

- Liver • Vascular • Hepatic artery • Portal vein • Hepatic vein

KEY POINTS

- Vascular disorders of the liver may be categorized as pathologies of inflow, outflow, or aberrant arteriovenous connections.
- Vascular abnormalities may mimic other diseases or hint at the presence of disease elsewhere in the body.
- Understanding the distinct vascular physiology of the liver can help radiologists detect the unique imaging appearances of vascular liver diseases.

BACKGROUND

The liver has a unique and complex blood supply, which is instrumental to its roles in synthesis, metabolism, and clearance of chemical substrates. Liver vascular disorders often have important physiologic consequences, both inside and outside of the liver. In addition, these vascular disorders often have distinct appearances on imaging examinations that can mimic other pathologies. It is important for radiologists to have a solid understanding of both the baseline liver vasculature and to recognize its impact on disease processes.

Liver vascular disorders may be broadly placed into 3 categories: (1) abnormalities of outflow, (2) abnormalities of inflow, and (3) aberrant arteriovenous connections. Abnormalities of outflow include Budd-Chiari syndrome, sinusoidal obstruction syndrome, and congestive hepatopathy. Abnormalities of inflow include hepatic arterial aneurysms (including mycotic aneurysms and pseudoaneurysms), hepatic infarction, portal venous occlusion (due to bland or tumor thrombus), pylephlebitis, and portal hypertension. Aberrant arteriovenous connections include hereditary hemorrhagic telangiectasia and arterioportal shunting. Vascular shunts may lead to imaging abnormalities that simulate disease or hint at the presence of disease; vascular mimics of disease include third inflow phenomena, transient differences in parenchymal enhancement, shunting adjacent to focal parenchymal lesions, and portosystemic shunting. Other more uncommon conditions include peliosis hepatis. In the following sections, the authors review each of these disorders as well as common imaging features that may accompany them.

LIVER BLOOD SUPPLY AND ITS IMPACT ON IMAGING

The dual blood supply of the liver aids its myriad functions including biosynthesis, metabolism, and clearance. Up to 80% of the liver's blood supply arises from the portal vein, with the remainder from the main hepatic artery; other very small portions of the liver are supplied by separate venous systems.[1] This unique relationship lends itself to a buffer response, wherein the hepatic artery produces compensatory increased flow in response to alterations in portal venous flow.[2] The terminal arterioles and venules of these afferent systems

[a] Department of Radiology and Biomedical Imaging, University of California San Francisco, 505 Parnassus Avenue, Box 0628, San Francisco, CA 94143, USA; [b] Department of Radiology and Biomedical Imaging, University of California San Francisco, Box 0628, 1001 Potrero Avenue, SFGH 5, 1X55, San Francisco, CA 94143, USA; [c] Department of Radiology, Zuckerberg San Francisco General Hospital, San Francisco, CA 94110, USA
* Corresponding author. Department of Radiology and Biomedical Imaging, University of California San Francisco, Box 0628, 1001 Potrero Avenue, SFGH 5, 1X55, San Francisco, CA 94143.
E-mail address: Michael.ohliger@ucsf.edu

Radiol Clin N Am 60 (2022) 857–871
https://doi.org/10.1016/j.rcl.2022.05.008

become intertwined with the efferent bile ductules at the level of the portal triad. Blood from these systems courses through the hepatic sinusoids and collects within efferent hepatic venules, with subsequent passage into the larger hepatic veins and inferior vena cava (IVC). Avenues of communication between the arterial and portal systems are also present; most notably, the peribiliary plexus provides communications between the right gastric, pancreaticoduodenal, and cholecystic venous branches.[3]

Multiple imaging modalities play a role in evaluating vascular anomalies of the liver. Ultrasound is inexpensive, widely available, and through color Doppler is excellent at assessing blood flow. Computed tomography (CT) and magnetic resonance (MR), particularly in the angiographic contrast phases, are also extensively used for assessing vascular disorders. Catheter angiography has been considered the reference standard in evaluation of hepatic arterial anatomy but is limited by invasiveness. CT and MR protocols are often tailored to reflect sequential phases of contrast enhancement that are influenced by the liver's dual blood supply, which may be subdivided into early and late arterial phases, portal venous phase, and delayed phase. There is little enhancement of normal liver parenchyma during early and late arterial phases. Peak enhancement of the arterial vessels occurs during the *early arterial phase*, which begins approximately 15 seconds after injection of contrast and lasts for 7 to 12 seconds. This phase is useful for assessment of hepatic arteries or aberrant vascularity associated with liver lesions. The *late arterial phase* begins approximately 30 seconds after injection of contrast and lasts for about 12 seconds. During this phase, there is arterial and early portal venous enhancement, but no hepatic venous enhancement. This phase provides a high degree of contrast between hypervascular lesions and background hepatic parenchyma. Peak parenchymal enhancement is observed during the portal venous phase, which begins approximately 60 to 70 seconds after injection. Finally, more delayed phases may aid in the detection of fibrosis or hypovascular lesions.[4,5] Other variables that may affect hepatic vascular and parenchymal appearance include the type of contrast material used, rate of contrast injection, and imaging modality.[3–5]

The conventional hepatic arterial anatomy involves the main hepatic artery arising from the celiac axis and the proper hepatic artery giving rise to the right and left hepatic arteries. This arrangement is only observed in 55% of the population.[6] There are several anatomic variants associated with the hepatic artery. Michels described a classification of 10 different hepatic arterial variants, as gleaned from more than 200 cadaveric dissections; this classification also uses critical terminology in differentiating replaced from accessory arteries.[7,8] The most common variants include replaced right hepatic artery arising from the superior mesenteric artery, replaced left hepatic artery arising from the left gastric artery, and accessory left hepatic artery from the left gastric artery (**Fig. 1**).[9,10]

DISORDERS OF HEPATIC OUTFLOW
Budd-Chiari Syndrome

Budd-Chiari syndrome (BCS) refers to a group of conditions characterized by a partial or complete hepatic venous outflow obstruction. BCS is more common in women and is classified generally by the cause of the obstruction. Primary BCS refers to hepatic venous outflow obstruction originating from endoluminal thrombosis, whereas secondary BCS refers to outflow obstruction from extrinsic compression of the venous system by lesions such as tumors, abscesses, or cysts.[11] Hypercoagulable states and myeloproliferative disorders are the most common causes of primary BCS. The site of obstruction may be the small hepatic veins, large hepatic veins, IVC, or a combination thereof. BCS is considered symptomatic when signs of abdominal pain, ascites, hepatomegaly, encephalopathy, and gastrointestinal bleeding are present. The disease may be acute (duration less than 1 month, with hepatic necrosis and ascites and without collateral formation), subacute (insidious onset between 1 and 6 months, ascites, minimal hepatic necrosis, and formation of portal and hepatic venous collaterals), and chronic (duration of more than 6 months with complications of cirrhosis superimposed on subacute findings). Fulminant disease is characterized by hepatic encephalopathy within 8 weeks of development of jaundice. Therapeutic options include anticoagulation and portosystemic shunting, although liver transplantation is indicated when there is progression of liver dysfunction.[11–14]

The imaging findings of BCS depend on its duration. At ultrasound, acute findings include hepatosplenomegaly and lack of visualization and thrombosis of the hepatic veins or the IVC (**Fig. 2**A, B). On CT, the caudate lobe may be enlarged, and the parenchyma may demonstrate diminished and heterogenous enhancement (**Fig. 2**C). Thrombosed hepatic veins may be seen, and ascites and splenomegaly are usually present.[15] In the subacute and chronic stages, collateral vessels are present, which may be located either within the hepatic parenchyma or

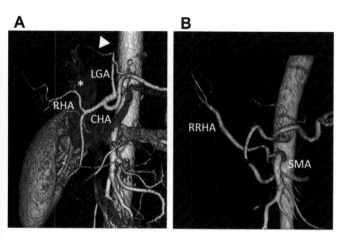

Fig. 1. Three-dimensional volume rendering from CT scans showing common hepatic artery variants. (A) Accessory left hepatic artery (arrowhead) arising from the left gastric artery (LGA). The normal common hepatic artery (CHA) and right hepatic artery (RHA) arise from the celiac artery. Separate left hepatic artery branch feeding segment IV (asterisk) is in standard position, arising from the proper hepatic artery. (B) Replaced right hepatic artery (RRHA) arising from the superior mesenteric artery (SMA).

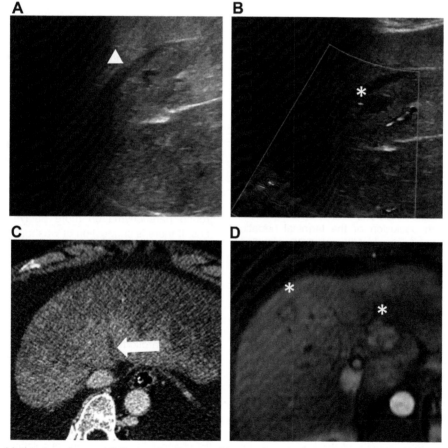

ig. 2. Budd-Chiari syndrome. (A) Gray-scale ultrasound image shows echogenic material in the left hepatic vein arrowhead). (B) Color Doppler ultrasound image in the same patient shows lack of flow in the left hepatic vein asterisk). (C) In a different patient with fulminant liver failure, contrast-enhanced CT shows heterogeneous nhancement of the liver and ascites, with nonenhancement of the hepatic veins (arrow = middle hepatic ein). (D) T₁-weighted spoiled gradient echo MR imaging with fat saturation following intravenous contrast in different patient, with Budd-Chiari syndrome, regenerative nodules (asterisk).

within subcutaneous tissues. Arterially hyperenhancing regenerative nodules may also be present; these nodules are also termed "focal nodular hyperplasia-like nodules," are usually smaller than 2 cm in diameter, and reflect a physiologically compensatory increase in hepatic arterial flow (**Fig. 2**D). On MR, heterogeneously increased signal on T_2-weighted images within the liver periphery may be seen, with increased enhancement of the caudate lobe on postcontrast acquisitions. Thrombi within the hepatic veins or IVC may best be seen on postcontrast sequences or on $T\_2^{\wedge*}$-weighted gradient echo sequences.[15–17] Regenerative nodules on MR imaging have intrinsically high signal on T_1-weighted images, and isointense or hypointense compared with hepatic parenchyma on T_2-weighted images, and demonstrate avid enhancement postcontrast. On both modalities, the periphery of the liver demonstrates decreased enhancement on late arterial phases, with the caudate demonstrating more pronounced enhancement, secondary to increased postsinusoidal pressure from venous obstruction. On portal venous phase, this pattern is reversed, with relatively decreased enhancement of the caudate lobe secondary to separate venous drainage and with enhancement of the periphery due to contrast accumulation within capsular veins; this has been described as the "flip-flop" pattern of enhancement.[18]

Sinusoidal Obstruction Syndrome

Hepatic sinusoidal obstruction syndrome (SOS), also known as veno-occlusive disease, is histologically characterized by injury to the hepatic sinusoidal cells with occlusion of the terminal hepatic venules and sinusoids.[19] Although SOS was first described in patients who had ingested monocrotaline-containing bush tea, more common contemporary associations include high-dose chemotherapy, stem cell transplantation, and high-dose radiation therapy.[20,21] SOS is diagnosed clinically according to the Baltimore and modified Seattle diagnostic criteria: painful hepatomegaly, hyperbilirubinemia, fluid retention, weight gain, and jaundice. Treatment options include supportive measures such as minimizing exposure to inciting toxins and paracentesis, as well as fibrinolysis with or without anticoagulant therapy.

Imaging findings of SOS include hepatosplenomegaly with heterogeneity of the hepatic parenchyma, narrowing of the hepatic veins and IVC, periportal edema, gallbladder wall edema, and ascites.[22] A decrease in velocity or reversal of the portal venous flow has been described with later stages of SOS; unfortunately, this finding has limited specificity early in the disease.[23] Irregular parenchymal lesions with peritumoral enhancement and central low attenuation/signal intensity may also be seen, which may resemble focal nodular hyperplasia.[24] These imaging findings are not pathognomonic and are best interpreted within the context of the clinical examination.

Congestive Hepatopathy

The liver receives approximately 25% of a person's cardiac output. Therefore, derangements in cardiovascular physiology may generate persistent hepatic venous congestion, which is termed as congestive hepatopathy. The most common cause of congestive hepatopathy is right heart disease, although any process that interferes with normal function of the IVC or hepatic veins may result in the congestive hepatopathy phenotype.[25] Increased venous pressure results in congestion and dilation of the hepatic sinusoids; there is subsequent exudation of proteins and fluid into the space of Disse, which impairs diffusion of nutrients and oxygen.[26] Long-standing congestion may lead to liver fibrosis and cirrhosis. Sonographic features include engorged hepatic veins and hepatomegaly; Doppler ultrasound features include increased portal and hepatic vein pulsatility. Imaging features include distention of the hepatic veins and IVC, reflux of contrast into the IVC and hepatic veins, periportal edema, and heterogenous and mottled parenchymal appearance, with decreased peripheral enhancement; this has been termed the "nutmeg liver."[27] Chronic congestion may lead to the formation of hyperenhancing hepatic nodules that become similar in enhancement to background parenchyma on more delayed acquisitions. If there is suggestion of washout compared with background parenchyma, a biopsy may ultimately be needed to differentiate these nodules from hepatocellular carcinoma.[27,28]

DISORDERS OF HEPATIC INFLOW
Hepatic Infarct

Hepatic infarction refers to coagulative necrosis caused by ischemia and may be secondary to diminished inflow from either the hepatic artery or the portal vein. Infarcts are uncommon in the liver because of its dual blood supply.[29] A study on hepatic infarcts by Saegusa and colleagues suggested that development of infarcts may also be caused by disturbances in portal venous circulation.[30] Conditions that may predispose for hepatic arterial occlusion are hepatobiliary surgery, especially liver transplantation, hepatic arterial aneurysms, intrahepatic chemoembolization, hypercoagulable state, sepsis, vasculitis, or trauma.[18] On imaging, a wedge-shaped defect within the parenchyma is identified, with heterogenous internal enhancement pattern (**Fig. 3** and **Fig. 4**). Bile lake formation may occur as a late complication of arterial ischemia, subsequent to biliary necrosis (**Fig. 5**).[18,31]

Portal Vein Thrombosis

Portal vein thrombosis (PVT) may be bland or neoplastic. Bland thrombosis may have many causes, with cirrhosis and underlying malignancy most common. Infection (omphalitis) is the most common cause in children.[11] Clinical features include abdominal pain and splenomegaly. Ultrasound with Doppler is the first-line modality in assessment for PVT. Sonographic features include heterogeneously echogenic thrombus within the portal venous lumen and lack of flow on Doppler evaluation if an occlusive thrombus is present. An important pitfall is the lack of flow on Doppler

evaluation, but without detection of thrombus; in this case, slow flow should be considered.[32,33] Acute bland thrombus is characterized by a centrally nonenhancing filling defect within the main portal vein or its branches, with increased attention on noncontrast CT images, and hyperintense or isointense signal on T1-weighted sequences in comparison to skeletal muscle. Enhancment after IV contrast administration may be seen within the periphery of the thrombus, thought related to trace flow or mural inflammation.[34] If the thrombus extends to the mesenteric venous arcade, venous intestinal infarction may occur. When the thrombus is long-standing, the portal vein may become diminutive, with cavernous transformation and the formation of periportal collateral vessels. Other findings in patients with portal vein thrombus include ascites, splenomegaly, and portosystemic shunts as part of the constellation of portal hypertension. Collateral vessels may sometimes

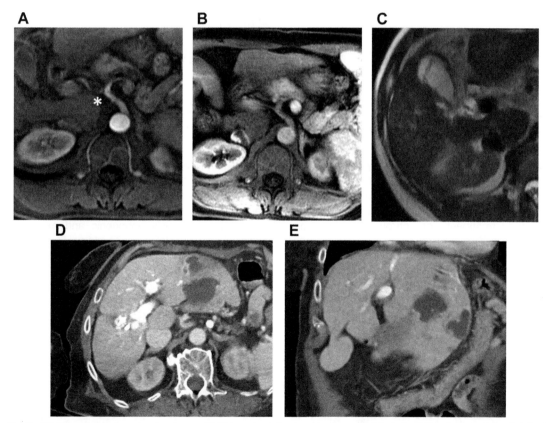

Fig. 3. (*A*) T1-weighted contrast enhanced MR imaging obtained in the arterial phase following transarterial chemoembolization (TACE) for hepatocellular carcinoma shows diminished caliber of the common hepatic artery (*asterisk*) compatible with dissection. (*B*) For reference, a scan obtained before the procedure shows normal hepatic artery. (*C*) T2-weighted MR imaging shows gallbladder edema with irregularity of the wall. (*D*) In a different patient, contrast-enhanced CT performed 4 weeks after TACE shows fluid-filled structures in the left hepatic lobe concerning for biloma as a consequence of biliary necrosis. (*E*) Similar findings shown on coronal contrast-enhanced CT.

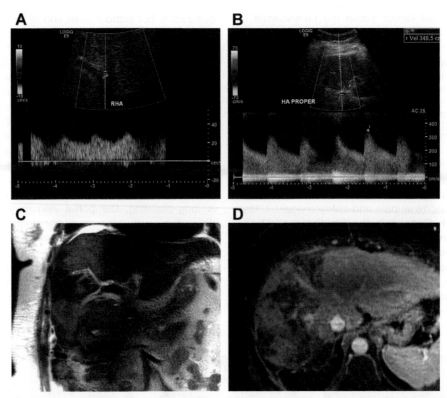

Fig. 4. Hepatic infarct in a patient with a history of liver transplant. (*A*) Color and spectral Doppler image of the right hepatic artery shows increased diastolic flow with parvus et tardus waveform. (*B*) For comparison, a normal waveform in the common hepatic artery. (*C*) Coronal T2-weighted image shows high signal in the right hepatic lobe in a geographic pattern consistent with infarct. (*D*) Axial postcontrast T1-weighted image shows liver parenchymal nonenhancement in a geographic pattern, confirming the diagnosis of infarct.

demonstrate a tumefactive appearance, referred to as a portal cavernoma.[34] Acute bland portal venous thrombosis may be treated with anticoagulation, but there is no consensus with regard to the treatment of chronic portal vein thrombosis.[11]

Portal vein tumor thrombus (PVTT) refers to neoplastic invasion of the portal venous system and is seen in up to 44% of hepatocellular carcinoma cases.[35] This finding portends a poor prognosis and precludes surgical resection as well as transplantation.[36] On sonography, PVTT appears as a heterogeneously echogenic and expansile mass within the portal vein with internal flow on color and spectral Doppler (**Fig. 6**). Continuity between the PVTT and a parenchymal tumor may

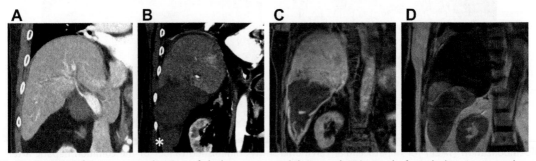

Fig. 5. Hepatic infarct as a complication of cholecystectomy. (*A*) Coronal CT image before cholecystectomy shows normal enhancement. (*B*) After presenting with abdominal pain following cholecystectomy, the inferior portion of the right hepatic lobe is nonenhancing. High-density material inferior to the liver capsule (*asterisk*) is compatible with hemorrhage. (*C*) Coronal T1-weighted contrast-enhanced MR imaging shows nonenhancement of the inferior right hepatic lobe. (*D*) Coronal T2-weighted MR imaging image shows heterogeneous signal intensity.

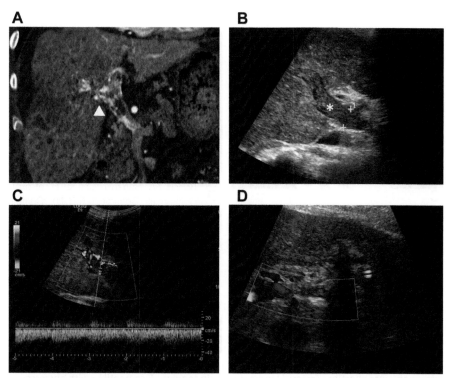

Fig. 6. Portal vein thrombus. (*A*) Contrast-enhanced CT showing enhancing tumor thrombus in the portal vein (*arrowhead*) of a patient with liver cirrhosis. (*B*) Gray-scale ultrasound shows expansile material filling the main portal vein (*asterisk*). (*C*) Color Doppler ultrasound images in the same patient show an arterial vascular wave form within the thrombus. (*D*) Color Doppler ultrasound images of the left portal vein in a different patient with bland thrombus shows absence of flow.

also be seen.[37] Contrast-enhanced ultrasound can also play a role in distinguishing between PVT and PVTT, with early and avid enhancement of the tumor thrombus and washout on portal venous phase.[37,38] Features of PVTT on CT and MR include presence of heterogenous endoluminal mass that expands the portal vein, with enhancement on postcontrast acquisitions. A role for diffusion-weighted imaging in MR has also been described in discriminating between PVT and PVTT.[39–42]

Pylephlebitis

Pylephlebitis refers to septic thrombophlebitis of the portal venous system. Infections from the intestinal tract may seed the portal vein, with diverticulitis as the most common cause, followed by appendicitis, inflammatory bowel disease, and other intraabdominal infections.[43,44] Infections are typically polymicrobial, with *Bacteroides fragilis* being the most common single micro-organism cultured.[45] Imaging findings include thrombus within the branches of the portal vein with transient parenchymal differences due to the arterial buffer response, as well as intrahepatic abscesses (Fig. 7). Treatment consists of combined anticoagulation and antibiotic therapy.[46]

Portal Hypertension

Portal hypertension refers to pathologically increased resistance to portal venous flow, with circumvention of blood throughout different portosystemic collateral vessels.[47] Clinically significant portal hypertension is defined as an increase of the portal-hepatic pressure gradient to more than 10 mm Hg. The most common cause of portal hypertension is chronic liver disease (cirrhosis), followed by hepatic schistosomiasis.[47] Ultrasound is the first-line modality in assessing for portal hypertension. Sonographic features include portal vein enlargement with hepatofugal flow, decreased portal venous velocity, and development of portosystemic collaterals.[48] CT and MR features of portal hypertension include distention of the main portal vein with portosystemic collaterals, as well as ascites and splenomegaly.[49]

Hepatic Artery Aneurysms

Hepatic artery aneurysms are the second most common type of visceral arterial aneurysms (following splenic artery aneurysms) and are more common in men.[50] The common hepatic artery is most often involved, followed by the right

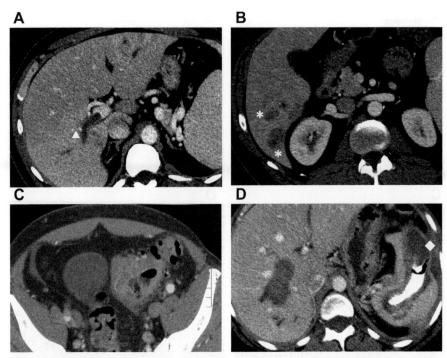

Fig. 7. Pylephlebitis. (*A*) Contrast-enhanced CT showing a filling defect in the right posterior portal vein (*arrowhead*). (*B*) Heterogeneous collections (*asterisk*) more distally in segment 6 compatible with abscesses. (*C*) Axial images through the sigmoid colon in the same patient with inflammatory changes concerning for sigmoid diverticulitis, presumably the source of the abscesses. (*D*) In a different patient with a history of inflected splenic cyst (previously drained, diamond), there is heterogeneous expansile material filling the posterior right portal vein, concerning for infection.

and left hepatic arteries. Most of the hepatic artery aneurysms may be attributed to atherosclerosis. Before the widespread use of antibiotics, mycotic hepatic artery aneurysms were common and often secondary to streptococcus or staphylococcus endocarditis. Mycotic aneurysms now account for only 0.1% of all arterial aneurysms. Hepatic artery pseudoaneurysms may develop secondary to trauma, surgery, or indwelling biliary catheter. The arterial intimal layer is damaged, with subsequent formation of a saccular outpouching. These aneurysms may rarely be caused by iatrogenic causes as well, including radiofrequency ablation and hepatobiliary or vascular surgery.

Hepatic artery aneurysms are usually asymptomatic and are often incidentally discovered on cross-sectional imaging. When symptomatic, a triad of epigastric pain, obstructive jaundice, and hemobilia, referred to as Quincke triad, may be seen in up to one-third of patients and is secondary to erosion of the aneurysm through the biliary tree.[51] On CT, a focal outpouching may be seen within the hepatic artery (**Fig. 8**). Treatment is indicated if the size of the aneurysm exceeds 2 cm or if the patient is symptomatic. Treatment also varies by location of the aneurysm: intrahepatic aneurysms are amenable to

coil embolization, whereas direct surgical repair is recommended for most extrahepatic aneurysms. Coil embolization is recommended for intrahepatic pseudoaneurysms.[52,53]

Vasculitis

Vasculitis refers to inflammation and necrosis of vessel walls. These disorders are classified by the Chapel Hill classification by the size of the vessel involved, number of organs involved, and by association with systemic disease, among other categories. Polyarteritis nodosa refers to necrotizing arteritis of medium-sized vessels; the liver is the third most common site of involvement, after the kidneys and gastrointestinal tract. On imaging, multiple microaneurysms may be seen. Other imaging appearances include vessel wall thickening and perivascular stranding, as well as hepatic parenchymal infarctions.[54,55]

ABNORMAL ARTERIAL-VENOUS CONNECTIONS
Hereditary Hemorrhagic Telangiectasia

Hereditary hemorrhagic telangiectasia (HHT), also known as Osler-Weber-Rendu syndrome, is a multisystem disorder of blood vessel maturation

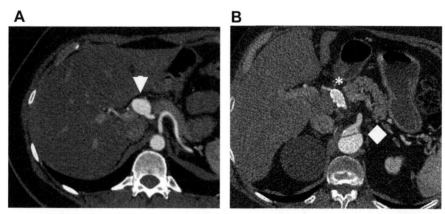

Fig. 8. Hepatic artery aneurysm. (*A*) Focal dilatation of the common hepatic artery (*arrowhead*). (*B*) In a different patient with Marfan syndrome, fusiform dilatation of the common hepatic artery (*asterisk*) with surrounding calcification and a dissection flap (*diamond*) within the abdominal aorta.

leading to abnormal arteriovenous connections. Symptoms depend on the location of these connections. The most common symptom is recurrent nosebleeds, but arteriovenous malformations (AVMs) may affect the brain, lungs, liver, and gastrointestinal tract.[56] Clinical diagnosis is made according the Curaçao criteria, which includes recurrent nose bleeds, skin telangiectasias, visceral arteriovenous malformations, and a history of HHT in a first-degree relative.[57] Liver involvement is common in HHT, although liver AVMs are frequently asymptomatic. When AVMs are symptomatic, the symptoms depend on the type of shunting. Predominantly arterial-portal shunting leads to symptoms of portal hypertension, including varices, splenomegaly, and liver nodularity ("pseudocirrhosis"). Predominantly arterial-systemic shunting leads to high-output heart failure. Imaging features of liver AVMs are variable and can be detected on ultrasound, CT, or MR imaging.[58] Ultrasound can show large ectatic intrahepatic vessels, with dilated hepatic artery and elevated hepatic arterial velocity (**Fig. 9**A, B). On CT or MR imaging, there is early filling of either the portal vein or hepatic vein, with diffuse multifocal areas of shunting throughout the liver (**Fig. 9**C, D). Of note, multifocal and diffuse shunting is characteristic of HHT.[59,60] Liver-related complications include biliary ischemia, which may be manifest as dilated intrahepatic bile ducts or bilomas. Focal liver lesions may develop, most commonly focal nodular hyperplasia.[61]

Arterioportal Shunts

An arterioportal shunt is a connection between a branch of the hepatic artery and the portal venous system. The underlying causes of these arterioportal shunts are myriad and include underlying portal or hepatic venous obstruction, inflammatory or infectious lesions, neoplasms, and trauma (including iatrogenic causes such as liver biopsies; **Figs. 10** and **11**).[62] These shunts may be seen with hepatocellular carcinoma in up to 63% of patients.[63] The connections may be through transsinusoidal, peribiliary vascular plexus, transvasal, or transtumoral routes. In the transsinusoidal route, retrograde flow from the hepatic arteries to the portal veins is secondary to increased hepatic venous pressures. The peribiliary vascular plexus figures prominently in cirrhosis: due to the underlying fibrosis and architectural distortion, the hepatic veins are diminutive, with subsequent compensatory engorgement of the peribiliary vascular plexus due to increased hepatic arterial flow. In the transvasal route, there is pronounced flow within the hypertrophied vasa vasorum. In the transtumoral route, the numerous vessels within the tumoral capsule related to angiogenesis act as conduits between arterial and portal venous systems.[64,65] CT and MR features include early and prolonged enhancement of the portal vein as well as transient enhancement peripheral to the tumor and dilated intrahepatic vessels during arterial phase imaging.[62]

The significance of arterioportal shunts lies in their potential to simulate pathology or hint at an underlying derangement. A lesion such as neoplasm or abscess may place mass effect on an adjacent portal venule, with resultant increased perfusion adjacent the lesion. Notably, these shunts may also lead to development of portal hypertension.[62]

Abernethy Malformation

Abernethy malformation is a generic eponym describing congenital extrahepatic portosystemic

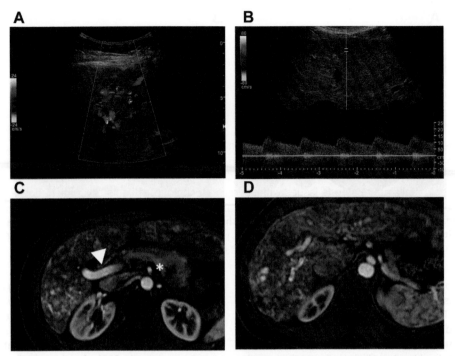

Fig. 9. Hereditary hemorrhagic telangiectasia (HHT). (A) Color Doppler ultrasound images demonstrating diffusely increased vascularity of the left lobe secondary to large diffuse arterial-venous malformations. (B) Spectral doppler wave form shows pulsatility with increased diastolic flow compatible with arterial-venous connection. (C) T1-weighted contrast-enhanced MR imaging in the arterial phase showing an abnormally dilated proper hepatic artery (arrowhead). For reference, a normal-sized superior mesenteric artery is visible (asterisk). (D) In the same patient, heterogeneous multifocal hyperenhancement throughout the liver compatible with numerous diffuse arteriovenous shunts.

shunts. These shunts can be divided into 2 types. In type 1, the portal vein is absent, with the superior mesenteric vein and splenic vein draining separately into the IVC (type 1a) or draining into the IVC (or other systemic vessel) as a single vessel (type 1b).[66] In type 2, a hypoplastic portal vein is present (Fig. 12). These shunts may become clinically significant, causing hepatopulmonary syndrome, metabolic dysfunction, and hepatic encephalopathy, and may be associated with other anomalies, including cardiac and skeletal anomalies. A multitude of hepatic lesions

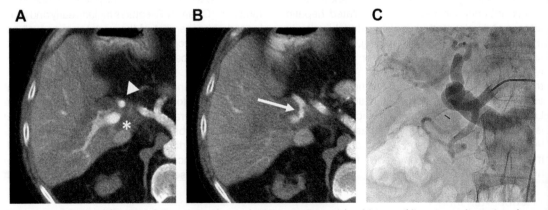

Fig. 10. Arterioportal fistula. (A) Contrast-enhanced CT in a patient with a history of liver transplantation shows similar level of enhancement of the hepatic artery (arrowhead) and portal vein (asterisk). (B) On a different axial slice, a fistulous connection can be seen (arrow). (C) Catheter angiogram showing selective injection of the proper hepatic artery with immediate opacification of the main portal vein, confirming arterioportal fistula.

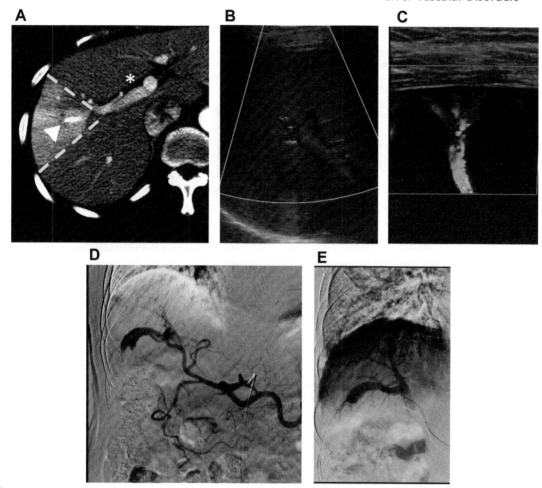

Fig. 11. (A) Axial contrast-enhanced CT obtained in the late arterial phase in a patient presenting with pain following liver biopsy shows ectasia of the hepatic artery (*arrowhead*), early filling of the portal vein (*asterisk*), as well as wedge-shaped segmental early enhancement of the liver peripheral to the ectatic artery (denoted by dashed *yellow lines*). This suggests arterial-portal fistula. (B) Color Doppler ultrasound image of the right portal vein shows turbulent flow in the posterior branch. (C) Color Doppler ultrasound image more peripherally in the right hepatic lobe shows dilated portal vein with turbulent flow. (D) Conventional angiogram in the same patient following injection into the celiac artery shows a pseudoaneurysm in the right hepatic artery and shunting of blood toward the portal vein. (E) Selective angiography more distally in the right hepatic artery shows early filling of the portal vein.

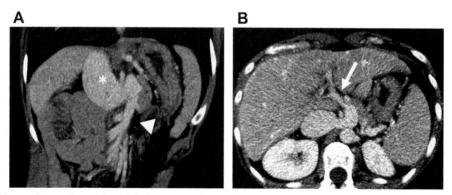

Fig. 12. Abernethy malformation. (A) Contrast-enhanced CT reconstructed in an oblique plane shows a direct connection between the superior mesenteric vein (SMV, *arrowhead*) and inferior vena cava (IVC, *asterisk*). (B) There is also a direct connection between the SMV and a diminutive portal vein (*arrow*), suggesting a type II Abernethy malformation.

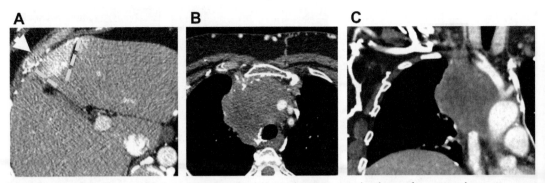

Fig. 13. Collateral inflow to the liver. (*A*) Contrast-enhanced CT in an early phase of contrast shows numerous collateral vessels in the abdominal wall (*arrow*) and wedge-shaped hyperenhancement in segment IV (*yellow dashed lines*). (*B*) Contrast-enhanced CT through the upper mediastinum shows a large mass, which was eventually proved to be a lymphoma. (*C*) Coronal reformation of the chest shows that the mass obstructs the superior vena cava, leading to subcutaneous collateral vessels and the early inflow seen on the liver slices in (*A*).

may be seen, including regenerative nodules and hepatic adenomas.[67]

Peliosis

Peliosis refers to dilated blood-filled sinusoids and lacunae formation within the hepatic parenchyma. This benign condition may be attributed to several causes, including drugs such as corticosteroids as well as toxins.[68,69] Notably, there has been an association described with Bartonella henselae and Bartonella quintana infections within the setting of AIDS.[70]

On imaging with noncontrast CT, peliosis is characterized by multiple low-attenuating lesions. On noncontrast MR, the appearance of these lesions depends on the age of blood products within the lacunae, with a common appearance of hyperintensity on T_2-weighted sequences and with hypointensity or isointensity on T_1-weighted sequences. Underlying hemorrhagic necrosis may result in intrinsic T_1 hyperintensity. Multiple imaging appearances have been described on postcontrast CT, including lesions appearing as hypoattenuating compared with adjacent parenchyma on late arterial phase acquisitions, with subsequent isoattenuating appearance on more delayed acquisitions, as well as enhancement proceeding from the center of the lesion to the periphery, the so-called centrifugal pattern. A centripetal pattern of enhancement has also been described. These patterns are also observed on postcontrast MR sequences as well.[71–73]

Pseudolesions

Cholecystic veins course underneath the liver bed and extend through the triangle of Calot and form a confluence at the porta hepatis. Other third inflow venous systems include the parabiliary venous system, epigastric-paraumbilical venous system,

and aberrant gastric veins.[64] Inflow from these venous systems mixes with unopacified blood from the portal venous system, resulting in pseudolesions in characteristic locations. These inflow systems are also reflected in focal fatty change or sparing in the characteristic location of the dorsal aspect of segment IV (**Fig. 13**).[74] Sources of alternative flow within the liver may also hint at pathologies elsewhere within the body. Focally increased blood flow within segment IV can be seen with superior vena cava obstruction, with collateralized vessels within the thorax forming an avenue to the left portal vein.[75,76]

SUMMARY

The underlying hepatic vascular physiology as well as a diverse imaging spectrum of vascular disorders of the liver was reviewed in this article, including pathologies related to outflow, inflow, and arteriovenous connections. Outflow abnormalities include Budd-Chiari syndrome, sinusoidal obstruction syndrome, and congestive hepatopathy. Inflow abnormalities include hepatic infarction, portal venous bland and tumor thrombus, pylephlebitis, hepatic arterial aneurysms, and vasculitis. Aberrant arteriovenous connections include hereditary hemorrhagic telangiectasia, arterioportal shunts, and Abernethy malformation. Other vascular disorders and mimics of disease include peliosis, shunting secondary to parenchymal mass lesions, and enhancing quadrate lobe secondary to superior vena cava obstruction. By understanding their varied multimodality imaging appearances, the radiologist is well positioned to improve patient care.

DISCLOSURE

Both authors have nothing to disclose.

REFERENCES

1. Vollmar B, Menger MD. The hepatic microcirculation: mechanistic contributions and therapeutic targets in liver injury and repair. Physiol Rev 2009; 89(4):1269–339.
2. Eipel C, Abshagen K, Vollmar B. Regulation of hepatic blood flow: the hepatic arterial buffer response revisited. World J Gastroenterol 2010;16(48):6046–57.
3. Itai Y, Matsui O. Blood flow and liver imaging. Radiology 1997;202(2):306–14.
4. Foley WD, Mallisee TA, Hohenwalter MD, et al. Multiphase hepatic CT with a multirow detector CT scanner. AJR Am J Roentgenol 2000;175(3):679–85.
5. Oto A, Tamm EP, Szklaruk J. Multidetector row CT of the liver. Radiol Clin North Am 2005;43(5): 827–48, vii.
6. Winter TC 3rd, Nghiem HV, Freeny PC, et al. Hepatic arterial anatomy: demonstration of normal supply and vascular variants with three-dimensional CT angiography. Radiographics 1995;15(4):771–80.
7. Michels NA. Newer anatomy of the liver and its variant blood supply and collateral circulation. Am J Surg 1966;112(3):337–47.
8. Noussios G, Dimitriou I, Chatzis I, et al. The Main Anatomic variations of the hepatic artery and their importance in surgical practice: review of the literature. J Clin Med Res 2017;9(4):248–52.
9. Sahani D, Mehta A, Blake M, et al. Preoperative hepatic vascular evaluation with CT and MR angiography: implications for surgery. Radiographics 2004;24(5):1367–80.
10. Catalano OA, Singh AH, Uppot RN, et al. Vascular and biliary variants in the liver: implications for liver surgery. Radiographics 2008;28(2):359–78.
11. Aqel BA. Vascular diseases of the liver. In: Talley N, Lindor K, Vargas H, editors. Practical gastroenterology and hepatology: liver and biliary disease. Hoboken NJ: Wiley-Blackwell; 2010. p. 261–74.
12. Janssen HL, Garcia-Pagan JC, Elias E, et al. European Group for the Study of Vascular Disorders of the Liver. Budd-Chiari syndrome: a review by an expert panel. J Hepatol 2003;38(3):364–71.
13. Menon KV, Shah V, Kamath PS. The Budd-Chiari syndrome. N Engl J Med 2004;350(6):578–85.
14. Inchingolo R, Posa A, Mariappan M, et al. Transjugular intrahepatic portosystemic shunt for Budd-Chiari syndrome: A comprehensive review. World J Gastroenterol 2020;26(34):5060–73.
15. Brancatelli G, Vilgrain V, Federle MP, et al. Budd-Chiari syndrome: spectrum of imaging findings. AJR Am J Roentgenol 2007;188(2):W168–76.
16. Bansal V, Gupta P, Sinha S, et al. Budd-Chiari syndrome: imaging review. Br J Radiol 2018;91(1092): 20180441.
17. Cura M, Haskal Z, Lopera J. Diagnostic and interventional radiology for Budd-Chiari syndrome. Radiographics 2009;29(3):669–81.
18. Torabi M, Hosseinzadeh K, Federle MP. CT of nonneoplastic hepatic vascular and perfusion disorders. Radiographics 2008;28(7):1967–82.
19. Wadleigh M, Ho V, Momtaz P, et al. Hepatic veno-occlusive disease: pathogenesis, diagnosis and treatment. Curr Opin Hematol 2003;10(6): 451–62.
20. Fan CQ, Crawford JM. Sinusoidal obstruction syndrome (hepatic veno-occlusive disease). J Clin Exp Hepatol 2014;4(4):332–46.
21. Mohty M, Malard F, Abecassis M, et al. Revised diagnosis and severity criteria for sinusoidal obstruction syndrome/veno-occlusive disease in adult patients: a new classification from the European Society for Blood and Marrow Transplantation. Bone Marrow Transpl 2016;51(7):906–12.
22. Erturk SM, Mortelé KJ, Binkert CA, et al. CT features of hepatic venoocclusive disease and hepatic graft-versus-host disease in patients after hematopoietic stem cell transplantation. AJR Am J Roentgenol 2006;186(6):1497–501.
23. Mahgerefteh SY, Sosna J, Bogot N, et al. Radiologic imaging and intervention for gastrointestinal and hepatic complications of hematopoietic stem cell transplantation. Radiology 2011;258(3):660–71.
24. Zhang Y, Yan Y, Song B. Noninvasive imaging diagnosis of sinusoidal obstruction syndrome: a pictorial review. Insights Imaging 2019;10(1):110.
25. Hilscher M, Sanchez W. Congestive hepatopathy. Clin Liver Dis (Hoboken) 2016;8(3):68–71.
26. Giallourakis CC, Rosenberg PM, Friedman LS. The liver in heart failure. Clin Liver Dis 2002;6(4): 947–67. viii-ix.
27. Wells ML, Venkatesh SK. Congestive hepatopathy. Abdom Radiol 2018;43:2037–51.
28. Wells ML, Fenstad ER, Poterucha JT, et al. Imaging Findings of Congestive Hepatopathy. Radiographics 2016;36(4):1024–37.
29. Carroll R. Infarction of the human liver. J Clin Pathol 1963;16(2):133–6.
30. Saegusa M, Takano Y, Okudaira M. Human hepatic infarction: histopathological and postmortem angiological studies. Liver 1993;13(5):239–45.
31. Elsayes KM, Shaaban AM, Rothan SM, et al. A comprehensive approach to hepatic vascular disease. Radiographics 2017;37(3):813–36.
32. Hertzberg BS, Middleton WD. Liver. In: Ultrasound: the requisites. Elsevier; 2016. p. 76–7.
33. Sacerdoti D, Serianni G, Gaiani S, et al. Thrombosis of the portal venous system. J Ultrasound 2007; 10(1):12–21.
34. Jha RC, Khera SS, Kalaria AD. Portal vein thrombosis: imaging the spectrum of disease with an

emphasis on MRI features. AJR Am J Roentgenol 2018;211(1):14–24.

35. Pawarode A, Voravud N, Sriuranpong V, et al. Natural history of untreated primary hepatocellular carcinoma: a retrospective study of 157 patients. Am J Clin Oncol 1998;21(4):386–91.

36. Takizawa D, Kakizaki S, Sohara N, et al. Hepatocellular carcinoma with portal vein tumor thrombosis: clinical characteristics, prognosis, and patient survival analysis. Dig Dis Sci 2007;52(11):3290–5.

37. Tarantino L, Francica G, Sordelli I, et al. Diagnosis of benign and malignant portal vein thrombosis in cirrhotic patients with hepatocellular carcinoma: color Doppler US, contrast-enhanced US, and fine-needle biopsy. Abdom Imaging 2006;31(5):537–44.

38. Danila M, Sporea I, Popescu A, et al. Portal vein thrombosis in liver cirrhosis - the added value of contrast enhanced ultrasonography. Med Ultrason 2016;18(2):218–33.

39. Catalano OA, Choy G, Zhu A, et al. Differentiation of malignant thrombus from bland thrombus of the portal vein in patients with hepatocellular carcinoma: application of diffusion-weighted MR imaging. Radiology 2010;254(1):154–62.

40. Karaosmanoglu AD, Onur MR, Uysal A, et al. Tumor in the veins: an abdominal perspective with an emphasis on CT and MR imaging. Insights Imaging 2020;11(1):52.

41. Gawande R, Jalaeian H, Niendorf E, et al. MRI in differentiating malignant versus benign portal vein thrombosis in patients with hepatocellular carcinoma: value of post contrast imaging with subtraction. Eur J Radiol 2019;118:88–95.

42. Kim JH, Lee JM, Yoon JH, et al. Portal vein thrombosis in patients with hepatocellular carcinoma: diagnostic accuracy of gadoxetic acid-enhanced MR imaging. Radiology 2016;279(3):773–83.

43. Choudhry AJ, Baghdadi YM, Amr MA, et al. Pylephlebitis: a Review of 95 Cases. J Gastrointest Surg 2016;20(3):656–61.

44. Wong K, Weisman DS, Patrice KA. Pylephlebitis: a rare complication of an intra-abdominal infection. J Community Hosp Intern Med Perspect 2013;3(2):1–4.

45. Kanellopoulou T, Alexopoulou A, Theodossiades G, et al. Pylephlebitis: an overview of non-cirrhotic cases and factors related to outcome. Scand J Infect Dis 2010;42(11–12):804–11.

46. Balthazar EJ, Gollapudi P. Septic thrombophlebitis of the mesenteric and portal veins: CT imaging. J Comput Assist Tomogr 2000;24(5):755–60.

47. Berzigotti A, Seijo S, Reverter E, et al. Assessing portal hypertension in liver diseases. Expert Rev Gastroenterol Hepatol 2013;7(2):141–55.

48. Robinson KA, Middleton WD, Al-Sukaiti R, et al. Doppler sonography of portal hypertension. Ultrasound Q 2009;25(1):3–13.

49. Bandali MF, Mirakhur A, Lee EW, et al. Portal hypertension: Imaging of portosystemic collateral pathways and associated image-guided therapy. World J Gastroenterol 2017;23(10):1735–46.

50. Abbas MA, Fowl RJ, Stone WM, et al. Hepatic artery aneurysm: factors that predict complications. J Vasc Surg 2003;38(1):41–5.

51. Jamtani I, Nugroho A, Irfan W, et al. Revisiting Quincke's triad: a case of idiopathic hepatic artery aneurysm presenting with obstructive jaundice. Ann Vasc Surg 2021;71:536.e1–4.

52. Lal RB, Strohl JA, Piazza S, et al. Hepatic artery aneurysm. J Cardiovasc Surg (Torino) 1989;30(3):509–13.

53. Jesinger RA, Thoreson AA, Lamba R. Abdominal and pelvic aneurysms and pseudoaneurysms: imaging review with clinical, radiologic, and treatment correlation. Radiographics 2013;33(3):E71–96.

54. Patel AP, Cantos A, Butani D. Mycotic aneurysm of the hepatic artery: a case report and its management. J Clin Imaging Sci 2020;10:41.

55. Ha HK, Lee SH, Rha SE, et al. Radiologic features of vasculitis involving the gastrointestinal tract. Radiographics 2000;20(3):779–94.

56. Hetts SW, Shieh JT, Ohliger MA, et al. Hereditary hemorrhagic telangiectasia: the convergence of genotype, phenotype, and imaging in modern diagnosis and management of a multisystem disease. Radiology 2021;300(1):17–30.

57. Shovlin CL, Guttmacher AE, Buscarini E, et al. Diagnostic criteria for hereditary hemorrhagic telangiectasia (Rendu-Osler-Weber syndrome). Am J Med Genet 2000;91(1):66–7.

58. Buscarini E, Gandolfi S, Alicante S, et al. Liver involvement in hereditary hemorrhagic telangiectasia. Abdom Radiol (NY) 2018;43(8):1920–30.

59. Memeo M, Stabile Ianora AA, Scardapane A, et al. Hepatic involvement in hereditary hemorrhagic telangiectasia: CT findings. Abdom Imaging 2004;29(2):211–20.

60. Siddiki H, Doherty MG, Fletcher JG, et al. Abdominal findings in hereditary hemorrhagic telangiectasia: pictorial essay on 2D and 3D findings with isotropic multiphase CT. Radiographics 2008;28(1):171–84.

61. Harwin J, Sugi MD, Hetts SW, et al. The role of liver imaging in hereditary hemorrhagic telangiectasia. J Clin Med 2020;9(11):3750.

62. Lane MJ, Jeffrey RB Jr, Katz DS. Spontaneous intrahepatic vascular shunts. AJR Am J Roentgenol 2000;174(1):125–31.

63. Itai Y, Furui S, Ohtomo K, et al. Dynamic CT features of arterioportal shunts in hepatocellular carcinoma. AJR Am J Roentgenol 1986;146(4):723–7.

64. Choi BI, Chung JW, Itai Y, et al. Hepatic abnormalities related to blood flow: evaluation with dual-phase helical CT. Abdom Imaging 1999;24(4):340–56.

65. Yu JS, Rofsky NM. Magnetic resonance imaging of arterioportal shunts in the liver. Top Magn Reson Imaging 2002;13(3):165–76.

66. Ghuman SS, Gupta S, Buxi TB, et al. The Abernethy malformation-myriad imaging manifestations of a single entity. Indian J Radiol Imaging 2016;26(3): 364–72.

67. Ranchi-Abella S, Branchereau S, Lambert V, et al. Complications of congenital portosystemic shunts in children: therapeutic options and outcomes. J Pediatr Gastroenterol Nutr 2010;51(3):322–30.

68. Dai YN, Ren ZZ, Song WY, et al. Peliosis hepatis: 2 case reports of a rare liver disorder and its differential diagnosis. Medicine (Baltimore) 2017;96(13): e6471.

69. Elsing C, Placke J, Herrmann T. Alcohol binging causes peliosis hepatis during azathioprine therapy in Crohn's disease. World J Gastroenterol 2007; 13(34):4646–8.

70. Sanz-Canalejas L, Gómez-Mampaso E, Cantón-Moreno R, et al. Peliosis hepatis due to disseminated tuberculosis in a patient with AIDS. Infection 2014;42(1):185–9.

71. Iannaccone R, Federle MP, Brancatelli G, et al. Peliosis hepatis: spectrum of imaging findings. AJR Am J Roentgenol 2006;187(1):W43–52.

72. Yoshida M, Utsunomiya D, Takada S, et al. The imaging findings of Peliosis hepatis on gadoxetic acid enhanced MRI. Radiol Case Rep 2020;15(8): 1261–5.

73. Battal B, Kocaoglu M, Atay AA, et al. Multifocal peliosis hepatis: MR and diffusion-weighted MR-imaging findings of an atypical case. Ups J Med Sci 2010;115(2):153–6.

74. Yoshimitsu K, Honda H, Kuroiwa T, et al. Unusual hemodynamics and pseudolesions of the noncirrhotic liver at CT. Radiographics 2001;21 Spec:S81–96.

75. Bryan RG Jr, Oliveira GR, Walker TG. Hot quadrate. J Vasc Interv Radiol 2013;24(12):1835.

76. Aloufi FF, Alabdulkarim FM, Alshahrani MA. The focal hepatic hot spot ("hot quadrate") sign. Abdom Radiol (NY) 2017;42(4):1289–90.

Moving?

Make sure your subscription moves with you!

To notify us of your new address, find your **Clinics Account Number** (located on your mailing label above your name), and contact customer service at:

Email: journalscustomerservice-usa@elsevier.com

800-654-2452 (subscribers in the U.S. & Canada)
314-447-8871 (subscribers outside of the U.S. & Canada)

Fax number: 314-447-8029

Elsevier Health Sciences Division
Subscription Customer Service
3251 Riverport Lane
Maryland Heights, MO 63043

*To ensure uninterrupted delivery of your subscription, please notify us at least 4 weeks in advance of move.

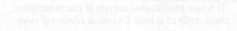

Printed and bound by CPI Group (UK) Ltd, Croydon, CR0 4YY

08/05/2025

01864704-0020